MRCP Part

D1145455

400 BOFs

5/4 — 25/4
last
return

Wrightington Wigan & Leigh
NHS Trust Library

G 0 3 2 7 9
G03279

MRCP Part 1

400 BOFs

Imran Mannan BSc (Hons) MBBS MRCP
Core Medical Trainee, Barts Health NHS Trust, London, UK

Vincent Cheung MA (Cantab) MBBS MRCP
Core Medical Trainee, Barts Health NHS Trust, London, UK

Claire Grout MA (Cantab) MB BChir MRCP
Core Medical Trainee, Barts Health NHS Trust, London, UK

Benjamin Mullish MA (Cantab) MB BChir MRCP
Core Medical Trainee, Barts Health NHS Trust, London, UK

Edited by
Aruna Dias BSc MBBS MRCP
Consultant Gastroenterologist,
Newham University Hospital, UK

Eric Beck BSc (Hons) MBBS FRCP FRCPG FRCPE
Former Chairman of MRCP(UK) Part 2 Board
and former Member of the MRCP(UK) Part 1 Board
University College London, UK

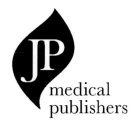
JP
medical
publishers

London • St Louis • Panama City • New Delhi

© 2013 JP Medical Ltd.
Published by JP Medical Ltd
83 Victoria Street, London, SW1H 0HW, UK
Tel: +44 (0)20 3170 8910   Fax: +44 (0)20 3008 6180
Email: info@jpmedpub.com   Web: www.jpmedpub.com

The rights of Imran Mannan, Vincent Cheung, Claire Grout, Benjamin Mullish, Aruna Dias and Eric Beck to be identified as authors of this work have been asserted by them in accordance with the Copyright, Designs and Patents Act 1988.

All rights reserved. No part of this publication may be reproduced, stored or transmitted in any form or by any means, electronic, mechanical, photocopying, recording or otherwise, except as permitted by the UK Copyright, Designs and Patents Act 1988, without the prior permission in writing of the publishers. Permissions may be sought directly from JP Medical Ltd at the address printed above.

All brand names and product names used in this book are trade names, service marks, trademarks or registered trademarks of their respective owners. The publisher is not associated with any product or vendor mentioned in this book.

Medical knowledge and practice change constantly. This book is designed to provide accurate, authoritative information about the subject matter in question. However readers are advised to check the most current information available on procedures included and check information from the manufacturer of each product to be administered, to verify the recommended dose, formula, method and duration of administration, adverse effects and contraindications. It is the responsibility of the practitioner to take all appropriate safety precautions. Neither the publisher nor the authors assume any liability for any injury and/or damage to persons or property arising from or related to use of material in this book.

This book is sold on the understanding that the publisher is not engaged in providing professional medical services. If such advice or services are required, the services of a competent medical professional should be sought.

Every effort has been made where necessary to contact holders of copyright to obtain permission to reproduce copyright material. If any have been inadvertently overlooked, the publisher will be pleased to make the necessary arrangements at the first opportunity.

ISBN: 978-1-907816-44-4

British Library Cataloguing in Publication Data
A catalogue record for this book is available from the British Library

Library of Congress Cataloging in Publication Data
A catalog record for this book is available from the Library of Congress

JP Medical Ltd is a subsidiary of Jaypee Brothers Medical Publishers (P) Ltd, New Delhi, India

Publisher: Richard Furn
Commissioning Editor: Hannah Applin
Senior Editorial Assistant: Katrina Rimmer
Editorial Assistant: Thomas Fletcher
Design: Designers Collective Ltd

Indexed, copy edited, typeset, printed and bound in India.

Preface

Passing the MRCP(UK) exam is internationally recognised as a significant achievement, reflecting the acquisition of the knowledge, skills and attributes required by trainee physicians to progress to higher specialist training. However, it is not an achievement that comes easily. Having recently taken the exam ourselves, we know first hand the difficulties of trying to balance revision with working in a busy job with demanding on-calls, whilst at the same time attempting to keep some semblance of a normal social and family life.

Another difficulty in preparing for MRCP(UK) (and particularly for Part 1) is that it is not clear how and what to study. Does every available guideline need to be scrutinised in exquisite detail? Should huge lists of rare complications be memorised for every disease encountered? Clearly there is no single, sure-fire 'correct way' of preparing for the exam – all of us have met very knowledgeable doctors who have taken several attempts to pass.

With this book we highlight the key areas of how and what to study, so that candidates can use it to revise and prepare for the exam as effectively as possible. We have attempted to do this in a number of different ways.

Firstly, the questions are in the same style as the exam and, like the exam, include normal values. They reflect the breadth of knowledge and level of difficulty of the exam. This will help candidates to appreciate what to expect on the actual day. It will quickly become obvious that some questions are more difficult than others – this again is a reflection of the exam itself.

Secondly, based on our own experiences of the exam, in the answers we have tried to put an emphasis on and simplify the most difficult topics, sharing key memory aids that we have found useful ourselves – including tables, mnemonics and illustrations.

Thirdly, we have tried to provide thorough but not overly-detailed explanations, with answers that not only explain why one option is correct but also justify why other options are not.

Fourthly, many questions have an accompanying reference, to direct further reading around the topic.

Whilst this book is principally aimed at those preparing for the MRCP(UK) Part 1, we hope it will also be of interest to junior doctors more generally. We have written questions that reflect typical challenging situations that might be encountered on a typical acute 'medical take', or dilemmas that might be faced in the clinic.

We hope that you find this book useful – and, hopefully, enjoyable to use. Best of luck for the exam!

Imran Mannan
Vincent Cheung
Claire Grout
Benjamin Mullish
December 2012

Contents

Contents

Exam revision advice

Format

The MRCP(UK) exam consists of three parts. Part 1 is a written exam, whilst Part 2 is split into a written and a clinical exam (PACES).

The MRCP(UK) Part 1 exam has a two-paper format. Each paper lasts 3 hours and consists of 100 multiple choice questions. All questions take a best of five (BOF) approach, where the single most appropriate answer must be selected from a list of five options. Questions cover the full range of medical specialties and include clinical science. The composition of the papers is shown in **Table 1**.

There is no specific syllabus for the MRCP(UK) Part 1 exam, but the Royal Colleges recommend

Table 1

Specialty	Number of questions*
Cardiology	15
Clinical pharmacology, therapeutics and toxicology	20
Clinical sciences**	25
Dermatology	8
Endocrinology	15
Gastroenterology	15
Haematology and oncology	15
Neurology	15
Ophthalmology	4
Psychiatry	8
Renal medicine	15
Respiratory medicine	15
Rheumatology	15
Tropical medicine, infectious and sexually transmitted diseases	15
Total	**200**

*This should be taken as an indication of the likely number of questions – the actual number may vary slightly.
**Clinical sciences comprise:

Cell, molecular and membrane biology	2
Clinical anatomy	3
Clinical biochemistry and metabolism	4
Clinical physiology	4
Genetics	3
Immunology	4
Statistics, epidemiology and evidence-based medicine	5

Table 1 Composition of the MRCP Part 1 exam.

that candidates refer to the Specialty Training Curriculum for General Internal Medicine, prepared by the Joint Royal Colleges of Physicians Training Board.

The MRCP(UK) Part 1 exam is now marked using a process called equating. Using the equating system means that rather than being given an overall percentage score, candidates will instead be given an 'overall scaled score'. This score is a number between 0 and 999, which is calculated from the number of questions a candidate has answered correctly (out of the maximum possible) and takes into account the relative difficulty of the exam. Since no two exams contain the same questions, it is inevitable that some papers may be slightly harder (or easier) than others, and equating is a statistical process that addresses this. At present, the equated score required to pass MRCP(UK) Part 1 is 521.

Candidates are strongly advised to visit the MRCP(UK) website for further details of the exam.

How to use this book to prepare for MRCP(UK) Part 1

The book has been set out in chapters that reflect the specialties covered by the MRCP(UK) Part 1 exam. The number of questions per specialty is directly proportional to the weight each specialty area will carry in the actual exam. Each chapter contains questions covering a broad range of topics within each specialty, and questions range in difficulty between relatively easy and very difficult, as in the exam itself. Each question is followed by an explanation to explain why that answer is the most appropriate and why the other options are not correct. Where illustrations enhance the explanations these have been included (though interpretation of images is not a re-quirement for the Part 1 exam). As in the exam, when a question includes a list of laboratory values we have included the normal values in parentheses.

Having recently sat the exam ourselves, our advice is to approach revision specialty by specialty. Remember to think laterally when revising, e.g. a question on vasculitis could appear in the renal, rheumatology, respiratory, neurology or dermatology sections. Tackle the questions as you would in the exam, by reading the rubric carefully and thinking about what the correct answer might be before reading the A–E options. Next, select which of the options best fits the answer that you were thinking of. There are no 'trick' questions, but there are definitely questions that are not as straightforward as they may initially appear. Use the information in the answer to confirm and ex-pand upon what you already know, or to help understand and remember why a certain answer is more appropriate than others. The references are provided throughout to enable you to clarify any uncertainties or to expand upon your knowledge if the topic particularly interests you. Remember, the key to success is practice, practice, practice!

Useful websites

MRCP(UK): http://www.mrcpuk.org/Pages/Home.aspx

Specialty Training Curriculum for General Internal Medicine from the Joint Royal Colleges of Physicians Training Board: http://www.jrcptb.org.uk/specialties/ST3-SpR/Documents/2009%20GIM%20curriculum.PDF

Acknowledgements

We are very grateful to Dr Aruna Dias, Consultant Gastroenterologist and Physician, Newham University Hospital, for his constant help and support throughout all stages of writing and editing this book. We would like to thank Dr Eric Beck for giving his time to provide helpful editorial input. We are very appreciative of the dedication and commitment of Hannah Applin at JP Medical Publishing.

We would also like to thank a number of people for their helpful comments and providing images for this book:

Dr Steve Ellis, Consultant Radiologist, Barts Health NHS Trust.

Dr Wendy Mills, Consultant Haematologist and James Butler, Section Head of Haematology, Pathology Department, Barts Health NHS Trust.

Dr Sam Khandhadia, Clinical Research Fellow, Eye Unit, University Hospitals Southampton.

IM, VC, CG, BM

Dedication

In memory of my mother, and for my father and brother.

Imran Mannan

For my mother, father, brother and girlfriend for their endless love and support.

Vincent Cheung

For my mum, dad and husband for their constant support and faith in me.

Claire Grout

For my mother for always being there, and in memory of my father.

Benjamin Mullish

Chapter 1

Cardiology

1. A 75-year-old man with asthma attended the emergency department complaining of palpitations. They came on suddenly 2 hours ago. He had a past medical history including congestive cardiac failure. On examination, his pulse was 180 beats per minute, irregular and blood pressure was 120/75 mmHg. A 12-lead ECG showed him to be in atrial fibrillation.

   What is the most appropriate initial treatment?

   A   Amiodarone
   B   Atenolol
   C   DC cardioversion
   D   Flecainide
   E   Sotalol

2. A 27-year-old man attended the emergency department in the middle of the night with a history of sudden onset central, crushing chest pain which radiated into his left arm. It occurred whilst he was dancing at a night club. ECG showed ST elevation in the inferior leads.

   Which one of the following drugs should be avoided during the acute treatment of this patient?

   A   Atenolol
   B   Glyceryl trinitrate (GTN)
   C   Low molecular weight heparin (LMWH)
   D   Oxygen
   E   Ramipril

3. A 73-year-old man attended his general practitioner complaining of increasingly frequent episodes of dizziness on standing. On examination, he was noted to have a slow rising pulse and a systolic murmur that radiated to the carotids.

   What is the most likely underlying cause of this man's dizziness?

   A   Aortic regurgitation
   B   Aortic sclerosis
   C   Aortic stenosis
   D   Mitral regurgitation
   E   Tricuspid regurgitation

4. A 59-year-old woman presented to the emergency department having collapsed whilst waiting at a bus stop. An ECG showed a prolonged QT interval.

    Which one of the following is the most likely underlying cause for her ECG changes?

    A   Hypercalcaemia
    B   Hypermagnesaemia
    C   Hyperthermia
    D   Hyperthyroidism
    E   Hypokalaemia

5. A 22-year-old man attended the emergency department with a history of central chest pain whilst playing football. Of note, his uncle had died suddenly on the football field aged 25.

    What is the most likely underlying diagnosis?

    A   Anxiety
    B   Hypertrophic cardiomyopathy
    C   Myocardial infarction
    D   Oesophageal reflux
    E   Pulmonary embolus

6. A 52-year-old man, a taxi driver, attended the emergency department with a history of sudden onset central chest pain, and was found to have an anterior myocardial infarction (MI) on ECG. He underwent angioplasty with the insertion of a single stent. He was fit for discharge 48 hours later.

    How long should this patient refrain from driving?

    A   Can drive immediately following discharge
    B   1 week
    C   4 weeks
    D   3 months
    E   6 months

7. A 40-year-old man presented to the emergency department with a history of fevers and rigors for the preceding 2 weeks. On examination, he was pyrexial and tachycardic, and was noted to have splinter haemorrhages on his right middle and index fingers. A diagnosis of infective endocarditis was suspected and an echocardiogram requested.

    Where on the echocardiogram are vegetations most likely to occur?

    A   Aortic and mitral valves
    B   Aortic valve
    C   Mitral valve
    D   Pulmonary valve
    E   Tricuspid valve

8. A 68-year-old man presented to the emergency department with a history of fever and weight loss. He was admitted and underwent a full septic screen. He was diagnosed with infective endocarditis and 48 hours later his blood cultures grew *Streptococcus bovis.*

What is the most appropriate next investigation?

A   Bronchoscopy
B   Chest X-ray
C   Colonoscopy
D   Repeat blood cultures
E   Repeat echocardiogram

9. A 54-year-old woman presented to the emergency department 10 weeks after having a metallic mitral valve replacement. She was feeling lethargic. On examination, she had a pyrexia of 38.2°C, with a blood pressure of 112/75 mmHg and a pulse of 112 beats per minute. On auscultation, she had a metallic first heart sound, and a late diastolic murmur heard over the apex. As part of the investigations, blood cultures were taken from multiple veins.

What is the most likely growth that would be expected from the blood cultures?

A   *Candida* species
B   Coagulase-negative *Staphylococcus*
C   Gram-negative bacilli
D   No growth
E   *Staphylococcus aureus*

10. A 24-year old woman presented to her general practitioner with a 3-week history of palpitations. Each episode was short lived and self terminated. Her ECG showed right bundle branch block and right axis deviation with a prolonged PR interval.

What is the most likely underlying diagnosis?

A   Aortic coarctation
B   Ostium primum
C   Ostium secundum
D   Patent ductus arteriosus
E   Ventricular septal defect

11. A 67-year-old man presented to the emergency department with central crushing chest pain.

Which one of the following ECG changes would not be an indication for thrombolysis?

A   New onset left bundle branch block (LBBB)
B   Posterior infarction
C   ST elevation greater than 1 mm in two or more contiguous chest leads
D   ST elevation greater than 2 mm in two or more contiguous chest leads
E   ST elevation greater than 1 mm in two or more contiguous limb leads

12. A 65-year-old man was known to be in atrial fibrillation. He did not want to be cardioverted. He had no other past medical history, and was a non-smoker.

    What is the most appropriate anticoagulation therapy?

    A   Aspirin
    B   Clopidogrel
    C   No anticoagulation
    D   Phenindione
    E   Warfarin

13. A 74-year-old man had been diagnosed with left ventricular failure. He got breathless when walking briskly uphill, but was able to conduct day-to-day activities free of symptoms.

    What grade of heart failure does he have (according to the New York Heart Association classification of heart failure)?

    A   Grade 0
    B   Grade 1
    C   Grade 2
    D   Grade 3
    E   Grade 4

14. A 38-year-old Afro-Caribbean woman was reviewed by her general practitioner regarding her recently diagnosed hypertension. Despite lifestyle modifications such as salt restriction, increased exercise and weight loss, her blood pressure remained elevated at 162/73 mmHg.

    What is the most appropriate next step in management?

    A   Ramipril
    B   Bisoprolol
    C   Isosorbide mononitrate
    D   Orlistat
    E   Verapamil

15. A 68-year-old man was admitted to the emergency department with a 1-hour history of central crushing chest pain.

    Which cardiac enzyme is the first to rise in myocardial infarction?

    A   Creatine kinase (CK)
    B   Creatine kinase-MB (CK-MB)
    C   Lactate dehydrogenase (LDH)
    D   Myoglobin
    E   Troponin T

16. A 23-year-old man attended his general practitioner complaining of palpitations. He first noticed the episodes 3 months ago and had had four further episodes. The general practitioner performed an ECG and informed the patient he would be referred to the cardiology clinic for consideration of radiofrequency ablation.

What abnormality had been identified on the ECG?

A   Peaked T waves
B   Prolonged PR interval
C   Shortened QT interval
D   U waves
E   Widened QRS intervals with a slurred upstroke

17. A 68-year-old woman was admitted to the emergency department with a diagnosis of an inferior ST elevation myocardial infarction.

What ECG changes would be seen?

A   ST elevation V1 and V2
B   ST elevation I, aVL, V5, V6
C   ST elevation V2–V6
D   ST elevation V5 and V6
E   ST elevation in II, III and aVF

18. A 64-year-old man presented to the emergency department with a history of dyspnoea on climbing the stairs and increased frequency of angina over the past few months. On examination, he was found to have an elevated jugular venous pressure and a positive Kussmaul's sign. His chest was clear on auscultation, but heart sounds were difficult to hear. Chest X-ray showed some areas of calcification at the cardiac border.

What is the most likely underlying diagnosis?

A   Asbestosis
B   Cardiac tamponade
C   Congestive cardiac failure
D   Constrictive pericarditis
E   Superior vena cava obstruction

19. A 73-year-old man presented to the emergency department 1 month after being discharged following percutaneous coronary intervention for an anterior myocardial infarction. He was currently complaining of fevers and central sharp chest pain that was worse on inspiration. Admission blood tests show an elevated erythrocyte sedimentation rate.

What is the most likely underlying diagnosis?

A   Cardiac rupture
B   Dressler's syndrome
C   Drug allergy
D   Pulmonary embolus
E   Reinfarction

20. A 58-year-old man was known to have aortic stenosis. He was asymptomatic and was sent by his general practitioner for a routine echocardiogram. The results showed a pressure gradient across the aortic valve of 40 mmHg.

What is the most appropriate treatment option?

A Aortic valvuloplasty
B Emergency aortic valve replacement
C No further follow-up or intervention required
D Regular follow-up in cardiology outpatients
E Routine valve replacement

21. A 68-year-old man admitted to the emergency department with central tearing chest pain, was found to have an aortic dissection involving the ascending aorta. He had a history of hypertension and chronic obstructive pulmonary disease (COPD), for which he used regular inhalers. His pulse was 135 beats per minute and blood pressure 155/84 mmHg.

What is the most appropriate next step in management?

A Intravenous calcium channel blockers
B Intravenous calcium channel blockers plus surgery
C Intravenous labetalol
D Intravenous labetalol plus surgery
E Oral bisoprolol

22. A 56-year-old man, who was on the coronary care unit following percutaneous coronary intervention for an inferior myocardial infarction was noted to have a pulse of 46 beats per minute. His blood pressure was 127/52 mmHg and he was mobilising around his bed space with no problems. A 12-lead ECG revealed complete heart block.

What is the most appropriate initial management?

A Atropine
B DC cardioversion
C Observation
D Permanent pacemaker insertion
E Temporary pacing wire insertion

23. A 28-year-old woman was brought into the emergency department with a blood pressure 85/36 mmHg and pulse rate 35 beats per minute. Empty packets of her mother's bisoprolol tablets were found beside her by the ambulance crew.

What is the most appropriate next step in management?

A Flumazenil
B Glucagon
C Naloxone
D *N*-acetyl cysteine
E Physostigmine

24. A 54-year-old man was brought into the emergency department complaining of sudden onset dyspnoea, and was diagnosed as having an episode of pulmonary oedema. ECG and cardiac enzymes were normal.

What is the most useful diagnostic investigation?

A   Cardiac MRI
B   CT angiogram
C   ECG
D   MR angiogram
E   Stress test

25. Which one of the following is a cause of right axis deviation on a 12-lead ECG?

A   Hyperkalaemia
B   Left anterior hemi-block
C   Left bundle branch block
D   Left posterior hemi-block
E   Ostium primum

26. A 28-year-old woman, who was 28 weeks pregnant, was found to have a blood pressure of 172/92 mmHg. Urinalysis: ++ protein.

What is the most appropriate treatment?

A   Amlodipine
B   Atenolol
C   Lifestyle advice
D   Methyldopa
E   Propranolol

27. Which one of the following features is severe left ventricular failure most likely to be associated with?
A   Collapsing pulse
B   Jerky pulse
C   Pulsus alternans
D   Pulsus bisferiens
E   Slow rising pulse

28. A 26-year-old woman presented to the emergency department with severe diarrhoea and vomiting.

Investigations:

sodium	136 mmol/L (137–144)
potassium	2.9 mmol/L (3.5–4.9)
urea	8.2 mmol/L (2.5–7.0)
creatinine	116 µmol/L (60–110)

What ECG changes would be consistent with these results?

A   Prolonged QT interval
B   Prolonged PR interval
C   Shortened QT interval
D   Tall T waves
E   U waves

29. A 29-year-old man presented to the emergency department with a history of palpitations. He took a salbutamol inhaler as required for asthma, and had no known allergies. His blood pressure was 128/62 mmHg. Electrocardiogram showed a regular narrow complex tachycardia with rate 128 beats per minute.

    What is the most appropriate next step in management?

    A   Adenosine
    B   Amiodarone
    C   DC cardioversion
    D   Vagal manoeuvres
    E   Verapamil

30. A 67-year-old man attended his general practitioner for a medication review. Twelve months ago, he underwent percutaneous coronary intervention for an ST elevation myocardial infarction. He had no other medical problems and no drug allergies.

    What medication should be on his repeat prescription?

    A   Angiotensin-converting enzyme (ACE) inhibitor + aspirin + bisoprolol + statin
    B   ACE inhibitor + aspirin + bisoprolol + clopidogrel + statin
    C   Aspirin + bisoprolol + clopidogrel + statin
    D   Aspirin + clopidogrel + statin
    E   Aspirin + statin

Answers

1. A Amiodarone

Flecainide is the drug most likely to restore sinus rhythm in atrial fibrillation (AF). However, the CAST trial suggests that it should be avoided in left ventricular failure and can be arrhythmogenic post-myocardial infarction. Amiodarone is an antiarrhythmic agent that spans all categories of the Vaughan Williams classification and can be used to terminate acute supraventricular and ventricular arrhythmias. It is of added benefit in this patient as it is the least negatively inotropic arrhythmic, second to digoxin. Beta-blockers should be avoided as the patient has a history of asthma. DC cardioversion is indicated in the acute stage if the patient is haemodynamically unstable. It may also be used in the chronic setting following six weeks of anticoagulation.

Cardiac Arrhythmia Suppression Trial (CAST) Investigators. Preliminary report: effect of encainide and flecainide on mortality in a randomized trial of arrhythmia suppression after myocardial infarction. N Engl J Med 1989; 321:406–412.
The Cardiac Arrhythmia Suppression Trial-II Investigators. Effect of antiarrhythmic agent moricizine on survival after myocardial infarction: the Cardiac Arrhythmia Suppression Trial-II. N Engl J Med 1992; 327:227–233.

2. A Atenolol

This man is having an myocardial infarction (MI), most likely secondary to cocaine use. Cocaine is a potent sympathomimetic agent. It acts by preventing the reuptake, and therefore accumulation of dopamine and noradrenalin at the synaptic junctions. Its positive effect on the α-adrenoceptors results in significant vasoconstriction, leading to hypertension, tachycardia and increased myocardial contractility. This in turn leads to increased oxygen demand of the myofibrils, but because of vasoconstriction of the coronary arteries, that oxygen demand is not met and ischaemia results. Beta-blockers aggravate the vasospasm and worsen the ischaemia. The treatment of choice in cocaine-induced MI is glyceryl trinitrate and calcium channel blockers.

Note that low molecular weight heparin (LMWH) should be used with caution in patients with long-term cocaine abuse, due to the increased risk of intracranial haemorrhage.

McCord, J et al. Management of cocaine-associated chest pain and myocardial infarction. Circulation 2008; 117:1897–1907.

3. C Aortic stenosis

Table 1.1 summarises the main features and associations of valvular heart disease.

4. E Hypokalaemia

Prolonged QT interval is associated with syncope and sudden death from ventricular tachycardia. There are multiple causes:

Table 1.1

Murmur	On auscultation	Associations
Aortic stenosis	Ejection systolic Loudest over the aortic area Radiates to carotids	Slow rising pulse Dizziness and collapse Displaced apex beat
Aortic sclerosis	Ejection systolic murmur Loudest over the aortic area No carotid radiation	Secondary to age related calcification of the valve No associated symptoms
Aortic regurgitation	Early diastolic murmur Heard over the lower left sternal edge in held expiration	Collapsing pulse
Mitral regurgitation	Pan-systolic murmur Loudest at the apex Radiates to the axilla	Associated with atrial fibrillation Displaced apex beat
Mitral stenosis	Mid-diastolic murmur Loudest at the apex when auscultating with the bell	Atrial fibrillation Evidence of pulmonary hypertension
Tricuspid regurgitation	Pan-systolic murmur Loudest at the lower left sternal edge on held inspiration No radiation	Giant V waves in jugular venous pressure Right ventricular heave

Table 1.1 Summary of valvular heart disease.

- Familial:
  - Romano-Ward syndrome (AD) – this is the most common inherited form of long QT syndrome
  - Jervell–Lang-Nielsen syndrome (AR) – this causes a profound hearing loss from birth as well as long QT syndrome
- Metabolic:
  - Hypocalcaemia
  - Hypokalaemia
  - Hypomagnesaemia
  - Hypothermia
  - Hypothyroidism
- Drugs:
  - Amiodarone
  - Erythromycin
  - Phenothiazines
  - Quinine
  - Sotalol
  - Terfenadine
  - Tricyclic antidepressants (TCAs)

- Ischaemic heart disease
- Myocarditis

Webster A, Brady W, Morris F; Recognising signs of danger: ECG changes resulting from an abnormal serum. Emerg Med J 2002; 19(1):74–77.

5. B Hypertrophic cardiomyopathy

As this man is young and active and has a family history of sudden death, you should be suspicious of an underlying genetic condition. Hypertrophic cardiomyopathy is therefore the most likely from the options available.

Hypertrophic cardiomyopathy is an autosomal dominant condition that affects the cardiac myocytes. Many patients are asymptomatic, but it can present with chest pain, palpitations, dyspnoea or sudden death. Investigations include ECG in the first instance, followed by echocardiogram. Treatment can be medical or surgical. Medications used include beta-blockers, calcium channel blockers or antiarrhythmics, such as amiodarone. In patients with significant outflow obstruction as a result of septal hypertrophy, surgical myomectomy or septal ablation may be considered. In those at risk of sudden death (previous history of cardiac arrest or failure to control symptoms with medications) and implantable cardioverter defibrillator should be inserted.

Elliott P, McKenna WJ. Hypertrophic cardiomyopathy. Lancet 2004; 363(9424):1881–1891.
Spirito P, Autore C. Management of hypertrophic cardiomyopathy. BMJ 2006; 332(7552):1251–1255.
Ramaraj R. Hypertrophic cardiomyopathy: etiology, diagnosis, and treatment. Cardiol Rev 2008; 16(4):172–180.

6. B 1 week

The UK Driver and Vehicle Licensing Agency (DVLA) has very clear regulations regarding driving following interventional procedures for cardiac conditions.

In an acute coronary syndrome (unstable angina, non-ST segment elevation myocardial infarction [NSTEMI], ST segment elevation myocardial infarction [STEMI]) that is successfully treated with coronary angioplasty, driving may recommence within 1 week. If angioplasty is not successful, driving may recommence after 4 weeks, providing there is no other disqualifying condition.

If a patient undergoes elective primary coronary angioplasty, driving may commence after 1 week.

If a patient undergoes coronary artery bypass grafting (CABG), driving must cease for at least 4 weeks.

The DVLA need not be notified in any of the above situations.

Driver and Vehicle and Licensing Agency UK. Guide to the current medical standards of fitness to drive. DVLA 2012. http://www.dft.gov.uk

7. C Mitral valve

The mitral valve is the most commonly affected valve in infective endocarditis followed, in reducing order of frequency, by the aortic valve, the aortic and mitral valves, the tricuspid valve and rarely the pulmonary valve.

The vegetations occur on the low pressure surface of the valve. On the mitral valve, vegetations occur on the aortic surface, whereas vegetations occur on the ventricular surface of the aortic valve.

Approximately 70% of cases of endocarditis on native valves are caused by *Streptococcus* species including viridans *Streptococcus*, *Streptococcus bovis* and *Enterococcus* species. 25% are caused by staphylococcal infections which are more aggressive and have a more acute course.

Beynon RP, Bahl VK, Prendergast BD. Infective endocarditis. BMJ 2006; 333:334.
Hoen B. Epidemiology and antibiotic treatment of infective endocarditis: an update. Heart 2006; 92(11): 1694–1700.

8. C Colonoscopy

Streptococcus bovis is associated with colorectal cancer and adenoma. 25–80% of patients with *S. bovis* bacteraemia have a colorectal cancer. Therefore, once the patient is well enough to tolerate the procedure, a colonoscopy should be performed.

Abdulamir AS, Hafidh RR, Abu Bakar F. The association of *Streptococcus bovis/gallolyticus* with colorectal tumors: the nature and the underlying mechanisms of its etiological role. J Exp Clin Cancer Res 2011; 30:11.

9. E *Staphylococcus aureus*

10–20% of all cases of infective endocarditis are associated with prosthetic valves. Eventually 5% of all prosthetic valves will become infected. Early prosthetic valve endocarditis occurs within 60 days of implantation and is associated with coagulase-negative staphylococcal organisms, *Candida* species and gram-negative bacilli. Late infection occurs 60 days or more after implantation, and tends to be associated with *Staphylococcus aureus*. α-haemolytic streptococci and enterococci are also implicated.

Metallic valves are more likely to become infected within the first 3 months of implantation and bioprosthetic valves are more likely to be infected 1 year after implantation.

Mandell GL, Bennett JE, Dolin R, (eds). Mandel, Douglas and Bennett's Principles and Practice and Infectious Diseases, 7th edition. Elsevier; 2009:1022–1044.
Wang A, et al. Contemporary clinical profile and outcome of prosthetic valve endocarditis. JAMA 2007; 297(12):1354–61.

10. C Ostium secundum

Clinical features of an atrial septal defect (ASD) include wide fixed splitting of the second heart sound, loud P2 and a pulmonary systolic flow murmur. Complications include pulmonary hypertension, Eisenmenger's syndrome, cardiac failure and infective endocarditis. The different characteristics of the different atrial septal defects are outlined in **Table 1.2a**. **Table 1.2b** outlines the features of other congenital heart diseases.

Table 1.2a

	%	Anatomy	Characterised ECG changes	Associations	Complications
Ostium secundum	70%	Defect of fossa ovale	Partial RBBB and right axis deviation Prolonged PR on ECG	Mitral valve prolapse	Atrial fibrillation
Ostium primum	15%	Defect sited above the AV valves	RBBB, Left axis deviation, 1st degree heart block	Mitral regurgitation, Down's syndrome, Klinefelter's, Noonan's	
Sinus venosus	15%	Defect in the upper part of the septum		Anomalous pulmonary venous drainage	

RBBB, right bundle branch block.

Table 1.2a Atrial septal defects.

Table 1.2b

	Clinical features	Associations
Ventricular septal defect (VSD) (25–30%)	Parasternal thrill Single S2 Pansystolic murmur loudest at lower left sternal edge Left to right shunt	Atrial fibrillation Ventricular arrhythmias Pulmonary hypertension Eisenmenger's syndrome
Patent ductus arteriosus (15%)	Continuous machinery murmur Collapsing pulse Left to right shunt	Women > men Closed with indomethacin Kept open with prostaglandins
Tetralogy of Fallot (10%)	Pulmonary stenosis – ejection systolic murmur in pulmonary area Right ventricular heave Right to left shunt through VSD – central cyanosis	Paradoxical embolus Polycythaemia Ventricular arrhythmias
Aortic coarctation (5%)	Ejection systolic infraclavicular murmur Radiofemoral delay Collateral artery formation	Berry aneurysms Turners syndrome Bicuspid aortic valve Rib notching seen on chest X-ray

Table 1.2b Other congenital heart diseases.

11. C ST elevation greater than 1 mm in two or more contiguous chest leads

Indications for thrombolysis include:

- New onset left bundle branch block
- ST elevation greater then 2 mm in two or more contiguous chest leads
- ST elevation greater than 1 mm in two or more contiguous limb leads
- Posterior infarction

Contraindications to thrombolysis include:

- Bleeding/trauma
- Recent surgery (sever liver disease)
- Oesophageal varices
- Head injury/cerebral neoplasm
- Recent haemorrhagic stroke
- Blood pressure > 200/120 mmHg
- Suspected aortic dissection

National Institute for Clinical Excellence (NICE). The clinical effectiveness and cost effectiveness of drugs for early thrombolysis in the treatment of acute myocardial infarction. Clinical Guideline TA52. London: NICE, 2002. The Task Force for the Management of Atrial Fibrillation of the European Society of Cardiology. Acute Myocardial Infarction in patients presenting with ST-segment elevation (Management of): ESC Clinical Practice Guidelines. Eur Heart J 2008; 29:2909–2945.

12. E Warfarin

The European Society of Cardiology published new guidelines to replace the CHAD2 scoring system in 2010. This is referred to as the CHA_2DS_2 VASc scoring system and is outlined in **Table 1.3** and **Table 1.4**. Using this system our patient scores 1 point (age), and therefore the preferred method of anticoagulation is warfarin over aspirin.

The Task Force for the Management of Atrial Fibrillation of the European Society of Cardiology. Guidelines for the management of atrial fibrillation. Eur Heart J 2010; 31: 2369–2429.

Table 1.3	
Risk factors	**Points**
Congestive heart failure/LV dysfunction	1
Hypertension	1
Age > 75	2
Diabetes	1
Stroke/transient ischaemic attack/thromboembolism	2
Vascular disease	1
Age 65–74 years	1
Sex (female)	1

Table 1.3 CHA_2DS_2 VAS Score.

Table 1.4

Score	Preferred anticoagulation
2+	Warfarin
1	Warfarin preferred to aspirin
0	No therapy preferred to aspirin

Table 1.4 Suggested anticoagulation.

13. C Grade 2

The New York Heart Association Classification of heart failure is:

Grade 1: No breathlessness, no effect on daily life

Grade 2: Breathless on severe exertion

Grade 3: Breathless on mild exertion

Grade 4: Breathless at rest, severely limited

NB there is no Grade 0

The Criteria Committee of the New York Heart Association. Nomenclature and Criteria for Diagnosis of Diseases of the Heart and Great Vessels, 9th edition. Little, Brown & Co; 1994:253–256.

14. E Verapamil

The **ABCD** rule is helpful here:

Angiotensin converting enzyme inhibitors ⎫ More successful in young patients

Beta-blockers ⎭

Calcium channel blockers ⎫ More successful in older patients and the Afro-Carribean population

Diuretics ⎭

Although this patient is young, she is Afro-Caribbean, and therefore she should be started on a calcium channel blocker or a diuretic; hence verapamil is the correct answer. Beta-blockers have been linked with diabetes, and they should no longer be used as first-line agents.

If single-agent therapy is not effective then further agents may be added.

Orlistat is an anti-obesity drug; it has anti-lipase activity and reduces absorption of dietary fat from the gut.

Brown MJ, et al. Better blood pressure control: how to combine drugs. J Hum Hyperten 2003; 17(2):81–86.

15. D Myoglobin

Myoglobin rises first in myocardial infarction. **Table 1.5** outlines the behaviour of the different cardiac enzymes.

Table 1.5			
	First rises	**Peak level**	**Normalises**
CK	4–8 hours	16–24 hours	3–4 days
CK-MB	2–6 hours	16–20 hours	2–3 days
LDH	24–48 hours	72 hours	8–10 days
Myoglobin	1–2 hours	6–8 hours	1–2 days
Troponin T	4–6 hours	12–24 hours	7–10 days

Table 1.5 Pattern of enzyme levels in myocardial infarction.

16. E Widened QRS intervals with a slurred upstroke

This patient most likely has Wolff–Parkinson–White syndrome which predisposes to supraventricular tachycardias, as a result of an accessory antrioventricular conduction pathway.

Classic ECG changes include:

- Short PR interval
- Widened QRS interval with slurred upstroke (delta waves – as depicted in **Figure 1.1**)
- Left axis deviation if there is a left sided accessory pathway
- Right axis deviation if there is a right sided accessory pathway

Definitive treatment is with radiofrequency ablation of the accessory pathway.

Jackman WM, et al. Catheter ablation of accessory atrioventricular pathways (Wolff- Parkinson-White syndrome) by radiofrequency current. N Engl J Med 1991; 324(23):1605–1611.

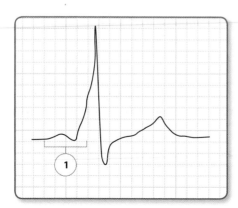

Figure 1.1 Delta wave in Wolff–Parkinson–White syndrome. 1: Slurred upstroke of the QRS complex – delta wave. (Reproduced from James S and Nelson K. Pocket Tutor ECG Interpretation. London: JP Medical Ltd, 2011.)

17. E ST elevation in II, III and aVF

An inferior myocardial infarction involves the right coronary artery and ECG changes involve leads II, III and aVF. **Table 1.6** outlines the ECG changes associated with occlusion of the different coronary arteries.

Table 1.6		
	ECG changes	**Artery**
Anteroseptal	V1–V4	Left anterior descending
Anterolateral	V4–V6, I, aVL	Left anterior descending
Inferior	II, III, aVF	Right coronary
Lateral	I, aVL, V5, V6	Left circumflex
Posterior	Tall R waves V1 and V2	Left circumflex Right coronary

Table 1.6 ECG changes associated with myocardial infarction.

18. D Constrictive pericarditis

Constrictive pericarditis classically presents as worsening dyspnoea over time.

Clinical findings include:

- Elevated jugular venous pressure (JVP)
- Muffled heart sounds
- Tachycardia
- Hypotension
- Positive Kussmaul's sign (rise in JVP on inspiration)
- Pericardial calcification seen on chest X-ray

Causes include:

- Post infective
- Recurrent pericarditis
- Connective tissue disease
- Tuberculosis
- Radiotherapy
- Uraemic pericarditis

The presentation of cardiac tamponade may be similar, but dyspnoea often worsens rapidly, and Kussmaul's sign is usually negative. There is also an absent Y descent in the JVP.

Asbestosis may present in a similar fashion, but fine crackles would be heard on auscultation of the chest (pulmonary fibrosis) and Kussmaul's sign would not be present.

Superior vena caval obstruction is identified by an elevated JVP with absent A and V waves. There is often associated facial swelling with dilated veins across the arms, neck and anterior chest wall.

In congestive cardiac failure the JVP is elevated and there is peripheral oedema. There is also evidence of left heart failure, with pulmonary oedema (bibasal crackles heard on chest examination).

19. B Dressler's syndrome

Dressler's syndrome (pericarditis and pleural effusions) occurs 2 weeks to 2 months after myocardial infarction or cardiac surgery. It presents with fever, pleurisy and pericarditis. Blood tests show an elevated erythrocyte sedimentation rate (ESR) with anaemia, and anticardiac muscle antibodies are identified in some cases. Treatment is with non-steroidal anti-inflammatory drugs (NSAIDs).

Reinfarction would not normally be associated with fevers. Myocardial rupture post myocardial infarction can occur between 1 day to 3 weeks after the original event, but usually occurs at 3–5 days. It is a rare complication, and classically presents as a catastrophic event.

Pulmonary embolus should be considered as a differential diagnosis, but would not normally be associated with an elevated ESR.

A drug reaction, secondary to any new medications started following the myocardial infarction, may present with fevers, but would not be expected to cause chest pain. Drug reactions may also present with skin rashes, dyspnoea or lymphoedema, or as a fixed drug eruption.

Wessman DE, Stafford CM. The postcardiac injury syndrome: case report and review of the literature. South Med J 2006; 99(3):309–314.

20. D Regular follow-up in cardiology outpatients

Currently aortic valve replacement in aortic stenosis is only considered for those who are symptomatic, or have a gradient of >50 mmHg with left ventricular dysfunction. Valvuloplasty may be considered in those unfit for surgery, but who are symptomatic.

The patient should be followed up in clinic as his left ventricular function and pressure gradient across the valve should be monitored for consideration of surgery in the future.

There is no indication within the scenario for emergency valve replacement to be undertaken (e.g. infective endocarditis, not responding to antibiotic therapy).

Bonow RO, et al. Focused update incorporated into the ACC/AHA 2006 guidelines for the management of patients with valvular heart disease. Circulation 2008; 118:e523.

21. B Intravenous calcium channel blockers plus surgery

Aortic dissections can be divided into two categories. Type A affects the ascending aorta and definitive treatment is surgical repair. The mainstay of management is for blood pressure to be controlled with intravenous agents whilst awaiting surgery. The aim of surgery is to prevent cardiac tamponade and aortic rupture.

Type B dissections do not involve the ascending aorta and are usually managed by strict blood pressure control with intravenous agents. Beta-blockers are usually used, but calcium channel antagonists are used in patients with chronic obstructive pulmonary disease (COPD).

Other conditions associated with aortic dissection include:

- Systemic hypertension
- Marfan's syndrome
- Noonan's syndrome
- Turner's syndrome
- Trauma
- Aortic coarctation
- Congenital bicuspid aortic valve
- Giant cell arteritis
- Cocaine abuse

Siegal EM. Acute aortic dissection. J Hosp Med 2006; 1(2):94–105.

22. C Observation

Complete heart block following an inferior myocardial infarction (MI) occurs due to ischaemic damage to the antrioventricular node (supplied by the right coronary artery in 90% of people). It often spontaneously resolves, and as this patient is haemodynamically stable, observation is all that is currently required.

Complete heart block following an anterior MI is an indication for pace-maker insertion.

Figure 1.2 shows an ECG showing an inferior myocardial infarction.

23. B Glucagon

Glucagon is the agent of choice to treat beta-blocker overdose. **Table 1.7** outlines the antidotes for common poisons.

24. D MR angiogram

This man probably has renal artery stenosis as an underlying cause of his pulmonary oedema, since his ECG and cardiac enzymes were normal, pointing away from a cardiac cause. The gold standard for investigation of renal artery stenosis is MR angiogram of the renal arteries, as it does not involve nephrotoxic contrast agents, or radiation exposure.

Tan KT, et al. Magnetic resonance angiography for the diagnosis of renal artery stenosis: a meta-analysis. Clin Radiol 2002; 57(7):617–624.

25. D Left posterior hemi-block

Causes of right axis deviation:

- Right ventricular hypertrophy

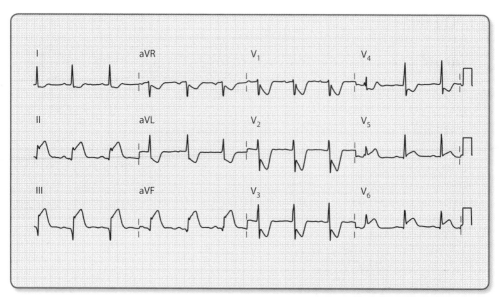

Figure 1.2 ECG showing an inferior myocardial infarction. (Reproduced from James S and Nelson K. Pocket Tutor ECG Interpretation. London: JP Medical Ltd, 2011.)

Table 1.7	
Poisons	**Antidotes**
Benzodiazepines	Flumazenil
Beta-blockers	Glucagon
Opiates	Naloxone
Paracetamol	N-acetyl cysteine
Anticholinergics	Physostigmine

Table 1.7 Common poisons and antidotes.

- Left posterior hemi-block
- Chronic lung disease
- Pulmonary embolus
- Ostium secundum

Causes of left axis deviation:

- Left anterior hemi-block
- Left bundle branch block
- Hyperkalaemia
- Ostium primum

26. D Methyldopa

This woman has a diagnosis of severe pre-eclampsia. Pre-eclampsia is associated with proteinuria, hypertension and intrauterine growth retardation. Methyldopa is the first line agent to treat elevated blood pressures, but labetalol and nifedipine may also be used. Intravenous agents are used in cases of severe hypertension. Delivery of the baby is the definitive treatment, but the timing of this is made on a case-by-case basis.

NB Labetalol use in maternal hypertension is not known to be harmful. Other beta-blockers are associated with intrauterine growth restriction, neonatal hypoglycaemia, and bradycardia.

Risk factors associated with pre-eclampsia include:

* Family history
* Primigravidas
* Prolonged interval between pregnancies
* Change in partner
* Teenage pregnancy
* Donor insemination
* Chronic hypertension
* Renal isease

27. C Pulsus alternans

Left ventricular failure is associated with pulsus alternans. **Table 1.8** outlines the pulse characteristics associated with various heart conditions.

28. E U waves

The blood results show hypokalaemia. U waves would be expected on the ECG. **Table 1.9** outlines the ECG changes associated with various electrolyte abnormalities.

Table 1.8	
Heart condition	**Pulse**
Tamponade	Pulsus paradoxus (>10 mmHg drop in systolic blood pressure during inspiration)
Aortic stenosis	Slow rising pulse
Aortic regurgitation	Collapsing pulse
Left ventricular failure	Pulsus alternans (alternation of force of pulse)
Mixed aortic valve disease	Pulsus bisferiens (double pulse)
Hypertrophic cardiomyopathy (HOCM)	Jerky pulse

Table 1.8 Pulse characters.

Table 1.9

Electrolyte abnormality	ECG change
Hypokalaemia	U Waves
Hyperkalaemia	Tall T waves $\rightarrow$ widened QRS complexes
Hypocalcaemia	Prolonged QT interval
Hypercalcaemia	Shortened QT interval
Hypomagnesaemia	T wave flattening ST depression U waves
Hypermagnesaemia	Prolonged PR interval Widened QRS complexes

Table 1.9 Electrolyte abnormalities and associated ECG changes.

29. D Vagal manoeuvres

In a haemodynamically stable patient with supraventricular tachycardia (as illustrated in **Figure 1.3**) vagal manoeuvres such as expiration against a closed glottis, are the first-line intervention. If this fails then adenosine should be given. However, adenosine is contraindicated in asthmatics and verapamil is the preferred alternative.

DC cardioversion should be used if the patient is haemodynamically unstable.

Beta-blockers may be considered if adenosine is unsuccessful in reverting to sinus rhythm.

Resuscitation Council UK. Resuscitation UK guidelines. http://www.resus.org.uk/pages/tachalgo.pdf 2010 (Last accessed may 2012)

30. A Angiotensin-converting enzyme (ACE) inhibitor + aspirin + bisoprolol + statin

The National Institute of Health and Clinical Excellence (NICE) guidelines state that after an ST elevation myocardial infarction (MI) all patients should be offered long term therapy with aspirin, an ACE inhibitor, bisoprolol and a statin.

After an ST elevation MI clopidogrel and aspirin should be given for 4 weeks. After this, only aspirin is required unless there are other indications for dual antiplatelet therapy (e.g. patients who receive a drug eluting stent during percutaneous intervention (PCI) should receive dual antiplatelet therapy for 1 year. As the question refers to a review 12 months after the PCI, even if the patient did receive a drug eluting stent, dual antiplatelet therapy is no longer required).

For patients who have had an acute MI and who have symptoms or signs of heart failure and left ventricular systolic dysfunction, treatment with an aldosterone

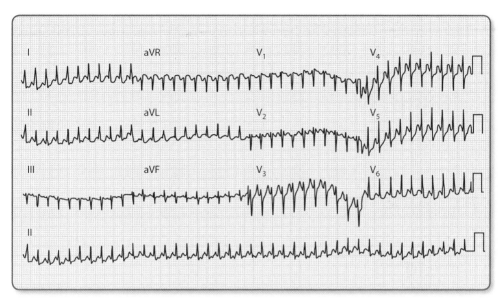

Figure 1.3 ECG from a patient with Supraventricular tachycardia (SVT). (Reproduced from James S and Nelson K. Pocket Tutor ECG Interpretation. London: JP Medical Ltd, 2011.)

antagonist should be initiated within 3–14 days of the MI, preferably after ACE inhibitor therapy.

Clopidogrel in combination with low-dose aspirin is recommended in the management of non-ST-segment-elevation MI in people who are at moderate to high risk of MI or death. This combination should be continued for 12 months.

National Institute for Clinical Excellence (NICE). MI: secondary prevention. Secondary prevention in primary and secondary care for patients following a myocardial infarction. Clinical Guideline CG48. London: NICE, 2007.

Chapter 2

Clinical pharmacology, therapeutics and toxicology

1. What is the mechanism of action of ciclosporin?

   A   Calcineurin inhibitor
   B   CD20 inhibitor
   C   Dihydrofolate reductase inhibitor
   D   Inosine monophosphate dehydrogenase inhibitor
   E   Purine synthesis inhibitor

2. Which one of the following drugs exhibit zero-order kinetics?

   A   Amiodarone
   B   Digoxin
   C   Heparin
   D   Isoniazid
   E   Rifampicin

3. What is the mechanism of action of simvastatin?

   A   Activates lipoprotein lipase
   B   Bile acid sequestrant
   C   Blocks breakdown of fats in adipose tissue
   D   Inhibits absorption of cholesterol from the intestines
   E   Inhibits hepatic cholesterol synthesis

4. A 28-year-old pregnant woman is seen in clinic to review her antidepressant medications.

   Which one of the following drugs is absolutely contraindicated during breastfeeding?

   A   Amitriptyline
   B   Fluoxetine
   C   Lithium
   D   Mirtazapine
   E   Paroxetine

5. A 28-year-old pregnant woman presented to the emergency department with shortness of breath, fever, cough and green sputum.

    What is the most appropriate medication?

    A   Amikacin
    B   Amoxicillin
    C   Ciprofloxacin
    D   Clarithromycin
    E   Doxycycline

6. Which one of these drugs is the least nephrotoxic?

    A   Amphotericin
    B   Furosemide
    C   Gentamicin
    D   Ramipril
    E   Verapamil

7. Which one of the following conditions is least likely to be associated with steroids?

    A   Acne
    B   Cataract
    C   Depression
    D   Hypotension
    E   Myopathy

8. Which one of the following drugs is least likely to cause gynaecomastia?

    A   Cimetidine
    B   Digoxin
    C   Methyldopa
    D   Metronidazole
    E   Nicorandil

9. Which one of the following is not a recognised side effect of angiotensin-converting enzyme (ACE) inhibitors?

    A   Anaphylaxis
    B   Hepatitis
    C   Impotence
    D   Leucocytosis
    E   Renal impairment

10. Which one of the following is not a recognised side effect of ciclosporin?

    A   Hair growth
    B   Hypertension
    C   Hypokalaemia
    D   Nephrotoxicity
    E   Tremor

11. A 30-year-old woman was started on a drug for bipolar disorder. Four weeks later, she was reviewed in clinic and complained of polydipsia, polyuria and weight gain.

Which one of the following drugs is most likely to be the cause?

A   Amisulpride
B   Carbamazepine
C   Clozapine
D   Lamotrigine
E   Lithium

12. A 65-year-old man presented with a worsening blistering rash affecting his palms and the soles of his feet. Two weeks ago, he had started chemotherapy for colorectal cancer.

What is the most likely cause?

A   Bleomycin
B   Capecitabine
C   Cisplatin
D   Doxorubicin
E   Vincristine

13. A 60-year-old man with oesophageal cancer was taking morphine sulphate tablets 45 mg twice daily as analgesia.

Which dose of Oramorph liquid should he be taken for breakthrough pain?

A   5 mg
B   10 mg
C   15 mg
D   20 mg
E   25 mg

14. A 25-year-old man was brought to the emergency department with confusion and slurred speech. The ambulance crew had found him by his car. On examination, he was apyrexial, pulse was 126 beats per minute, and blood pressure 168/95 mmHg. He had dilated, slow reacting pupils, was hypotonic and had slow reflexes. Visual acuity and fields were normal.

Investigations:

serum sodium	139 mmol/L (137–144)
serum potassium	4.0 mmol/L (3.5–4.9)
serum corrected calcium	2.02 mmol/L (2.20–2.60)
serum urea	15 mmol/L (2.5–7.0)
serum creatinine	186 µmol/L (60–110)

What is the most appropriate management?

A   Desferrioxamine
B   Dicobalt edetate

    C   Ethanol
    D   Fomepizole
    E   Pyridoxine

15. A 75-year-old man with a history of epilepsy presented to the medical admissions unit with confusion. He had no other significant past medical history. He was apyrexial and physical examination was normal.

Investigations:

serum sodium	116 mmol/L (137–144)
plasma osmolality	250 mOsmol/kg (278–300)
urine sodium	24 mmol/L (<20)
urine osmolality	600 mOsmol/kg (350–1000)

Which one of the following drugs is most likely to be causing the problem?

    A   Carbamazepine
    B   Levetiracetam
    C   Phenytoin
    D   Valproate
    E   Vigbatrin

16. A 26-year-old man, a welder, presented to the emergency department with a 3-month history of colicky abdominal pain and a 6-week history of difficulty walking. On examination, he had conjunctival pallor. The abdomen was soft and generally tender but not peritonitic and there were no signs of chronic liver disease. He had bilateral foot drop but no weakness in the limbs.

Investigations:

haemoglobin	97 g/L (130–180)
mean cell volume	68 fL (80–96)
blood film	basophilic stippling of red blood cells

What is the most likely diagnosis?

    A   Arsenic poisoning
    B   Cyanide poisoning
    C   Iron poisoning
    D   Lead poisoning
    E   Selenium poisoning

17. A 35-year-old woman was brought into the emergency department with nausea, vomiting and tinnitus after ingesting a number of unknown tablets 1 hour ago. She had no significant medical history but smoked 30 cigarettes per day. On examination, her Glasgow Coma Score was 9/15. Her temperature was 38.2°C, pulse 95 beats per minute, blood pressure 120/76 mmHg, respiratory rate 30 breaths per minute and oxygen saturation 88% on air. She had coarse crackles up to the mid-zones in both lungs.

Investigations:

Arterial blood gas on air:

pH	7.49 (7.35–7.45)
pO_2	8.6 kPa (11.3–12.6)
pCO_2	2.6 kPa (4.7–6.0)
base excess	4.5 mmol/L (± 2)
bicarbonate	22 mmol/L (21–29)

What is the most appropriate next step in management?

A   Activated charcoal
B   Haemodialysis
C   Intravenous normal saline
D   Intravenous sodium bicarbonate
E   Intubation

18. A 78-year-old man was admitted with shortness of breath and coughing green sputum. He had a history of chronic obstructive pulmonary disease (COPD) for which he was on salbutamol and ipratropium bromide inhalers and oral aminophylline. He also had type 2 diabetes and was on metformin. He had evidence of lobar pneumonia and was treated with intravenous amoxicillin and clarithromycin. In addition he was given nebulisers, oral prednisolone and oxygen. Later that evening, he developed two generalised seizures that lasted about 1 minute each with some loss of consciousness. His temperature was 38.0°C, pulse 120 beats per minute, blood pressure 88/45 mmHg and respiratory rate 25 breaths per minute. He had bilateral wheeze and crackles in his right lower zone. Neurological examination was normal.

What is the most likely cause of his deterioration?

A   Amoxicillin
B   Clarithromycin
C   Metformin
D   Prednisolone
E   Salbutamol

19. Which one of the following is not associated with warfarin?

A   Alopecia
B   Oral ulcers
C   Photosensitivity
D   Purple toe syndrome
E   Skin necrosis

20. What is the mechanism of action of flecainide?

A   Activates potassium channels
B   Activates sodium channels
C   Blocks calcium channels

    D   Blocks potassium channels

    E   Blocks sodium channels

21. Which one of the following is not associated with valproate?

    A   Ataxia

    B   Hirsutism

    C   Oedema

    D   Pancreatitis

    E   Tremor

22. A 75-year-old woman presented to her general practitioner feeling generally unwell. She had blood tests taken.

Investigations:

serum sodium	137 mmol/L 137–144)
serum potassium	6.8 mmol/L (3.5–4.9)
serum creatinine	230 µmol/L (60–110)

Which one of the following drugs is the most likely cause?

    A   Amlodipine

    B   Bendroflumethiazide

    C   Cimetidine

    D   Ibuprofen

    E   Phenytoin

23. Which one of the following drugs can precipitate a myasthenic crisis in susceptible patients?

    A   Bendroflumethiazide

    B   Losartan

    C   Metformin

    D   Naproxen

    E   Propranolol

24. An 18-year-old girl was brought to the emergency department with an overdose of an unknown substance she took 8 hours ago. She complained of abdominal pain, nausea, loss of vision, hearing loss and tinnitus. On examination, her pulse was 120 beats per minute and blood pressure 78/55 mmHg.

Investigations:

ECG	sinus tachycardia, long QT interval

What is she most likely to have overdosed on?

    A   Methanol poisoning

    B   Paracetamol overdose

    C   Quinine poisoning

    D   Salicylate overdose

    E   Tricyclic antidepressant overdose

25. A 46-year-old man attended the emergency department with epistaxis. He was currently receiving warfarin for deep vein thrombosis. His international normalised ratio (INR) had always been within target range when seen in anticoagulation clinic. He also had epilepsy, and had been started on a new anticonvulsant when reviewed by a neurologist 3 weeks earlier. He took no other regular medication and drank no alcohol.

Investigations:

haemoglobin	145 g/L (130–180)
white cell count	7.8×10^9/L (4.0–11.0)
platelet count	250×10^9/L (150–400)
international normalised ratio	6.6 (< 1.4)

Which anticonvulsant is most likely to have caused this?

A   Carbamazepine
B   Lamotrigine
C   Levetiracetam
D   Phenytoin
E   Sodium valproate

26. A 31-year-old woman was ten weeks pregnant. She had a background of essential hypertension. Her blood pressure was 162/94 mmHg.

Which one of the following should not be used to treat her condition?

A   Doxazosin
B   Labetolol
C   Methyldopa
D   Nifedipine
E   Ramipril

27. Which molecule does rituximab target?

A   Bcr-Abl protein tyrosine kinase
B   CD20
C   CD52
D   Interleukin-1
E   Tumour necrosis factor-α (TNF-α)

28. A 30-year-old woman was found at home drowsy by her husband. She had a history of depression and was being treated with amitriptyline. On examination, her Glasgow Coma Score was 13/15, but the rest of her physical examination was normal.

Investigations:

ECG	heart rate 114 beats per minute, sinus rhythm
	QRS duration of 138 ms
	several brief runs of non-sustained ventricular tachycardia

What is the most appropriate next step in management?

A   Amiodarone
B   Flecainide
C   Procainamide
D   Quinidine
E   Sodium bicarbonate

29. Where in the nephron do thiazide diuretics act?

A   Collecting duct
B   Distal convoluted tubule
C   Macula densa
D   Proximal tubule
E   Thick ascending limb of the loop of Henlé

30. A 33-year-old man complained of several weeks of paraesthesia in his hands. His only past medical history was of pulmonary tuberculosis, diagnosed 2 months earlier, and for which he was currently receiving treatment.

What is the most likely cause?

A   Ethambutol
B   Isoniazid
C   Pyrazinamide
D   Rifampicin
E   Streptomycin

31. A 28-year-old man visited a travel clinic to obtain malaria prophylaxis for an upcoming holiday. He had a background of glucose-6-phosphate dehydrogenase deficiency.

Which one of the following should be avoided as antimalarial prophylaxis?

A   Atovaquone-proguanil
B   Doxycycline
C   Mefloquine
D   Primaquine
E   Proguanil

32. A 55-year-old woman was admitted to the hospital with severe vomiting and diarrhoea. She was treated for presumed viral gastroenteritis. She had a background of type 2 diabetes mellitus which was controlled with tablet medication.

Investigations:

serum sodium	36 mmol/L (137–144)
serum potassium	4.9 mmol/L (3.5–4.9)
serum urea	9.2 mmol/L (5.8 three months earlier) (2.5–7.0)
serum creatinine	188 µmol/L (104 three months earlier) (60–110)

Which one of the following medications should be mostly strongly avoided?

A   Acarbose
B   Gliclazide

   C   Metformin
   D   Pioglitazone
   E   Repaglinide

33. Which of the following antiarrhythmic medications is most strongly associated with pulmonary fibrosis?

   A   Amiodarone
   B   Digoxin
   C   Disopyramide
   D   Metoprolol
   E   Verapamil

34. A 21-year-old man was brought to the emergency department after his housemate found him drowsy at home. The housemate said that his friend had a history of depression, but had also recently been suffering from anxiety because of forthcoming examinations, and had been commenced on propranolol by his general practitioner a few days earlier. He also had a history of acute angle glaucoma but took no other regular medications. Examination revealed the patient had a Glasgow Coma Score of 14, pulse 40 beats per minute and regular, and blood pressure 80/48 mmHg.

What is the most appropriate next management step?

   A   Adrenaline
   B   Atropine
   C   Glucagon
   D   Salbutamol infusion
   E   Sodium bicarbonate

35. A 48-year-old woman presented with 3 weeks of worsening shortness of breath. She had recently been diagnosed with carcinoma of the breast and started on treatment by her oncologist, but had no other medical history of note. Examination of the chest revealed bibasal crackles. A transthoracic echocardiogram prior to treatment had been normal, but a repeat study now confirmed the diagnosis of impaired left ventricular systolic function.

Which drug is most likely to have caused her heart failure?

   A   Anastrazole
   B   Tamoxifen
   C   Trastuzumab
   D   Trilostane
   E   Zoledronic acid

36. What is the mechanism of action of aspirin?

   A   Antagonism of adenosine diphosphate (ADP) receptors
   B   Antagonism of glycoprotein IIb/IIIa receptors
   C   Direct inhibition of thrombin
   D   Inhibition of activated factor Xa
   E   Inhibition of arachidonic acid metabolism

37. Which one of the following medications would be contraindicated with the concomitant use of sildenafil?

    A   Aspirin
    B   Furosemide
    C   Isosorbide mononitrate
    D   Ramipril
    E   Simvastatin

38. A 54-year-old woman was brought to the emergency department by her husband after developing unusual movements. She had a past medical history of recent lumbar disc prolapse, and had been taking regular diazepam, morphine and metoclopramide for the past 1 month. Examination revealed the woman to be holding her neck in a hyperextended position and turned to the left, from which it was very difficult to move. Her pupils were equal and reactive to light and accommodation, but were both fixed in superior gaze. She was alert and orientated.

What is the most appropriate initial treatment?

    A   Cyclizine
    B   Flumazenil
    C   Lorazepam
    D   Naloxone
    E   Procyclidine

39. Which one of the following drugs is not associated with gingival hypertrophy?

    A   Ciclosporin
    B   Nifedipine
    C   Phenytoin
    D   Sodium valproate
    E   Sotalol

40. A 35-year-old man complained of 1 week of bruising with minimal trauma. He had a background of Crohn's disease for which he had taken azathioprine for the past 2 years. He also suffered from recurrent gout, and had recently been started on new medication for this.

Investigations:

	Now	Three months earlier
haemoglobin	98 g/L	132 g/L (130–180)
white cell count	2.7×10^9/L	4.3×10^9/L (4.0–11.0)
platelet count	44×10^9/L	184×10^9/L (150–400)
international normalised ratio	1.2	1.2 (< 1.4)
activated partial thromboplastin time	36s	36s (30–40)

What is the most likely cause?

    A   Allopurinol
    B   Colchicine
    C   Diclofenac
    D   Methylprednisolone
    E   Probenecid

Answers

1. A Calcineurin inhibitor

Table 2.1 summarises the mechanism of action of the common immunosuppressants.

Ciclosporin crosses the cell membrane and binds to cyclophilin. The ciclosporin-cyclophilin complex inhibits calcineurin, which normally dephosphorylates the transcription factor nuclear factor of activated T-lymphocytes (NF-AT). This prevents NF-AT translocating from the cytoplasm into the nucleus in an IL-2 mediated process and thus stops stimulation of the immune response. The mechanism of action of ciclosporin is summarised in **Figure 2.1**.

Tedesco D, Haragsim L. Cyclosporin: a review. J Transplant 2012; 2012:230386. Epub ahead of print
Kahan B. Ciclosporine. N Engl J Med 1989; 321:1725–1738.

Table 2.1

Drug	Mechanism of action
Azathioprine (pro-drug so its metabolite 6-mercaptopurine is the active agent)	Purine synthesis inhibitor
Ciclosporin	Calcineurin inhibitor
Methotrexate	Dihydrofolate reductase inhibitor
Mycophenolate mofetil	Inosine monophosphate dehydrogenase inhibitor
Rituximab	CD20 inhibitor
Tacrolimus	Calcineurin inhibitor

Table 2.1 Mechanism of action of immunosuppressants.

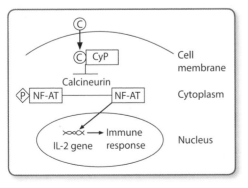

Figure 2.1 Mechanism of ciclosporin action. C, Ciclosporin; CyP, Cyclophilin; IL-2, Interleukin-2; NF-AT, Nuclear factor of activated T-cells.

2. C Heparin

Zero-order kinetics describes the process whereby the metabolism of a drug is independent of its concentration so a small increase in the dose of a drug can lead to a dramatic increase in serum concentration, thus causing toxicity. This occurs because of saturation of the hepatic metabolizing enzymes or of the excretory transport process. Zero-order kinetics can be summarised on a rate–concentration graph as shown in **Figure 2.2**.

Drugs displaying zero-order kinetics can be remembered by the mnemonic **HEPS**:

Heparin
Ethanol
Phenytoin
Salicylates

Craig S. Phenytoin poisoning. Neurocrit Care 2005; 3(2):161–170.

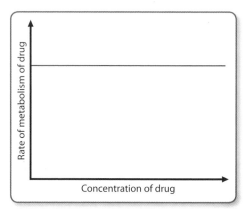

Figure 2.2 Zero-order kinetics.

3. E Inhibits hepatic cholesterol synthesis

Table 2.2 summarises the mechanism of action of the main lipid-lowering agents.

Camelia S, Anca S. Statins: mechanism of action and effects. J Cell Mol Med 2001; 5 (4):378–387.

Table 2.2	
Drug	**Mechanism of action**
Cholestyramine	Bile acid sequestrant
Ezetimibe	Inhibits absorption of cholesterol from the intestines
Fibrates	Activates lipoprotein lipase through being a peroxisome proliferator-activated receptor alpha (PPAR-α) agonist
Nicotinic acid	Blocks breakdown of fats in adipose tissue
Statins	Inhibits hepatic cholesterol synthesis

Table 2.2 Mechanism of action of lipid-lowering agents

4. C Lithium

The British National Formulary (BNF) advises that the amount of tricyclic antidepressants secreted into breast milk is too small to cause harm but manufacturers advise avoiding during breastfeeding. It also advises avoiding selective serotonin reuptake inhibitors (SSRIs) and using mirtazapine only if potential benefit outweighs risk.

Drugs that cannot be taken safely during breastfeeding, can be remembered by the mnemonic **ALOGIC**:

Amiodarone (thyroid abnormalities)/**A**spirin (neonatal bleeding, Reye's syndrome)
Lithium (involuntary movements)
Oestrogens (feminisation of male infants)
Gold (haematological reactions and renal impairment)
Indomethacin (seizures)/**I**odides (thyroid abnormalities)
Cytotoxics/**C**hloramphenicol (both can cause blood dyscrasia)

Joint Formulary Committee. Chapter 4.2.3. Antimanic drugs. British National Formulary (BNF) 63, 63rd edition. London: Pharmaceutical Press, 2012.
Ito S, Blajchman A, Stephenson M, et al. Prospective follow-up of adverse reactions in breast-fed infants exposed to maternal medication. Am J Obstet Gynecol 1993; 168:1393–1399.

5. B Amoxicillin

Antibiotics contraindicated in pregnancy can be remembered by the mnemonic **FACTS**:

Fluoroquinolones (ciprofloxacin causes congenital malformations and limb defects)
Aminoglycosides (ototoxicity)
Clarithromycin (cardiovascular defects, cleft palate, intrauterine growth retardation)
Tetracycline (doxycycline causes adverse effects on fetal teeth and bones, congenital cataracts)
Sulphonamides (teratogenic in first trimester)

Joint Formulary Committee. Chapter 5.1. Antibacterial drugs. British National Formulary (BNF) 63, 63rd edition. London: Pharmaceutical Press, 2012.

6. E Verapamil

Nephrotoxic drugs can be remembered by the mnemonic **RENAL CA**:

Ramipril (angiotensin-converting enzyme [ACE] inhibitors)
g**E**ntamicin
Non-steroidal anti-inflammatory drugs (NSAIDs)
Amphotericin
Loop diuretics

Calcineurin inhibitors (ciclosporin, tacrolimus)
Angiotensin-II receptor blockers

Therapeutic drug monitoring may be used to prevent the effects of nephrotoxicity, e.g. gentamicin levels.

Perazella MA. Renal vulnerability to drug toxicity. Clin J Am Soc Nephrol 2009; 4(7):1275–1283.

7. D Hypotension

Side effects of steroids can be remembered by the mnemonic **AM CUSHINGOID**:

Acne
Myopathy (proximal)

Cushingoid facies/**C**ataract
Ulcers
Striae/**S**kin thinning
Hypertension/**H**airy/**H**ypokalaemia
Infection
Necrosis (avascular necrosis of femoral head)
Glycosuria
Obesity/**O**steoporosis
Immunosuppression/**I**nsomnia
Depression

Whitworth JA. Adrenocorticotrophin and steroid-induced hypertension in humans. Kidney Int Suppl 1992; 37:S34.

8. E Nicorandil

Drugs causing gynaecomastia can be remembered by the phrase 'Some Drugs Cause Awesome Mammaries':

Spironolactone
Digoxin
Cimetidine
Alcohol
Metronidazole/**M**ethyldopa

Johnson RE, Murad MH. Gynecomastia: pathophysiology, evaluation, and management. Mayo Clin Proc 2009; 84(11):1010–1015.

9. B Hepatitis

Side effects of angiotensin-converting enzymes (ACE) inhibitors can be remembered by the mnemonic **CAPTOPRIL**:

Cough
Anaphylaxis/**A**ngioedema
Palpitations
Taste
Orthostatic hypotension
Potassium elevated
Renal impairment
Impotence
Leucocytosis

Dykewicz MS. Cough and angioedema from angiotensin-converting enzyme inhibitors: new insights into mechanisms and management. Curr Opin Allergy Clin Immunol 2004; 4(4):267.
Reardon LC, Macpherson DS. Hyperkalemia in outpatients using angiotensin-converting enzyme inhibitors. How much should we worry? Arch Intern Med 1998; 158(1):26.

10. C Hypokalaemia

Ciclosporin is an immunosuppressant that reduces clonal proliferation of T cells by reducing interleukin-2 (IL-2) release through being a calcineurin inhibitor. The side effects of ciclosporin can be remembered by the 8 **H**s:

Harm to kidneys
Hepatotoxicity
Hirsutism
Hypercholesterolaemia
Hyperglycaemia
Hyperkalaemia
Hyperplasia of gums
Hypertension
Fluid retention and tremor are also common side effects.

Fleming DR, Ouseph R, Herrington J. Hyperkalemia associated with cyclosporine (CsA) use in bone marrow transplantation. Bone Marrow Transplant 1997; 19(3):289–291.

11. E Lithium

Side effects of lithium can be remembered by the mnemonic **LITHIUM**:

Leucocytosis
Insipidus diabetes (polydipsia, polyuria)
Tremor/Teratogenicity
Hypothyroidism
Interstitial nephritis
na**U**sea + vomiting
Miscellaneous–acne, weight gain, T wave flattening/inversion on ECG

Drugs that can precipitate lithium toxicity can be remembered by the mnemonic **CHABS**:

Calcium channel blockers/**C**arbamazepine
Haloperidol
Angiotensin-converting enzyme (ACE) inhibitors/**A**ngiotensin-II receptor blockers
Bendroflumethiazide
Selective serotonin reuptake inhibitors (SSRIs)/**S**umatriptan

Table 2.3 shows the side effects of the other antipsychotic medications in the question.

Juurlink DN, et al. Drug-induced lithium toxicity in the elderly: a population-based study. J Am Geriatr Soc 2004; 52(5):794–798.

12. B Capecitabine

This man has developed hand–foot syndrome from capecitabine. **Table 2.4** shows the side effects of the various cytotoxic agents.

Saif M. Capecitabine and hand-foot–syndrome. Expert Opin Drug Saf 2011; 10(2):159–169.

Table 2.3	
Drug	**Side effects**
Amisulpride	Akathisia, amenorrhoea, galactorrhoea, insomnia, prolonged QT interval, weight gain
Carbamazepine	'SAND'
	Syndrome of inappropriate ADH secretion (SIADH)
	Ataxia
	Nausea
	Dizziness/Diarrhoea
Clozapine	'CASH'
	Cardiomyopathy/Constipation
	Agranulocytosis
	Seizures
	Hypotension
Lamotrigine	'DIMS'
	Depression
	Influenza-like symptoms
	Maculopapular rash
	Stevens–Johnson syndrome
ADH, antidiuretic hormone.	

Table 2.3 Side effects of antipsychotic medications.

Table 2.4	
Drug	**Side effect**
Bleomycin	Lung fibrosis
Capecitabine	Hand–foot syndrome (desquamating rash)
Cisplatin	Interstitial nephritis, ototoxicity, peripheral neuropathy
Cyclophosphamide	Bone marrow suppression, haemorrhagic cystitis, secondary AML
Doxorubicin	Cardiomyopathy, skin rash
Etoposide	Bone marrow suppression, hypotension
Methotrexate	Mucositis, myelosuppression, liver fibrosis, pneumonitis
Vincristine	Peripheral neuropathy
AML, acute myeloid leukaemia.	

Table 2.4 Side effects of cytotoxic agents.

13. C 15 mg

The breakthrough dose should be 1/6th of the daily morphine dose

Therefore, in this case $(45 \times 2)/6 = 15$ mg

Scottish Intercollegiate Guidelines Network (SIGN). Control of pain in adults with cancer: a national clinical guideline. Edinburgh: SIGN, 2008.

14. D Fomepizole

This man has ethylene glycol toxicity through ingestion of antifreeze. Patients tend to present inebriated initially, with confusion, slurred speech, headache, dizziness, dilated slow reacting pupils, hypotonia, and reduced tendon reflexes. They then become hypertensive and tachycardic. Arterial blood gas analysis would show metabolic acidosis with a high anion gap. The characteristic picture on blood tests is renal impairment with hypocalcaemia.

In the past, ethanol was used as an antidote because it competes with ethylene glycol for the enzyme alcohol dehydrogenase, thus limiting the formation of toxic metabolites. However, the current first-line treatment is fomepizole (a competitive inhibitor of alcohol dehydrogenase), which has fewer adverse effects. High-dose thiamine and pyridoxine should also be used as they reduce the formation of oxalate from glyoxylic acid. Sodium bicarbonate can also contribute to correcting the acidosis and enhancing clearance of the active metabolites. Calcium may be needed to correct hypocalcaemia. In cases resistant to treatment, haemodialysis may be indicated.

Lepik, KJ et al. Adverse drug events associated with the antidotes for methanol and ethylene glycol poisoning: a comparison of ethanol and fomepizole. Ann Emerg Med 2009; 53(4):439.

15. A Carbamazepine

This patient has syndrome of inappropriate antidiuretic hormone (ADH) secretion (SIADH). The diagnosis requires:

- Concentrated urine (sodium >20 mmol/L and urine osmolality >500)
- Hyponatraemia (<125 mmol/L) or low plasma osmolality (<260)
- Absence of hypovolaemia or oedema

Drug causes of SIADH can be remembered by the mnemonic **DRS ABC**:

Diuretic (thiazide)
Rifampicin
SSRIs
Analgesics– opiates, non-steroidal anti-inflammatory drugs (NSAIDs)
Barbiturates
Carbamazepine/**C**hlorpromazine/**C**hlorpropamide/**C**yclophosphamide

Rose B. Pathophysiology and etiology of the syndrome of inappropriate antidiuretic hormone secretion (SIADH). In: Basow DS (ed), UpToDate. Waltham, MA: UpToDate, 2011. http://www.uptodate.com (Last accessed 1 May 2012).

16. C Lead poisoning

Features of lead poisoning can be remembered by the mnemonic **ABCDEFGH**:

Anaemic
Basophilic stippling
Colicky abdominal pain
Diarrhoea
Encephalopathy
Foot and/or wrist drop
Gum (lead line)
Hearing loss

Management of lead poisoning involves:

- Removing the patient from the source
- Oral DMSA (2–3 dimercaptosuccinic acid) or intravenous EDTA (sodium calcium edetate)
- Discussion with the local poisons unit

Table 2.5 summarises the features and treatment of the other types of poisoning.

Goldman R, Hu H. Adult lead poisoning. In: Basow DS (ed), UpToDate. Waltham, MA: UpToDate, 2012. http://www.uptodate.com (Last accessed 1 May 2012).

Table 2.5

Type of poisoning	Features	Treatment
Arsenic	Gastrointestinal – abdominal pain, watery diarrhoea, hepatitis	IV fluids
	Cardiovascular – hypotension, arrhythmias, prolonged QTc	Chelation with dimercaprol or DMSA
	Dermatological – Mee's lines (2 mm horizontal lines on the nails), pruritic rash, patchy alopecia	
Cyanide	Gastrointestinal – abdominal pain, vomiting, dysgeusia (abnormal taste)	IV fluids, thiamine and naloxone
	Neurological – headache, anxiety, seizures, tobacco amblyopia, Leber's hereditary optic neuropathy	Sodium thiosulfate and hydroxocobalamin
	Dermatological – cherry red flushing, cyanosis	
	Respiratory – pulmonary oedema	
Iron	Gastrointestinal – abdominal pain, vomiting, diarrhoea, melaena, haematemesis, hepatotoxicity, bowel obstruction	IV fluids
	Shock and metabolic acidosis	Desferrioxamine
Selenium	Gastrointestinal – abdominal pain, vomiting, 'garlic' breath	IV fluids
	Dermatological – alopecia, hair discolouration	
	Neurological – peripheral neuropathy, tremor	
	Diaphoresis	

Table 2.5 Heavy metal poisoning.

17. B Haemodialysis

This is a difficult case of salicylate poisoning. This patient has the common features of nausea, vomiting, tinnitus, fever and early respiratory alkalosis due to tachypnoea (which is usually followed by metabolic acidosis). However, she also has the severe features of hyperthermia, altered mental status (Glasgow Coma Score 9) and non-cardiogenic pulmonary oedema.

In the absence of cerebral or pulmonary oedema, treatment involves supplemental oxygen, aggressive fluid resuscitation with IV fluids and IV sodium bicarbonate. Intubation of the salicylate-poisoned patient is dangerous and should be avoided if at all possible as aspirin can act on the respiratory centre of the medulla to increase the respiratory rate and cause a huge increase in minute ventilation.

Indications for haemodialysis include:

- Altered mental status
- Clinical deterioration despite aggressive and appropriate supportive care
- Fluid overload that prohibits use of sodium bicarbonate
- Plasma salicylate concentration >100 mg/dL (7.2 mmol/L) in acute overdose
- Pulmonary or cerebral oedema
- Renal insufficiency that interferes with salicylate excretion

Greenberg MI, Hendrickson RG, Hofman M. Deleterious effects of endotracheal intubation in salicylate poisoning. Ann Emerg Med 2003; 41(4):583.
Boyer E. Aspirin poisoning in adults. In: Basow DS (ed), UpToDate. Waltham, MA: UpToDate, 2011. http://www.uptodate.com (Last accessed 1 May 2012).

18. B Clarithromycin

This man has theophylline toxicity with the clarithromycin. Features of toxicity include:

- Nausea, vomiting, epigastric pain
- Severe acidosis, hypokalaemia, hyperglycaemia, and hypercalcaemia
- Tachycardia, arrhythmias
- Confusion, seizures

Theophylline toxicity is precipitated by drugs that inhibit cytochrome P450 (CYP1A2, CYP2E1 and CYP3A4) and, thus, decrease theophylline clearance, e.g. cimetidine, ciprofloxacin, clarithromycin, erythromycin and verapamil.

Management involves repeated doses of oral activated charcoal and fluid resuscitation with potassium supplementation. Charcoal haemoperfusion provides a higher theophylline clearance rate than hemodialysis.

Rieder MJ, Spino M. The theophylline-erythromycin interaction. J Asthma 1988; 25(4):195–204.
Shannon MW. Comparative efficacy of hemodialysis and hemoperfusion in severe theophylline intoxication. Acad Emerg Med 1997; 4(7):674.

19. C Photosensitivity

The side effects of warfarin can be remembered by the mnemonic **SHOP**:

- **S**kin necrosis
- **H**aemorrhage/**H**air loss

- Oral ulcers
- Purple toe syndrome (dark, purplish, mottled discolouration of the plantar and lateral surfaces of the toes due to cholesterol microembolisation).

Krahn MJ, Pettigrew NM, Cuddy TE. Unusual side effects due to warfarin. Can J Cardiol 1998;14(1):90–93

20. E Blocks sodium channels

Table 2.6 shows the classification of the various antiarrhythmic agents according to the Vaughan Williams classification and their mode of action.

Vaughan Williams EM. A classification of antiarrhythmic actions reassessed after a decade of new drugs. J Clin Pharmacol 1984;24:129–147.

Table 2.6

Class	Drugs	Mode of action
Ia	Disopyramide, procainamide, quinidine	Blocks sodium channels
Ib	Lidocaine, mexiletine	Blocks sodium channels
Ic	Flecainide, moricizine, propafenone	Blocks sodium channels
II	Bisoprolol, carvedilol, propranolol	Beta-blocker
III	Amiodarone*, bretylium, dronedarone, dofetilide ibutilide, sotalol#	Blocks potassium channels
IV	Diltiazem, verapamil	Calcium channel blocker

*Amiodarone has Class I, II, and III activity. #Sotalol is also a beta-blocker.

Table 2.6 Vaughan Williams classification of antiarrhythmic agents.

21. B Hirsutism

Side effects of sodium valproate can be remembered by the mnemonic **VALPROATE**:

Vomiting/Visual disturbances (diplopia, amblyopia)
Ataxia
Liver impairment (hepatitis)
Pancreatitis/Pancytopenia
Retention of fat (i.e. weight gain)
Oedema
Alopecia
Tremor
Enzyme inhibitor (cytochrome P450)

Perucca E. Pharmacological and therapeutic properties of valproate: a summary after 35 years of clinical experience. CNS Drugs. 2002;16(10):695–714.

22. D Ibuprofen

Non-steroidal anti-inflammatory drugs (NSAIDs) can induce two different types of acute kidney injury:

1. Haemodynamically-mediated inhibition of prostaglandin synthesis causes reversible renal ischaemia
2. Acute interstitial nephritis that is often accompanied by the nephrotic syndrome

Bendroflumethiazide can cause hypokalaemia and hyponatraemia. Amlodipine, cimetidine and phenytoin do not cause potassium or sodium disturbances.

An easy way to remember drugs causing hyperkalaemia is with the mnemonic **CAD K+ BANK**:

Calcineurin inhibitors (ciclosporin, tacrolimus)
ACE inhibitors
Digoxin

K+–sparing diuretics, e.g. spironolactone

Beta-blockers
Angiotensin-II receptor blockers
NSAIDs
K+ supplements

Perazella MA. Drug-induced hyperkalemia: old culprits and new offenders. Am J Med 2000; 109(4):307–314.

23. E Propranolol

Myasthenic crisis is a life-threatening condition where weakness from myasthenia gravis (MG) is severe enough to necessitate intubation or to delay extubation following surgery. This should be suspected in MG patients with worsening dyspnoea (especially on lying supine), severe dysphagia, hypophonia, tachypnoea, use of accessory muscles of breathing, paradoxical abdominal breathing and low baseline vital capacity.

Table 2.7 shows the various drugs that can increase weakness in myasthenia.

Table 2.7	
Class of drug	**Examples**
Antibiotics	Aminoglycosides, fluoroquinolones, macrolides, tetracyclines
Cardiovascular 'BPPV'	Beta-blockers, lidocaine, Propafenone, Procainamide, quinidine, Verapamil
Neurological	Gabapentin, phenytoin
Psychiatric	Chlorpromazine, lithium, phenothiazines
Rheumatological	Chloroquine, penicillamine

Table 2.7 Drugs that can increase weakness in myasthenia gravis.

Patients with myasthenic crisis should be treated in an intensive care setting with close monitoring of their vital capacity (VC). Elective intubation should be considered when the VC is < 20 mL/kg body weight or there are signs of respiratory distress. Treatment involves plasmapheresis or intravenous immunoglobulin (literature suggests no advantage of one over the other). As the therapeutic effects of plasmapheresis and IV Ig last only weeks, high-dose steroids (prednisolone 60–80 mg OD) should be started. Other immunomodulating agents like azathioprine, mycophenolate mofetil and ciclosporin can be considered if steroids are contraindicated or there is a poor clinical response.

Bird S. Myasthenic crisis. In: Basow DS (ed), UpToDate. Waltham, MA: UpToDate, 2011. http://www. uptodate.com (Last accessed 1 May 2012).

24. C Quinine poisoning

The collection of symptoms described here (blindness, gastrointestinal disturbances, deafness, tinnitus) are those of cinchonism, a pathological state caused by quinine or quinidine overdose. Arrhythmias, hypoglycaemia and hypotension (due to alpha-blockade) can occur. Blindness is the defining feature and tends to occur at 6–24 hours after ingestion. Most symptoms resolve once quinine is withdrawn. Treatment is principally supportive and repeated dose-activated charcoal has been shown to increase quinine clearance.

Prescott LF, Hamilton AR, Heyworth R. Treatment of quinine overdosage with repeated oral charcoal. Br J Clin Pharmacol 1989; 27:95–97.

25. E Sodium valproate

Of the anticonvulsants listed, only sodium valproate has a strong association with cytochrome P450 inhibition. As such, when co-administered with warfarin, there is the possibility of international normalised ratio (INR) levels increasing beyond the therapeutic range and so a risk of significant bleeding.

Table 2.8 lists the main inhibitors/inducers of cytochrome P450 enzymes.

Table 2.8	
Hepatic cytochrome P450 inhibitors	**Hepatic cytochrome P450 inducers**
• Allopurinol • Acute alcohol intake • Antidepressants – especially selective serotonin reuptake inhibitors (e.g. fluoxetine) • Clarithromycin – plus other macrolides • Cimetidine – plus other H2 antagonists, and proton pump inhibitors (e.g. omeprazole) • Ciprofloxacin – plus other fluoroquinolones • Imidazoles, e.g. fluconazole • Isoniazid • Sodium valproate	• Carbamazepine • Chronic alcohol intake • Phenytoin • Phenobarbitone • Primidone • Sulfinpyrazone • Smoking • St John's Wort • Rifampicin • Griseofulvin

Table 2.8 Cytochrome P450 inhibitors and inducers.

26. E Ramipril

There is evidence that the use of angiotensin-converting enzymes (ACE) inhibitors by pregnant women at any stage of pregnancy is associated with fetal malformations and complications in labour. These malformations are particularly related to the cardiovascular system, neurological system and urinary tract. Angiotensin receptor blockers (ARBs) appear to have a similar effect. All the other options listed have a role in the management of hypertension in pregnancy.

Lindheimer MD, Taler SJ, Cunningham FG. Hypertension in pregnancy. J Am Soc Hypertens 2008; 2(6): 484–494.

27. B CD20

As increasing understanding of the molecular basis of disease occurs, monoclonal antibodies are developing an ever-wider role in medicine. For example, the recent understanding that B cell clones that produce autoantibody are key to the disease process in rheumatoid arthritis prompted the development of B cell depleting therapies; CD20 is a B cell specific antigen that is antagonised by rituximab. Rituximab is now recognised as an effective agent in the treatment of rheumatoid arthritis unresponsive to conventional agents, along with other conditions where B cell activity may contribute to disease (e.g. diffuse large B cell Non-Hodgkin's lymphoma).

The Bcr-Abl protein tyrosine kinase is the target for imatinib, a monoclonal antibody used particularly in the treatment of chronic myeloid leukaemia. CD52 is present on mature lymphocytes, and is the target for alemtuzumab, a monoclonal antibody used in the treatment of certain lymphomas and as immunosuppression in organ transplantation. Anakinra is a drug that antagonises interleukin-1 which has shown some efficacy in the treatment of rheumatoid arthritis. TNF-α is a major target for new therapies, with monoclonal antibodies that inhibit TNF-α (e.g. infliximab) and soluble TNF-α receptors (e.g. etanercept) both being of use in clinical practice. Anti-TNF-α therapy has shown efficacy in treating a wide range of diseases with a complex immunological basis, including rheumatoid arthritis, Crohn's disease and psoriasis.

28. E Sodium bicarbonate

The clinical features of tricyclic antidepressant (TCA) overdose may be divided into three categories:

- Neurological: reduction in Glasgow Coma Score, confusion, seizure, dilated pupils, urinary retention.
- Cardiovascular: prolonged PR and QT intervals, widening of the QRS complex, sinus tachycardia, hypotension.
- Other: intestinal ileus, flushing.

Patients with TCA overdose who develop evidence of cardiac toxicity (including QRS complexes >100 milliseconds and/or the development of ventricular arrhythmias) require rapid treatment, with sodium bicarbonate being the mainstay of therapy. Sodium bicarbonate narrows the width of the QRS interval and reduces the risk of further ventricular arrhythmia. If improvement is only minimal with a bolus of sodium bicarbonate, then it may be administered as an infusion.

Antiarrhythmic medications from Vaughan Williams class Ia (such as procainimide and quinidine) and Ic (such as flecainide) are absolutely contraindicated in the management of TCA overdose. This is because these drugs act by closing myocardial sodium channels, which is similar to the mechanism by which TCAs produce cardiac toxicity. Although amiodarone has a role in the management of ventricular arrhythmia, neither has any evidence supporting their use in the setting of TCA overdose.

29. B Distal convoluted tubule

Table 2.9 summarises the site and mechanism of action of diuretics, and their associated side effects.

30. B Isoniazid

Peripheral neuropathy is a well-characterised side effect of isoniazid. It reflects the drug's ability to deplete stores of pyridoxine (vitamin B_6). The neuropathy is easily

Table 2.9

Class of diuretic	Examples	Site and mechanism of action	Side effects
Loop diuretics	Furosemide, bumetanide	Block the $Na^+/K^+/2Cl^-$ transporter of the apical membrane in the thick ascending limb of the loop of Henle	Electrolyte depletion ($\downarrow Na^+$, K^+, Mg^{2+}, H^+, Ca^{2+}) Dyslipidaemia Deafness (at very high doses)
Thiazide diuretics	Bendroflumethiazide, hydrochlorothiazide, indapamide, metolazone	Block the Na^+/Cl^- co-transporter of the apical membrane of the distal convoluted tubule	Electrolyte disturbance ($\downarrow Na^+$, K^+, Mg^{2+}, H^+, but $\uparrow Ca^{2+}$) Hyperglycaemia $\uparrow$Urate (risk of gout) May also cause impotence
Potassium-sparing diuretics	Spironolactone, eplerenone	Antagonises aldosterone receptors in the distal tubule	$\uparrow K^+$ Gynaecomastia Menstrual disturbance
	Amiloride	Blocks apical sodium reabsorption/potassium secretion in the collecting tubule	$\uparrow K^+$

Table 2.9 Site, mechanism of action and side effects of different diuretics.

treated with dietary supplementation of pyridoxine. In rare cases, isoniazid can also cause optic neuritis, which may progress to optic atrophy if untreated.

Table 2.10 summarises the main side effects of the most common antituberculous treatments.

Table 2.10	
Drug	**Side effects**
Isoniazid	The Hs: • Hand tingling and Hindrance of vision (i.e. neuropathy) • Hepatotoxicity • Haematological (agranulocytosis, haemolytic anaemia, etc) • Hypersensitivity reactions (e.g. drug-related fever) • Cytochrome P450 in Hibition
Rifampicin	TORCH: • Tubulointerstitial disease (acute nephritis) • Orange discolouration of secretions • Rash • Cytochrome P450 induction • Hepatotoxicity
Ethambutol	• Optic neuritis (assessment of vision required prior to commencing)
Pyrazinamide	• Hepatotoxicity
Streptomycin	• Nephrotoxicity • Ototoxicity • Peripheral neuropathy

Table 2.10 Side effects of antituberculous treatments.

Isoniazid elimination is principally through acetylation in the liver, which requires the action of an acetyltransferase enzyme. The speed of acetylation is determined by the genotype of acetyltransferase inherited. There are similar numbers of 'fast acetylators' and 'slow acetylators' in most populations. Peripheral neuropathy is caused by the isoniazid itself, whilst hepatotoxicity is caused by its acetylated metabolite, acetylhydrazine; as such, slow acetylators are more prone to peripheral neuropathy, whilst fast acetylators are more prone to hepatotoxicity. Other drugs where acetylation is an important part of their metabolism include hydralazine, procainamide and sulphonamides.

31. D Primaquine

Glucose-6-phosphate dehydrogenase (G6PD) acts within erythrocytes as part of the pathway in which oxidised glutathione is converted to its reduced form, a key means of protecting the red blood cell from damage by oxidising agents. Those lacking the enzyme are at risk of haemolytic crisis on exposure to any of a broad range of oxidising triggers. Such triggers include infection, metabolic derangements (e.g. diabetic ketoacidosis), foods (classically fava beans), and a range of medications.

Malaria prophylaxis is guided by the region to which the traveller is visiting, as this dictates the likely species and resistance patterns to which the traveller may be exposed. In this case, however, one major consideration is the traveller's G6PD deficiency, since several antimalarial agents are known triggers for G6PD haemolytic crises. Of the options given, primaquine has the most consistent association with haemolysis, so would be the least appropriate choice. Other antimalarial agents useful in the treatment but not prophylaxis of malaria – including quinine and chloroquine – may also trigger G6PD haemolytic crises.

Table 2.11 summarises the medications most commonly associated with haemolysis in G6PD.

Youngster I et al. Medications and glucose-6-phosphate deficiency: an evidence-based review. Drug Safety 2010;33(9):713–726.

Table 2.11	
Class of drug	**Examples**
Antibiotics	Nitrofurantoin Sulfonamides Chloramphenicol Isoniazid Streptomycin
Antimalarials	Primaquine Chloroquine Quinine
Antiplatelets	Aspirin
Rheumatic agents	Colchicine
Other	Vitamin K

Table 2.11 Typical drug causes of haemolysis in G6PD deficiency

32. C Metformin

Although rare, one well-established serious side effect of metformin therapy is lactate acidosis. Risk factors for lactate acidosis include renal failure, liver failure, and conditions predisposing to tissue hypoperfusion (e.g. dehydration, sepsis or shock). The exact level of renal failure at which metformin becomes contraindicated is not well-defined, but most clinicians would consider a plasma creatinine of between 130–150 µmol/L to be the limit of acceptability. This patient's acute kidney injury secondary to presumed dehydration means that metformin is strongly contraindicated here.

Acarbose would not be absolutely contraindicated here; however, given that its major side effect is loose stool, it would need to be used with considerable caution. Sulphonylureas (such as gliclazide), thiazolidinediones (such as pioglitazone) and prandial glucose regulators (such as repaglinide) may all require dose reductions in the context of acute renal failure in order to minimise the risk of hypoglycaemia, but would not necessarily be contraindicated.

Fitzgerald E, Mathieu S, Ball A. Metformin associated lactic acidosis. BMJ 2009; 339:b3660.

33. A Amiodarone

Pulmonary fibrosis has a wide range of aetiologies, and the diagnosis of 'drug-induced' pulmonary fibrosis should only be made as a diagnosis of exclusion, since there are no highly-specific radiological or histological features. A number of medications are well-established as causes of pulmonary fibrosis; from the options given, amiodarone is by far the most likely cause. The drugs most strongly associated with pulmonary fibrosis are summarised in **Table 2.12**.

In all cases of drug-induced pulmonary fibrosis, the appropriate initial treatment is cessation of the drug and replacement with an alternative where possible. If alveolitis is present, there may be an indication for corticosteroid therapy.

Amiodarone has a large number of side effects. These may be remembered as **SLATE TAN:**

- **S**kin discolouration – classically 'slate grey'; plus photosensitivity.

Table 2.12	
Class of drug	**Examples**
Antibiotics	Nitrofurantoin
	Sulfonamides
Cardiac	Amiodarone
	Procainamide
	Quinidine
Chemotherapy	Bleomycin
	Busulfan
	Carmustine
	Chlorambucil
	Cyclophosphamide
	Melphalan
	Methotrexate
	Mitomycin
Rheumatological	Gold
	Penicillamine
	Sulfasalazine

Table 2.12 Drug causes of pulmonary fibrosis.

- **L**FT derangement – drug-induced hepatitis.
- **A**taxia.
- **T**hyroid dysfunction – both hyper- and hypothyroidism may be found.
- **E**yes – reversible corneal microdeposits.
- **T**orsade de pointes – and other cardiac arrhythmias.
- **A**lveolitis – which may progress to pulmonary fibrosis.
- **N**europathy – peripheral neuropathy.

Camus, P et al. Drug-induced and iatrogenic infiltrative lung disease. Clin Chest Med 2004; 25(3):479– 519, vi.

34. C Glucagon

The history given is suggestive of the student taking a beta-blocker overdose. Characteristic clinical features include bradycardia, hypotension, a reduction in Glasgow Coma Score, bronchospasm and hypoglycaemia.

The initial management involves stabilisation of the patient, including the use of atropine and fluids to antagonise beta-blockade effects upon the circulatory system. Temporary pacing may be required in the case of severe bradycardia or heart block. Salbutamol inhalers may be used in the treatment of bronchospasm, but there is no evidence for the use of a salbutamol infusion.

Given the history of acute angle glaucoma, antimuscarinic agents such as atropine are contra-indicated. The next most appropriate treatment is intravenous glucagon. This hormone binds to receptors on the myocardium and through activation of the enzyme adenylate cyclase acts to increase intracellular concentrations of cyclic AMP (cyclic adenosine 3′, 5′-monophosphate). Cyclic AMP affects intracellular biochemical cascades that result in increased calcium release, in turn strengthening the force of cardiac contraction.

A number of other medical therapies may also be tried, including intravenous calcium salts. Vasoactive drugs (such as adrenaline) and haemodialysis are appropriate to consider if the patient remains hypotensive and bradycardic despite maximal medical therapy but would not be first-line treatments. Sodium bicarbonate has a role in treatment of those with beta-blocker overdose who develop arrhythmia, but not in other cases.

Kerns W. Management of beta-adrenergic blocker and calcium channel antagonist toxicity. Emerg Med Clin North Am 2007; 25(2):309–331.

35. C Trastuzumab

Trastuzumab is a monoclonal antibody therapy that targets human epidermal growth factor receptor-2 (HER-2), a protein expressed in up to 20% of breast carcinomas. Systolic heart failure is now well-recognised as a side effect of trastuzumab, with up to 27% of those who are prescribed the drug affected. Risk factors include age and pre-existing cardiac disease. Another major risk factor is the co-administration of anthracycline chemotherapy, as this in itself has well-established cardiotoxic side effects. The spectrum of disease may range from asymptomatic (with deteriorating left ventricular function only detected on echocardiogram) to clinically severe biventricular cardiac failure. Most oncologists will arrange a transthoracic echocardiogram prior to treatment, and repeat regularly during the course of therapy. Left ventricular function generally improves on stopping the drug. None of the other options given have a significant association with cardiotoxicity.

Hudis CA. Trastuzumab – mechanism of action and use in clinical practice. N Engl J Med 2007; 357(1):39–51.

36. E Inhibition of arachidonic acid metabolism

A combination of medications is used in the treatment of acute coronary syndrome for stabilisation of the ruptured atherosclerotic plaque. Each of these inhibits different molecules involved in the platelet aggregation and coagulation pathways. These are summarised in **Table 2.13**.

37. C Isosorbide mononitrate

Sildenafil, along with other type 5 phosphodiesterase inhibitors, slows the degradation of cyclic GMP. Cyclic GMP acts to potentiate the various actions

Table 2.13			
	Class of drug	**Examples**	**Mechanism of action**
Antiplatelets	Salicyclates	Aspirin	Irreversibly inhibits the enzyme cyclo-oxygenase (COX; particularly the COX-1 isoform, found in all cell membranes) that is responsible for the metabolism of arachidonic acid. COX-1 acts in platelet membranes to convert arachidonic acid to thromboxane A2 (TXA2), a molecule responsible for platelet aggregation
	Thienopyridines	Clopidogrel, ticlodipine, prasugrel	Inhibit ADP receptors, a component in platelet aggregation
	Dipyridamole*		Phosphodiesterase inhibitor with antiplatelet and vasodilator action
	Glycoprotein IIb/IIIa (GP IIb/IIIa) receptor antagonists	Abciximab, eptifibatide, tirofiban	Inhibit GP IIb/IIIa receptors, a component in platelet aggregation

Contd...

Contd...

Anticoagulants	Heparins	Either unfractionated, or low molecular weight (e.g. enoxaparin)	Activate antithrombin III, an inhibitor of thrombin
	Direct thrombin inhibitors (DTIs)	Lepirudin, dabigatran	Inhibit thrombin, a molecule that promotes coagulation (converts fibrinogen to fibrin) as well as platelet aggregation
	Factor Xa inhibitors	Fondaparinux, rivaroxaban	Inhibit factor Xa, a molecule responsible for conversion of prothrombin to thrombin
	Thrombolytics	Streptokinase, alteplase	Promote the formation of plasmin from its progenitor plasminogen; plasmin lyses the fibrin present in clots

* Dipyridamole principally indicated for secondary prevention of ischaemic stroke and venous thromboembolism prophylaxis rather than used in acute coronary syndrome.

Table 2.13 Mechanism of action of antiplatelets and anticoagulants used in acute coronary syndrome.

of nitric oxide, the major one of which is vasodilatation. This vasodilatation occurs amongst other sites in the corpus cavernosa of the penis, which is a crucial element of the initiation of an erection. Nitrate-based medications (such as isosorbide mononitrate (ISMN), as used in the symptomatic management of ischaemic heart disease) are metabolised to nitric oxide, and relieve angina through their actions of vasodilatation of collateral vessels that bypass narrowed coronary artery segments. When sildenafil is taken at the same time as nitrate-based medications, the two can interact and produce profound vasodilatation that may lead to hypotension and syncope (**Figure 2.3**). As such, option C is the correct answer. Nicorandil is a potassium channel opening drug that also has some nitrate-like activity, so it would also be contraindicated with the use of sildenafil.

None of the other options offered will interact significantly with sildenafil. Interestingly, trials have shown only minor additional reductions in blood pressure when sildenafil is prescribed at the same time as most conventional antihypertensives, and therefore antihypertensives are normally not a

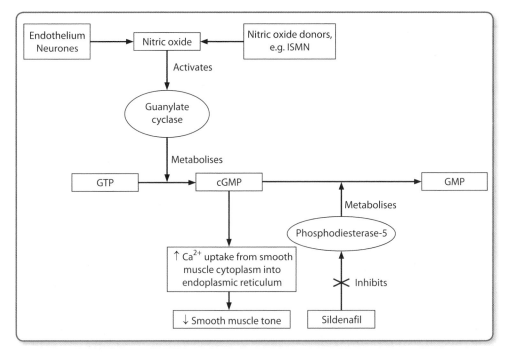

Figure 2.3 Interaction between sildenafil and nitrate-based medications. Sildenafil is a selective inhibitor of phosphodiesterase-5 (PDE-5), preventing degradation of cGMP, and therefore leading to vascular smooth muscle relaxation and erection. When nitrate-based medication is administered at the same time as sildenafil, there is increased cGMP formation and reduced degradation; this may result in profound vasodilatation and cause severe hypotension. cGMP, Cyclic guanosine monophosphate; GMP, Guanosine monophosphate; GTP, Guanosine triphosphate; ISMN, Isosorbide mononitride.

contraindication to their use. The only class of antihypertensive where particular care should be taken in order to avoid excessive hypotension are alpha-blockers.

Kloner RA. Cardiovascular effects of the 3 phosphodiesterase-5 inhibitors approve for the treatment of erectile dysfunction. Circulation 2004; 110 (19):3149–3155.

38. E Procyclidine

This woman's examination findings are highly suggestive of tardive dystonic activity in the neck and extraocular muscles. Tardive dystonia in the extraocular muscles is known as oculogyric crisis. Dystonia is an involuntary movement disorder associated with excessive activity in the extrapyramidal system. One major risk factor is prolonged use (>1 month) of medications that antagonise dopamine receptors, including antipsychotics (e.g. haloperidol) and antiemetics (e.g. metoclopramide). First-line emergency treatment of tardive dystonia is with anticholinergic medications, such as procyclidine or trihexyphenidyl.

There are no features of either opiate or benzodiazepine overdose, hence no indication for naloxone or flumazenil respectively. Lorazepam is an appropriate treatment for the termination of seizures, but the examination findings here are much more suggestive of tardive dystonia rather than complex seizure. Cyclizine exerts its antiemetic action principally via antagonism of histamine receptors, hence is a more appropriate choice than metoclopramide if an antiemetic is required for a prolonged period.

Kenney C, et al. Metoclopramide, an increasingly recognized cause of tardive dyskinesia. J Clinical Pharm 2008; 48(3):379–384.

39. E Sotalol

Ciclosporin, calcium channel blockers, and phenytoin are all associated with gingival hypertrophy when used for a prolonged period. Gingival hypertrophy in neonates has been reported in association with exposure to sodium valproate in utero. There is no strong association between the use of beta-blockers and gingival hypertrophy, making E the correct answer.

Dongari-Bagtzoglou A. Drug-associated gingival enlargement. J Periodontol 2004; 75: 1424–1431.

40. A Allopurinol

The patient has new onset pancytopenia probably as a result of drug-induced bone marrow suppression. This has most likely been caused by elevated plasma levels of azathioprine. Azathioprine is a prodrug that is metabolised to the active compound 6-mercaptopurine by red blood cells. A number of enzymes are involved in its subsequent metabolism and eventual excretion, including thiopurine methyltransferase (TPMT) and xanthine oxidase. Assays of TPMT concentrations are usually performed prior to starting azathioprine, with patients with low levels contraindicated from starting the drug.

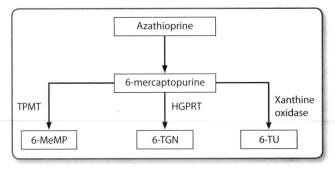

Figure 2.4 Interaction between azathioprine and allopurinol. 6-mercaptopurine is metabolised by the enzyme TPMT into the inactive metabolite 6-MeMP, and by the enzyme xanthine oxidase into the inactive metabolite 6-TU. It is also metabolised by the enzyme HGRPT into various active 6-TGN compounds. Some of these 6-TGN compounds are responsible for the desired immunosuppressive effect of the drug, but others have intense myelosuppressive activity. Inhibition of xanthine oxidase with allopurinol results in more 6-TGN formation, and increases the risk of excessive bone marrow suppression. HGPRT, Hypoxanthine-guanine-phosphoribosyl-transferase; 6-MeMP, 6-methylmercaptopurine; 6-TGN, 6-thioguanine nucleotides; TPMT, thiopurine methyltransferase; 6-TU, 6-thiouric acid.

Xanthine oxidase is also involved in the conversion of purine compounds to uric acid. Allopurinol acts by inhibiting xanthine oxidase, limiting uric acid formation and therefore preventing recurrent gout. However, when allopurinol and azathioprine are co-administered, allopurinol will limit azathioprine metabolism, making the patient prone to azathioprine toxicity (**Figure 2.4**).

All of the five drugs listed have a role in the management of gout. However of the options listed, only allopurinol limits azathioprine metabolism and hence increases the risk of bone marrow toxicity. As such, option A is the correct answer.

Gearry RB, et al. Azathioprine and allopurinol: A two-edged interaction. J Gastroenterol Hepatol 2010; 25(4):653–655.

Chapter 3

Clinical sciences

Cell, molecular and membrane biology

1. What happens during translation?

    A   Exons are removed from the genetic sequence and introns are expressed
    B   mRNA is synthesised from a DNA template
    C   Ribosomes synthesise proteins from tRNA
    D   RNA polymerase binds to a promotor code to initiate the process
    E   The anticodon of tRNA binds to the codon of mRNA

2. Which one of the following applies to the messenger RNA?

    A   Carries information from the cytoplasm to the nucleus
    B   Is synthesised in the cytoplasm
    C   Is synthesised in the nucleus
    D   Uracil replaces cytosine
    E   Uracil replaces guanine

3. Which part of the cell is responsible for the sorting and modification of proteins?

    A   Endoplasmic reticulum
    B   Golgi apparatus
    C   Lysosome
    D   Nucleus
    E   Ribosome

4. How does growth hormone exert its effects on cells?

    A   Activation of the adenylate cyclase signalling system
    B   Direct action with intracellular proteins
    C   Inhibition of the adenylate cyclase signalling system
    D   Phosphoinositide pathway
    E   Tyrosine kinase receptors

Clinical anatomy

5. Where are the ureters visible on an intravenous pyelogram?

    A   At the level of L1/L2, but lateral to the vertebral bodies
    B   Lying along the border of the psoas muscle
    C   Superimposed on the spinous processes of the lumbar spine

    D   Superimposed on the transverse processes of the lumbar spine
    E   Superimposed on the transverse processes of the thoracic spine

6. What level does the oesophagus pass through the diaphragm?

    A   T7
    B   T8
    C   T9
    D   T10
    E   T11

7. What is the arterial supply to the sigmoid colon?

    A   Inferior mesenteric artery
    B   Left gastroepiploic artery
    C   Marginal artery
    D   Superior mesenteric artery
    E   Superior rectal artery

8. A 25-year-old woman presented to her general practitioner complaining that she was having difficulty walking properly, and found that she was tripping over frequently. On examination, she was unable to dorsiflex or evert her right foot. These movements were preserved on the left.

    What is the most likely underlying lesion?

    A   Common peroneal nerve palsy
    B   Femoral nerve lesion
    C   L5 root lesion
    D   Tibial nerve palsy
    E   Sciatica

9. A 21-year-old woman attended her general practitioner complaining of pins and needles in her left forearm and hand. On examination, she had reduced sensation on the ulnar border of her 4th and 5th fingers.

    What is the most likely site of the underlying problem?

    A   Axillary nerve
    B   Medial nerve
    C   Musculocutaneous nerve
    D   Radial nerve
    E   Ulnar nerve

10. What is the main action of pectoralis major?

    A   Abducts the arm
    B   Abducts the arm and rotates it medially
    C   Extends, adducts and medially rotates the arm
    D   Medially rotates the arm
    E   Medially rotates and abducts the arm

Clinical biochemistry and metabolism

11. In which one of the following is increased serum cholesterol most likely to be seen?

    A   Alcohol excess
    B   Chronic renal failure
    C   Diabetes mellitus
    D   Nephrotic syndrome
    E   Use of thiazide diuretics

12. Which lipid condition are eruptive xanthomata characteristic of?

    A   Familial hypercholesterolemia
    B   Familial hyperchylomicronaemia
    C   Familial dysbetalipoproteinaemia
    D   Hypertriglyceridemia
    E   Lipoprotein lipase deficiency

13. A 78-year-old woman presented to her general practitioner complaining of abdominal pain and swelling. She had lost 10 kg in weight over the preceding 3 months. On examination, there was a palpable mass in the right iliac fossa that was felt to arise from the pelvis.

What is the most useful diagnostic test to follow-up her presumed malignancy after treatment?

    A   Alpha fetoprotein (AFP)
    B   Carcino-embryogenic antigen (CEA)
    C   Carbohydrate antigen 19-9 (CA19-9)
    D   Carbohydrate antigen 125 (CA 125)
    E   Human chorionic gonadotrophin (hCG)

14. A 48-year-old woman was referred to the hepatology clinic because of jaundice. Urinalysis was negative for bilirubin.

What is the most likely underlying cause?

    A   Alcoholic liver disease
    B   Gallstones
    C   Haemolytic anaemia
    D   Hepatitis A
    E   Paracetamol overdose

15. A 16-year-old boy was brought to his general practitioner because his parents were concerned about his disruptive behaviour, especially at school. He was noted to frequently rock and had very pale hair and blue eyes. A musty smell was also noted.

What is the most likely underlying diagnosis?

    A   Hypermethioninaemia
    B   Isovaleric acidaemia

C   Maple syrup urine disease
D   Phenylketonuria
E   Trimethylaminuria

16. Which one of following serum proteins decrease in concentration during pregnancy?

A   Albumin
B   Alkaline phosphatase (ALP)
C   Fibrinogen
D   Thyroxine binding globulin (TBG)
E   Transferrin

17. Which one of the following are dietary triglycerides are incorporated into?

A   Chylomicrons
B   High density lipoproteins
C   Lipoprotein lipases
D   Low density lipoproteins
E   Very low density lipoproteins

18. Which one of the following causes a narrow serum-ascites albumin gradient?

A   Chronic liver disease
B   Congestive cardiac failure
C   Hepatic metastases
D   Nephrotic syndrome
E   Spontaneous bacterial peritonitis

Clinical physiology

19. Which one of the following causes a left shift in the oxygen dissociation curve?

A   Acidosis
B   Decreased temperature
C   Exercise
D   Increased pCO_2
E   Increased temperature

20. Which one of the following causes an elevated carbon monoxide transfer factor?

A   Chronic obstructive pulmonary disease
B   Goodpasture's syndrome
C   Lower respiratory tract infection
D   Pneumothorax
E   Pulmonary oedema

21. A 76-year-old man, a smoker, was brought to the emergency department via ambulance. He had been having increasing difficulty breathing. Arterial blood gases on admission showed:

Investigations:

pH	7.29 (7.34–7.45)
pCO_2	9.2 kPa (4.7–6.0)
pO_2	18.1 kPa (11.3–12.6)
bicarbonate	22.1 mmol/L (21–29)

What is the most likely cause for this result?

A   High-flow oxygen therapy
B   Hyperventilation
C   Lactic acidosis
D   Renal failure
E   Vomiting

22. A 35-year-old woman attended the emergency department because of persistent vomiting for 3 weeks.

Which one of the following results is most consistent with her condition?

A   pH 7.37 (7.35–7.45), pO_2 14.2 kPa (11.3–12.6),
    pCO_2 5.1 kPa (4.7–6.0), bicarbonate 22 mmol/L (21–29)
B   pH 7.37, pO_2 14.2 kPa, pCO_2 5.1 kPa, bicarbonate 15 mmol/L
C   pH 7.49, pO_2 14.2 kPa, pCO_2 3.1 kPa, bicarbonate 32 mmol/L
D   pH 7.32, pO_2 14.2 kPa, pCO_2 6.8 kPa, bicarbonate 32 mmol/L
E   pH 7.49, pO_2 14.2 kPa, pCO_2 6.8 kPa, bicarbonate 32 mmol/L

23. Which one of the following causes a metabolic acidosis with a normal anion gap?

A   Acute renal failure
B   Diabetic ketoacidosis
C   Lactic acidosis
D   Renal tubular acidosis
E   Salicylate poisoning

24. Which one of the following drugs is most likely to be associated with a metabolic alkalosis?

A   Acetazolamide
B   Aspirin
C   Bendroflumethiazide
D   Metformin
E   Methanol

25. A 32-year-old woman presents to the emergency department and has the following arterial blood gas on air.

Investigations:

pH	7.49 (7.35–7.45)
pCO_2	2.9 kPa (4.7–6.0)
pO_2	16.2 kPa (4.7–6.0)
bicarbonate	22 mmol/L (21–29)

What condition is the result most consistent with?

A   Anxiety
B   Bendroflumethiazide use
C   Chronic obstructive pulmonary disease
D   Pulmonary embolus
E   Vomiting

26. A 64-year-old man, a breathless patient, attended for spirometry. His FEV1/FVC ratio was measured as 62% predicted.

What is the most likely underlying diagnosis?

A   Asbestosis
B   Chronic obstructive pulmonary disease (COPD)
C   Pleural effusion
D   Pulmonary oedema
E   Scoliosis

Genetics

27. The second child of a couple was diagnosed as having cystic fibrosis. Neither parent is affected by the disease.

What is the chance of their first child being a carrier?

A   0%
B   25%
C   50%
D   75%
E   100%

28. Which one of the following best describes the clinical features of neurofibromatosis type 1?

A   6 or more café-au-lait spots, axillary freckling and bilateral acoustic neuromas
B   6 or more café-au-lait spots, axillary freckling and lens opacities
C   6 or more café-au-lait spots, axillary freckling and Lisch nodules
D   6 or more café-au-lait spots, axillary freckling and peripheral schwannomas
E   6 or more café-au-lait spots, axillary freckling and tinnitus

29. Which one of the following is rheumatoid arthritis most strongly associated with?

A   HLA-A3
B   HLA-B27
C   HLA-DR2
D   HLA-DR3
E   HLA-DR4

30. A 35-year-old man attended his general practitioner complaining of joint pain and swelling. A finger prick glucose was recorded as 12.2 mmol/L (3-6 fasting) and his liver function tests were abnormal.

What is the most likely underyling genetic mutation?

A   Autosomal dominant chromosome 6
B   Autosomal recessive chromosome 6
C   Autosomal dominant chromosome 13
D   Autosomal recessive chromosome 13
E   Autosomal recessive chromosome 14

31. A 21-year-old woman presented to her general practitioner complaining of amenorrheoa. On examination, she was noted to have widely spaced nipples and an increased carrying angle of her arms.

What is the underlying genetic defect?

A   45 XO
B   47 XXX
C   Trisomy 13
D   Trisomy 18
E   Trisomy 21

32. During mitosis, what is the name of the stage when chromatids migrate to opposite poles of the cell?

A   Anaphase
B   Interphase
C   Metaphase
D   Prophase
E   Telophase

Immunology

33. Which complement component deficiency would lead to a susceptibility to pneumococcal infection?

A   C1
B   C1 inhibitor
C   C3
D   C7
E   C9

34. What type of hypersensitivity reaction is seen in Goodpasture's syndrome?

A   Type I
B   Type II
C   Type III
D   Type IV
E   Type V

35. Which one of the following vaccines consists of a killed organism?

- **A** Bacillus Calmette–Guérin (BCG)
- **B** Hepatitis B
- **C** Pertussis
- **D** Tetanus
- **E** Varicella

36. A 19-year-old woman attended the emergency department complaining of sudden onset severe abdominal pain and vomiting. On review of her records, it is noted she has attended the department on multiple occasions since she was a child, with the same condition. Her attendances had increased in frequency in recent years. She had had an appendicectomy at the age of 9 years and a maternal aunt died unexpectedly at the age of 37 years.

What is the most likely diagnosis?

- **A** Abdominal migraine
- **B** Hereditary angioedema
- **C** Mesenteric adenitis
- **D** Small bowel obstruction
- **E** Somatisation disorder

37. Which part of the antibody is responsible for binding antigen?

- **A** C-terminus heavy chain
- **B** C-terminus light chain
- **C** C-terminus heavy and light chain
- **D** N-terminus heavy and light chain
- **E** N-terminus light chain

38. In which condition is there a failure to produce bactericidal oxygen radicals during phagocyte activation?

- **A** Chédiak–Higashi syndrome
- **B** Chronic granulomatous disease
- **C** Common variable immunodeficiency
- **D** Hyper immunoglobulin M (IgM) syndrome
- **E** Severe combined immunodeficiency

39. Which one of the following conditions is nucleolar anti-nuclear antibody (ANA) pattern most likely to be seen?

- **A** CREST (Cyanosis, Raynaud's phenomenon, oEsophageal dysmotility, Sclerodactyly, Telangiectasia) syndrome
- **B** Polymyositis
- **C** Scleroderma
- **D** Systemic lupus erythematosus
- **E** Sjögren's syndrome

40. Which one of the following statements is not an action of the T cell?

- **A** Associate with major histocompatibility complex I (MHC I)

B   Classified according to the type of MHC molecule they associate with
C   Express CD4
D   Recognise native proteins
E   Selected in the thymus

Statistics, epidemiology and evidence-based medicine

41. In a population of 35,000 people, where 48% are female, 750 people develop ovarian cancer in 1 year.

What is the annual risk of developing ovarian cancer?

A   2.1%
B   2.5%
C   4.1%
D   4.5%
E   9.0%

42. In a population of 2500 people, two people a month are diagnosed with lung cancer.

What is the point prevalence of lung cancer at 6 months?

A   0.0048%
B   0.08%
C   0.32%
D   0.48%
E   0.96%

43. In a population of 1000 footballers, 30 players are diagnosed with torn cruciate ligaments over a period of 1 year. The incidence is spread equally throughout the 12-month period.

What is the incidence rate?

A   2.5/1000 players/year
B   30/1000 players/year
C   250/1000 players/year
D   360/1000 players/year
E   3000/10000 players/year

44. In an oncology centre 3000 people were treated for colonic cancer every year. Of these patients 1762 patients die over the year.

What is the survival rate for colonic cancer at this centre?

A   0.29
B   0.41
C   0.59
D   1.70
E   2.42

45. In a study, 1149 of 6328 smokers who were given nicotine gum stopped smoking. 893 out of 8380 smokers in the control group stopped smoking.

What is the absolute risk reduction?

A   0.017%
B   0.075%
C   1.70%
D   1.74%
E   7.50%

46. In a cohort study 2246 patients out of 7462 patients in a control group suffered a myocardial infarction, whereas 982 out of 9756 patients who were taking an angiotensin-converting enzyme inhibitor had myocardial infarctions.

What is the number needed to treat (NNT) with the medication to prevent one myocardial infarction?

A   1
B   5
C   14
D   46
E   500

47. Over a 5-year period 350 of 1268 smokers were diagnosed with lung cancer. Over the same time period 120 of 1972 non-smokers were also diagnosed with lung cancer.

What is the risk attributable to smoking?

A   0.22%
B   0.78%
C   4.5%
D   22%
E   78%

48. In a screening programme 5000 women were called to undergo mammography for breast screening. Of these 1342 were called back for further investigation with ultrasound guided biopsy. Biopsies subsequently revealed that 65% of these women had breast cancer. This cohort was then followed up and a further 25 women were diagnosed as having breast cancer, who had had previously negative mammography.

What is the sensitivity of the screening test?

A   2.8%
B   11.5%
C   65.0%
D   88.5%
E   97.2%

49. A population of 1000 undergo faecal occult blood testing as a screening test for bowel cancer. 463 test positive and go on for further investigation with colonoscopy. Of these 28% are found to have an underlying malignancy. On follow-up a further 42 patients are diagnosed with a bowel malignancy, who had previously had negative screening.

What is the positive predictive value of the screening test?

A   24%
B   28%
C   40%
D   60%
E   76%

50. Which one of the following is not criteria for judging whether to screen a population for a certain condition?

A   A large number of the population are affected
B   Available treatment is acceptable to the general public
C   Early treatment is beneficial
D   Facilities are available to perform the screening
E   The test is cost-effective

Answers

1. E The anticodon of tRNA binds to the codon of mRNA

Translation is the process in the cell by which ribosomes synthesise proteins from mRNA. It follows the process of transcription in which mRNA is synthesised from a DNA template.

Transcription:

- Synthesis of mRNA from a DNA template
- Occurs in the nucleus
- RNA polymerase binds to a specific base sequence in the DNA (promotor) and binds to it
- Complementary bases are assembled
- Transcription stops when the RNA polymerase reaches a termination code

Before translation can occur, further processing of the mRNA transcript must occur. There are sequences of DNA that do not code for proteins, known as introns, which must be removed. The significance of these sections is not well understood. The remaining parts of the code are known as exons, and these are the sections of the code that are expressed.

Translation (**Figure 3.1**):

- Ribosomes synthesise proteins from mRNA
- There is a specific tRNA for each amino acid
- 3 letter anticodon of tRNA bind to the 3 letter codon of mRNA

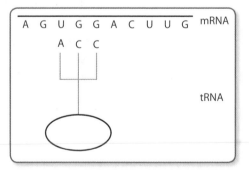

Figure 3.1 Translation.

2. C Is synthesised in the nucleus

mRNA is synthesised in the nucleus during transcription, and carries information from DNA into the cell cytoplasm. The base thymine in DNA is replaced by uracil in RNA.

3. B Golgi apparatus

The **Golgi apparatus** is responsible for the sorting and modification of proteins within the cell. The other structures' responsibilities are:
Nucleus: DNA storage and RNA transcription
Endoplasmic reticulum: protein synthesis (rough ER) and lipid synthesis (smooth ER)
Ribosomes: protein translation
Mitochondria: cellular respiration
Lysosomes: breakdown of macromolecules within the cell

4. E Tyrosine kinase receptors

Hormones are chemical messengers, released by endocrine glands and carried in the blood stream to their target cells. They exert their effect on cells via different signalling cascades (**Table 3.1**):

- Diffuse through cell membranes and act directly on intracellular proteins: steroids
- Adenylate cyclase signalling system: catecholamines
- Phosphoinositide pathway: catecholamines
- Tyrosine kinase receptors: growth factors

Lodish H, et al. Molecular Cell Biology, 4th edition. London: WH Freeman, 2000.
Voet D, Voet JG, Pratt CW. Fundamentals of Biochemistry: Life at the Molecular Level, 2nd edition. London: John Wiley & Sons, 2007.

Table 3.1

	Receptor tyrosine kinase	Adenylate cyclase	Phosphoinositide pathway
Hormone	Growth factors	Catecholamine	Catecholamine
Trans membrane receptor	Monomer	7 trans membrane segments	7 trans membrane segments
C terminus action	Tyrosine kinase activity	Release of bound GDP and GTP uptake	Phospholipase C
Downstream signalling	Ras	cAMP	IP3

cAMP, cyclic adenosine monophosphate; GDP, guanosine diphosphate; GTP, guanosine triphosphate; IP3, inositol triphosphate.

Table 3.1 Cell signalling pathways.

5. D Superimposed on the transverse processes of the lumbar spine

During an intravenous pyelogram, iodine containing contrast is injected intravenously, and concentrated and excreted by the kidneys. The urinary system is then opaque on X-rays. The ureters can be visualised superimposed on the transverse processes of the lumbar vertebrae. They cross the sacroiliac joints and enter the bladder at the level of the ischial spines.

6. D T10

The oesophagus crosses the diaphragm at T10.

The aorta crosses the diaphragm at T12.

The inferior vena cava crosses the diaphragm at T8.

7. A Inferior mesenteric artery

The superior mesenteric artery supplies the gut from the distal past of the duodenum to the distal third of the transverse colon. The inferior mesenteric artery then supplies the distal third of the transverse colon to the upper half of the anal canal. It then changes its name to the superior rectal artery. The marginal artery is the single arterial trunk formed by the anastomosis of the colic arteries. The left gastroepiploic artery supplies the greater curvature of the stomach. There is a watershed area at the splenic flexure, where, due to a lack of collateral blood supply, the area is vulnerable to ischaemic colitis.

8. A Common peroneal nerve palsy

The common peroneal nerve is the motor supply to tibialis anterior and the peronei muscles. Patients usually present with foot drop and are unable to dorsiflex or evert their foot. There is only minimal sensory loss over lateral aspect of the dorsum of the foot. Common causes of common peroneal nerve palsy include; trauma, vasculitis and diabetes mellitus.

In an L5 root lesion patients often present in a similar fashion, but on examination foot inversion is also lost, and knee flexion is weakened. There will be loss of sensation in the L5 dermatome.

The femoral nerve supplies the quadriceps muscles in the anterior thigh, and the tibial nerve supplies muscles in the calf responsible for plantar flexion of the foot (gastrocnemius, popliteus, soleus and plantaris muscles).

9. E Ulnar nerve

The ulnar nerve supplies sensation to the 5th finger and the ulnar border of the 4th finger, and motor supply to the small muscles of the hand (except the lateral two lumbricals, opponens pollicis, abductor pollicis and flexor pollicis brevis). It is easily damaged at the elbow, with external compression or bony deformities being the most common aetiology. Patients usually complain of numbness and tingling in the ring and little fingers, and may have also noticed some weakness of the hand. Nerve conduction studies are required for definitive diagnosis.

The median nerve is the most commonly affected nerve, usually as a result of carpal tunnel syndrome. Patients often present with pins and needles of the hand and weakness of grip. On examination, there is loss of sensation in the median nerve distribution, and there may be wasting of the thenar eminence.

Radial nerve lesions present as a wrist drop and result from compression of the radial nerve against the humerus. Sensation is lost over the anatomical snuffbox.

10. B Adducts the arm and rotates it medially

Pectoralis major adducts the arm and rotates it medially. Pectoralis minor pulls the shoulder downward and forward. Subscapularis medially rotates the arm. Latissimus dorsi extends, adducts and medially rotates the arm. Deltoid abducts the arm, with the help of the supraspinatus muscle.

11. D Nephrotic syndrome

Nephrotic syndrome and hypothyroidism usually have an elevated cholesterol level as the dominant lipid abnormality.

Alcohol excess, chronic renal failure, diabetes mellitus and use of thiazide diuretics are usually associated with an elevated triglyceride level.

12. D Hypertriglyceridemia

Eruptive xanthomata are characteristic of hypertriglyceridemia. Familial hypercholesterolemia may present with xanthelasma, tendon xanthoma and premature ischaemic heart disease. It is associated with over 500 mutations of the low-density lipoprotein (LDL) receptor gene.

Familial hypercholesterolemia presents with recurrent abdominal pain and pancreatitis. It may result from mutations of the lipoprotein lipase or *Apo C-II* genes. Lipoprotein lipase deficiency may also present with pancreatitis.

13. D Carbohydrate antigen 125 (CA 125)

This lady most likely has an ovarian tumour. The tumour marker associated with this is CA 125. Tumour markers are mainly used in the monitoring of treatment, but can be used in the screening, diagnosis and follow-up of cancers (**Table 3.2**).

14. C Haemolytic anaemia

Jaundice is a yellow discolouration of the skin or sclera, caused by an elevated bilirubin. Bilirubin is formed by breakdown of haemoglobin to form unconjugated bilirubin. This is conjugated in the liver and excreted into the small intestine via the bile ducts. It is converted into stercobilinogen in the bowel. This is either excreted with the stool, or reabsorbed and converted to urobilinogen by the liver, which is then excreted in the urine. **Table 3.3** outlines the different types of jaundice.

Table 3.2

Tumour marker	Tumour
Alpha fetoprotein (AFP)	Germ cell tumour Hepatocellular carcinoma
Human chorionic gonadotrophin (HCG)	Germ cell tumour Seminoma
Carbohydrate antigen 125 (CA 125)	Ovarian
Carbohydrate antigen 19-9 (CA 19-9)	Pancreatic
Carcino embryogenic antigen (CEA)	Colonic

Table 3.2 Tumour markers.

Table 3.3

	Prehepatic	Hepatocellular	Cholestatic
Bilirubin	Unconjugated (not water soluble) usually < 75 µmol/L	Conjugated (water soluble)	Conjugated (water soluble)
Urine	Bilirubin negative	Bilirubin positive	Bilirubin positive Dark urine with pale stools
LFTs	Elevated LDH	ALT and AST elevated ALP may be elevated later	ALP > 3 x upper limit of normal AST, ALT and LDH may also be elevated
Causes	Increase in Hb breakdown overloading the conjugating system, e.g. haemolysis	Damage to hepatocytes, e.g. by toxins or infection leading to failure of the conjugating system within the hepatocyte	Obstruction within the biliary system, e.g. gall stones/malignancy, and intrahepatic bile ducts

ALP, alkaline phosphatase; ALT, alanine transaminase; AST, aspartate transaminase; LDH, lactate dehydrogenase; LFTs, liver function tests.

Table 3.3 Types of jaundice.

15. D Phenylketonuria

This patient has phenylketonuria, an inborn error of metabolism. It is caused by absence of phenylalanine hydroxylase (PAH) enzyme activity, which converts dietary phenylalanine to tyrosine. The condition is usually identified in neonatal heel prick blood screening. Untreated problems include:

- Mental retardation
- Pale hair and blue eyes
- 'Mousey/musty' odour
- Skin rashes
- Seizures
- Behavioural difficulties
- Rhythmic rocking
- Writhing movements of hands and feet

Treatment is with a low phenylalanine diet, especially during childhood.

Steiner RD. Phenylketonuria. eMedicine 2011. http://emedicine.medscape.com/article/947781-overview (Last accessed May 2012).
Poustie VJ, Rutherford P. Dietary interventions for phenylketonuria. Cochrane Database Syst Rev. 2000; (2):CD001304.

16. A Albumin

Serum albumin concentrations fall during the pregnancy due to extracellular fluid expansion. Placental proteins, such as alkaline phosphatase (ALP) increase, as do transport proteins and hormone binding glycoproteins.

17. A Chylomicrons

Dietary lipid is absorbed in the small bowel and incorporated into chylomicrons. These are carried in the lymphatics and released into the circulation at the thoracic duct. Lipoprotein lipases then remove the triglycerides. The chylomicron remnants are removed by the liver. This is known as the **exogenous** lipid cycle (see **Figure 3.2**).

The liver synthesises very low density lipoproteins (VLDL) which are delipidated by lipoprotein lipase enzymes, forming intermediate density lipoproteins (IDL) and low

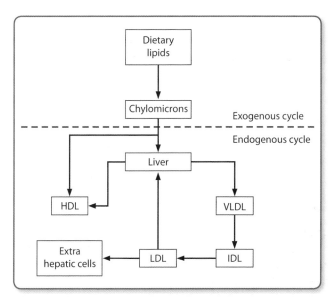

Figure 3.2 The endogenous and exogenous lipid cycles. HDL, high density lipoproteins; IDL, intermediate density lipoproteins; LDL, low density lipoproteins; VLDL, very low density lipoproteins.

density lipoproteins (LDL). LDLs are removed from the circulation by LDL receptors on extra hepatic cells, and at high levels are incorporated into atheromatous plaques.

High density lipoproteins (HDL) particles are derived from the liver and the gut, and act as cholesterol shuttles. They transport cholesterol to the liver, where it may be used in cell membrane formation and bile acid synthesis, or it may be excreted in the bile. HDL levels are thought to be protective against formation of atheromatous plaques, as more cholesterol is excreted via the liver, rather than being incorporated into atheromatous plaques by LDL. The lipid cycle involving HDL and LDL is known as the endogenous lipid cycle (**Figure 3.2**).

18. D Nephrotic syndrome

The serum-ascites albumin gradient (SAAG) is calculated by subtracting the ascitic fluid albumin concentration from the serum albumin concentration.

A wide SAAG >11 g/L is indicative of portal hypertension and occurs in:

- Chronic liver disease
- Congestive cardiac failure
- Hepatic metastases
- Veno-occlusive disease (e.g. Budd–Chiari)
- Spontaneous bacterial peritonitis

A narrow SAAG <11 g/L is found in patients with ascites, but no portal hypertension. Causes include:

- Peritoneal carcinomatosis
- Secondary peritonitis
- Low plasma oncotic pressure (e.g. nephrotic syndrome)

19. B Decreased temperature

The oxygen dissociation curve depicts the saturation of haemoglobin at varying pO_2 levels. Different conditions cause a shift in the curve, allowing for maximum uptake in the lungs and maximum oxygen release in the tissues – the Bohr Effect.

Causes of a right shift (allowing more oxygen release to the tissues, but reducing uptake):

- Increased pCO_2
- Acidosis
- Exercise
- Raised temperature
- Increased 2,3-diphosphoglycerate (2,3-DPG)

Causes of a left shift (increasing oxygen uptake on the lungs, but reducing the ability to unload O_2 at the tissues):

- Decreased pCO_2
- Alkalosis
- Reduced temperature

- Reduced 2,3-DPG
- Increased carbon monoxide concentrations

20. B Goodpasture's syndrome

An elevated transfer factor of the lung for carbon monoxide (TLCO) occurs due to pulmonary haemorrhage and is therefore seen in Goodpasture's syndrome. It may be falsely elevated in polycythaemia, and can be elevated in asthma, secondary to air trapping.

Reduced TLCO occurs in fibrosis, chronic obstructive pulmonary disease (COPD), pulmonary embolus and pulmonary hypertension and pneumonia. It may be falsely low in anaemia.

21. A High-flow oxygen therapy

This gentleman is a smoker and has been admitted with dyspnoea. It is highly likely he was given high-flow oxygen therapy in the ambulance, which has led to CO_2 retention and a respiratory acidosis (elevated pCO_2 with normal bicarbonate), secondary to underlying chronic obstructive pulmonary disease.

22. E pH 7.49, pO_2 14.2 kPa, pCO_2 6.8 kPa, bicarbonate 32 mmol/L

Persistent vomiting causes a metabolic alkalosis, secondary to loss of hydrogen ions in gastric fluid. This is seen by an elevated pH and high bicarbonate. As the patient has been vomiting persistently for several weeks, there will be a degree of respiratory compensation, and the pCO_2 would be expected to be elevated as a result of this.

23. D Renal tubular acidosis

Metabolic acidosis results from increased production of hydrogen ions, ingestion of hydrogen ions, impaired excretion of hydrogen ions or loss of bicarbonate from the gastrointestinal (GI) tract. They can be further differentiated by the anion gap. The anion gap is calculated by subtracting the concentration of chloride and bicarbonate ions from the concentration of sodium and potassium ions:

Anion gap = $([Na^+] + [K^+]) - ([Cl^-] + [HCO_3^-])$

Table 3.4 outlines the causes of metabolic acidosis with normal and elevated anion gaps.

24. C Bendroflumethiazide

Diuretics, such as bendroflumethiazide, are associated with a metabolic alkalosis due to loss of K^+ in the urine, and retention of H^+ inside cells to maintain electrochemical neutrality. Metformin has been rarely associated with lactic acidosis. Aspirin and methanol are both associated with a metabolic acidosis with raised anion gap. Acetazolamide is associated with a metabolic acidosis with a normal anion gap.

Table 3.4

Elevated anion gap	Normal anion gap
Renal disease: failure of excretion of H^+ ions	Chronic diarrhoea: loss of bicarbonate from the GI tract
Diabetic ketoacidosis: endogenous production of acetoacetic and B-hydroxybutyric acids	Intestinal fistula: loss of bicarbonate from the GI tract
Lactic acidosis: endogeneous production of lactate	Renal tubular acidosis: loss of bicarbonate in the urine and failure of H^+ secretion
Salicylate poisoning: ingestion of drugs metabolised to acids	

Table 3.4 Causes of metabolic acidosis.

25. A Anxiety

The gas result shows a respiratory alkalosis, most likely caused by hyperventilation in anticipation of the test being performed. If this was a significant pulmonary embolus then one would expect to see hypoxia as shown by low pO_2. Bendroflumethiazide and vomiting result in a metabolic alkalosis. Chronic obstructive pulmonary disease is usually associated with a respiratory acidosis.

26. B Chronic obstructive pulmonary disease (COPD)

Spirometry is performed to help determine the underlying aetiology of respiratory problems. Several basic measurements can be taken:

FEV1: Volume of air expelled in the first second of forced expiration

FVC (Forced vital capacity): volume of lungs from full inspiration to forced maximal expiration

FEV1/FVC ratio: A ratio of FEV1 to FVC

These values can then be used to determine if the underlying diagnosis is obstructive of restrictive. **Table 3.5** outlines the spirometry results associated with restrictive and obstructive defects.

Causes of obstructive defects include:

• COPD
• Asthma

Causes of restrictive defects include:

• Fibrosis
• Large pleural effusions
• Pulmonary oedema
• Scoliosis
• Neuromuscular disorders

Table 3.5

	FEV1	FVC	FEV1/FVC
Obstructive	< 80% predicted	Normal or reduced	< 70%
Restrictive	Reduced	< 80%	Normal

Table 3.5 Spirometry interpretation.

27. C 50%

Cystic fibrosis is an autosomal recessive condition, carried on Chromosome 7. It is caused by the ΔF508 mutation in 75% of cases. In order to suffer with the disease the patient must carry two copies of the defective gene. In this case, as neither parent has the disease, they must both be carriers (heterozygous genotype). As demonstrated in **Figure 3.3**, any child they have will have a 50% chance of being a carrier of the defective gene.

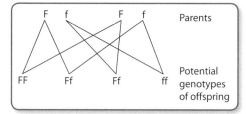

Parents

Potential genotypes of offspring

Figure 3.3 Inheritance of cystic fibrosis. F, dominant; f, recessive (defective). Two combinations are carriers (heterozygous), one unaffected (homozygous dominant) and one affected (homozygous recessive).

28. C 6 or more café-au-lait spots, axillary freckling, lisch nodules

Table 3.6 outlines the key features of neurofibromatosis types 1 and 2.

Table 3.6

	Neurofibromatosis 1	Neurofibromatosis 2
Clinical features	6 or more café-au-lait spots Axillary freckling Lisch nodules (iris hamartomas) Peripheral neurofibroma	Bilateral acoustic neuromas Peripheral schwannomas Lens opacities
Complications	Optic glioma Meningiomas Renal artery stenlosis Phaeochromocytoma Learning difficulties	Deafness Tinnitus Nerve compression Malignant change of tumours
Gene	Chromosome 17 – mutation or deletion of *NF1* gene Reduced neurofibromin 1 (tumour suppressor)	Chromosome 22 – mutation or deletion of *NF2* gene Reduced neurofibromin 2 (merlin) (tumour suppressor)

Table 3.6 Key features of neurofibromatosis types 1 and 2.

29. E HLA-DR4

Human leucocyte antigens (HLAs) are coded for by genes on chromosone 6. They are strongly assocaited with various conditions:

HLA-A3:   Haemochromatosis
HLA-B5:   Beçhet's disease
HLA-B27:   Psoriatic arthritis
            Enteropathic arthritis
            Ankylosing spondylitis
            Reiter's syndrome
HLA-DR2:   Goodpasture's syndrome
            Multiple sclerosis
HLA-DR3:   Coeliac disease
            Dermatitis herpetiformis
            Sjögren's syndrome
            Primary biliary cirrhosis
            Type 1 diabetes mellitus
            Myasthenia gravis
            Graves' disease
HLA-DR4:   Type 1 diabetes mellitus
            Rheumatoid arthitis

30. B Autosomal recessive chromosome 6

This patient has a diagnosis of hereditary haemochromatosis. Features include:

- Cirrhosis
- Chondrocalcinosis
- Pseudogout
- Skin bronzing
- Diabetes
- Cardiomyopathy
- Arrhythmias
- Testicular atrophy

Serum iron is elevated, and transferrin saturation is greater than 60%. Molecular genetic testing is now available, looking for the human haemochromatosis (HFE) protein gene mutation carried on chromosome 6 (autosomal recessive).

Treatment includes venesection and chelation therapy with desferioxamine.

Wilson's disease is an autosomal recessive condition, caused by a mutation on chromosome 13 of the *ATP 7B* gene. Total body and tissue copper levels rise due to a defective intrahepatic formation of ceruloplasmin. Features include:

- Hepatic dysfunction
- Hypoparathyroidism
- CNS involvement
- Kayser-Fleischer rings
- Arthropathy

31. A 45 XO

This patient has Turner's syndrome, karyotype 45 XO. It affects 1 in every 2500 female live births. **Table 3.7** outlines the typical features of other genetic defects.

32. A Anaphase

Interphase is the stage of growth that occurs prior to a cell entering mitosis. During prophase the chromatin condenses into chromosomes and the spindle forms at opposite poles of the cell. The nucler membrane breaks down. In metaphase the spindle completes formation and the chromatids line up along the spindle, equidistant from the two poles. During anaphase the sister chromatids migrate along the spindle to opposite poles of the cell. The two new daughters cells are

Table 3.7

	Karyotype	Clinical features
Turner's syndrome	45 XO	Short stature
		Streak ovaries
		Webbed neck
		Widely spaced nipples
		Increased carrying angle of the arms
		Cardiovascular complications in 25%
		Renal abnormalities in 30%
Triple X syndrome	47 XXX	Tall stature
		Normal fertility
		Mild developmental and behavioural difficulties
Edwards' syndrome	Trisomy 18	Prominent occiput
		Rockerbottom feet
		Congential heart disease
		Mental retardation
Patau's syndrome	Trisomy 13	Microcephaly
		Cleft lip and palate
		Polydactyly
		Congential heart disease
		CNS abnormalities
Down's syndrome	Trisomy 21	Moderate mental retardation
		Single palmar crease
		Protruding tongue
		Atrioventricular septal defect (AVSD)
		Early-onset Alzheimer's disease

Table 3.7 Typical features of genetic defects.

completed during telophase, with new nuclear membranes forming and final membrane division.

33. C C3

The complement cascade is a plasma protein sequence with three distinct pathways. During an infection no one pathway is thought to predominate. The classical pathway involves components C1, C4, C2 and C3 and is triggered by antibody-antigen complexes. The alternative pathway involves properdin, factor D, factor B and C3. It is activated by polysaccharides within the walls of gram-negative bacteria. The lectin binding pathway involves C2 and C4. It is activated by bacterial cell wall carbohydrates.

All three pathways have a common end point – the cleavage of C3 protein. This leads to the activation of the terminal membrane attack sequence, made up of components of C5, C6, C7, C8 and C9, which bind to cell membranes, causing cell lysis (**Figure 3.4**).

It is C3 deficiency within the complement cascade that predisposes to infection with encapsulated organisms (pneumococcus, meningococcus, haemophilus). Deficiencies of the terminal complement cascade (C5–C9) predisposes to dissemination of neisserial infection dissemination. Deficiencies of the classical pathway (C1, C4, C2) lead to systemic lupus erythematosus like disorders. Deficiency of C1 inhibitor leads to recurrent episodes of acute non-inflammatory oedema. This is known as hereditary angioedema, and is mediated by vasoactive C2 fragments.

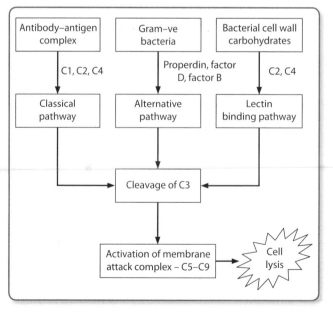

Figure 3.4
Complement cascade.

34. B Type II

In 1963 Gell and Coombs developed a four-group classification for hypersensitivity reactions:

- Type I: anaphylactic/immediate
  - Antigen + IgE
  - Release of vasoactive substances (histamine, leukotrienes, interleukins)
  - Reaction within 30 minutes
  - Asthma, atopy, drug reactions
- Type II: antibody dependent
  - Cell bound antigen + circulating IgG or IgM
  - Complement activation resulting in cell lysis
  - Transfusion reactions, rhesus incompatibility, Goodpasture's syndrome
- Type III: immune complex mediated
  - Free antigen + free antibody
  - Precipitation of antigen-antibody complexes and complement activation
  - Farmers lung, glomerulonephritis
- Type IV: cell mediated/delayed type
  - Antigen + memory T-cells
  - T cell activation
  - Reactions take up to 24 hours to develop
  - Tuberculin reaction, contact dermatitis, graft rejection

A further classification that has later been added is type V hypersensitivity. This is a further classification of type II hypersensitivy and is caused by an antibody reacting with a cell surface receptor (rather than a cell membrane component) and includes Graves' disease and myaesthenia gravis.

Rajan TV. The Gell–Coombs classification of hypersensitivity reactions: a re-interpretation. Trends Immunol 2003; 24 (7): 376–379.

35. C Pertussis

Killed organisms are used for pertussis vaccination. **Table 3.8** outlines the different types of vaccinations commonly used.

Table 3.8

Killed organism	Preformed antibody	Live attenuated	Subunit
Cholera	Botulism	BCG	Hepatitis B
Influenza	Diphtheria	Measles	*Haemophilus influenzae*
Pertussis	Hepatitis B	Mumps	*Neisseria meningitides*
Polio (Salk)	Rabies	Polio (Sabin)	*Streptococcus pneumoniae*
Rabies	Tetanus	Rubella	
Typhoid	Varicella	Vaccinia	

Table 3.8 Types of vaccine.

36. B Hereditary angioedema

Hereditary angioedema is a condition caused by reduced levels of, or poor function of C1 esterase inhibitor. It presents as recurrent episodes of angioedema, which typically affects the face, larynx or GI tract. Attacks can be spontaneous, or triggered by events such as trauma or infection. Angioedema of the GI tract presents as abdominal pain. Events may come on suddenly, but classically develop over several hours. Episodes usually begin in childhood, and escalate during teenage years. There is often a family history, but this may just be recorded as a sudden unexpected death, as no diagnosis was made.

Reduced levels of C1 esterase inhibitor lead to over activation of the complement cascade, and consumption of C2 and C4.

In type I hereditary angioedema low levels of C1 esterase inhibitor are identified. In type II there are normal levels, but functional assays show it to be inactive.

Type III is a recently documented form that mainly affects females. It is triggered by high oestrogen levels and is not related to C1 esterase inhibitor activity. It is linked to an increase in kininogenase activity leading to elevated levels of bradykinin.

Treatment of the acute episode includes immediate treatment with C1 inhibitor concentrate. Glucocorticoids and antihistamines are of no benefit. Appropriate airway management, analgesia and intravenous fluids are also an important part of treatment. If no C1 inhibitor concentrate is available, fresh frozen plasma may be used with caution, as it can worsen an attack. If a patient presets with only peripheral oedema, a watch and wait approach can be adopted.

Long term management includes attenuated androgens (e.g. danazol) or tranexamic acid. Investigations for diagnosis include C4 and C1 inhibitor levels and C1 inhibitor function.

Bowen T, et al. International consensus algorithm for the diagnosis, therapy and management. Allergy Asthma Clin Immunol 2010; 6(1):24.

Grigoriadou S, Longhurst HJ. Clinical Immunology Review Series: An approach to the patient with angio-oedema. Clin Exp Immunol 2009; 155(3):367–377.

37. D N-terminus heavy and light chain

An antibody is a protein molecule made up of four protein chains; two heavy chains and two light chains, as depicted in **Figure 3.5**. The heavy chains are identical in each antibody, and the light chains are identical. Each protein chain has a C and an N-terminus, as is the case with all protein molecules.

The heavy chain determines the class of the antibody.

It is the N-terminus of the heavy and light chains that makes up the antigen binding site. This is known as the variable domain as the amino acid sequence varies between different antibodies. The structure of the variable domain is unique to each antibody.

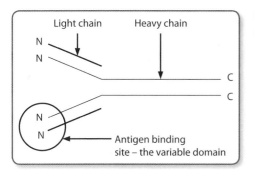

Figure 3.5 Basic structure of an antibody.

38. B Chronic granulomatous disease

Chronic granulomatous disease is a group of disorders resulting from failure of production of bactericidal oxygen radicals during phagocytic activation. It is an X-Linked recessive disorder and is an example of a primary immunodeficiency. Patients are prone to infections with *Staphylococcus aureus* or fungal infections.

Other primary immunodeficiency disorders include:

- Bruton's disease (X-linked agammaglobulinaemia): X-linked condition where there are absent circulating B cells, with normal T cells. Pro-B cells are unable to mature due to the absence of a gene coding for Bruton's tyrosine kinase.
- Hyper-IgM syndrome: patients have a high IgM level due to a failure of CD40 ligand expression on CD4 + T cells. Antigen stimulated B cells fail to make the switch from IgM to IgG or IgA production. Replacement immunoglobulin therapy is required.
- Selective IgA deficiency: this is characterised by undetectable serum IgA levels, and is the most common primary immunodeficiency. The aetiology is unknown.
- Chédiak–Higashi syndrome: an autosomal recessive condition, characterised by abnormal intracellular protein transport and abnormal synthesis of storage/secretory granules in a variety of cells. Patients are particularly susceptible to *Staphylococcus aureus, Streptococcus pyogenes,* and *Pneumococcus* species.
- Common variable immunodeficiency: a lack of B cells able to produce antibodies, resulting in frequent bacterial infections. Several genes have been identified, some autosomal dominant and some autosomal recessive.
- Severe combined immunodeficiency: major failure of both T-cell and B-cell lymphocyte function. Infants die before 2 years of age unless bone marrow transplant is undertaken. It results from a heterogeneous group of conditions affecting the immune system.

Rezaei N, Wing J, Aghamohammadi A, et al. B-cell-T-cell activation and interaction in common variable immunodeficiency. Hum Immunol 2010; 71(4):355–62.
van de Ven AA, et al. Lymphocyte characteristics in children with common variable immunodeficiency. Clin Immunol 2010; 135(1):63–71.

39. C Scleroderma

Anti-nuclear antibodies are a heterogeneous group of antibodies that bind to nuclear antigen. They are relatively non-specific and can occur in systemic lupus erythematosus (SLE), rheumatoid arthritis, Sjögren's syndrome, CREST, systemic sclerosis, systemic infections and mixed connective tissue disease (MCTD). They can also be drug induced or occur in healthy individuals. Anti-nuclear antibody (ANA) staining patterns can be a little more specific, but there is still a degree of overlap:

- Nucleolar: scleroderma
- Speckled: MCTD, SLE, Sjögren's syndrome, polymyositis
- Centromere: CREST
- Homogeneous: SLE

To generate a more specific diagnosis, antibodies to extractable nuclear antigens (ENA) can be tested for:

- Anti dsDNA: SLE (90%)
- Anti RNP: mixed connective tissue disease (MCTD)(>95%) SLE (40%)
- Anti Ro: Sjögren's syndrome (50%)
- Anti La: Sjögren's syndrome (50%)
- Anti SM: SLE (30%)
- Anti Jo1: polymyositis (30%)
- Anti Scl70: scleroderma (30)
- Anti TTG (Tissue transglutaminase): coeliac disease
- Anti gliadin: coeliac disease (less specific)
- Anti gastric parietal cell: pernicious anaemia
- Antinuclear cytoplasmic antibody: vasculitis
- Antimitochondrial: primary biliary cirrhosis
- Anti smooth muscle: autoimmune hepatitis

40. D Recognise native proteins

Lymphocytes are derived from a common lymphoid progenitor in the bone marrow. They then mature in the bone marrow (B cells) or thymus (T cells). Naïve T cells are then activated in secondary lymphoid organs (lymph nodes and spleen).

T lymphocytes cannot recognise native proteins, they can only recognise peptides when complexed with major histocompatability complex (MHC) molecules on antigen presenting cells.

T cells can be classified according to the class of MHC protein used in antigen presentation, the accessory molecule they express and their function, as outlined in **Table 3.9**.

T cells are selected in the thymus and then enter the circulation as mature naïve T cells.

Table 3.9

	T helper cells	Cytotoxic T cells
MHC protein	MHC-II	MHC-I
Accessory molecule	CD4	CD8
Function	Cytokine production Help for cytotoxic T cells	Cytokine production Cytotoxic lysis of viral infected cells.

Table 3.9 Classification of T cells.

41. D 4.5%

$$\text{Risk} = \frac{\text{Number of people who become diseased in a period}}{\text{Number of people in the population at risk at the beginning of the period}}$$

In this example, the population at risk are the females. The number of females in the population is 48% of 35,000 = 16,800. We know from the information in the question that 750 women develop ovarian cancer in a year, so the risk is:

$$750/16800 = 0.0446 = \textbf{4.5\%}.$$

42. D 0.48%

Point prevalence =

$$\frac{\text{Number of diseased persons in a defined population at one point in time}}{\text{Number of persons in the defined population at the same moment in time}}$$

In this example, as two people are diagnosed every month, by 6 months 12 people will have been diagnosed with lung cancer giving a point prevalence of $12/2500 = 0.0048 = 0.48\%$

43. B 30/1000 players/year

$$\text{Incidence rate} = \frac{\text{Number of persons who have developed disease in a given time}}{\text{Population at risk in a given time}}$$

In this example, we know that 30 of the 1000 players are injured every year, giving an incidence rate of 30/1000 players/year.

44. B 0.41

Survival rate = 1 – case fatality rate

In this example, the case fatality rate = 1762/3000 = 0.59. The survival rate is therefore 1 – 0.59 = **0.41.**

45. E 7.50%

Absolute risk reduction (ARR) = incidence rate in exposed – incidence in unexposed

ARR is a measure of absolute effect of exposure. It may be estimated in cohort studies, but not in case control studies.

In this example, the incidence rate in the exposed population = 1149/6328 = 0.1816.

The incidence rate in the unexposed population = 893/8380 = 0.1066.

Therefore, the absolute risk reduction = 0.1816 – 0.1066 = 0.075 = **7.5%**.

The figures in the question are sourced from Silagy (1994).

Silagy C, Mant D, Fowler G, et al. Meta-analysis on efficacy of nicotine replacement therapies in smoking cessation. Lancet 1994; 343:139–142.

46. B 5

Number needed to treat (NNT) =

$$\frac{100}{\% \text{ desired outcome in treated group} - \% \text{ desired outcome in control group}}$$

In this example, 30% (2246/7462) of patients in the control group had an myocardial infarction (MI) and 10% (982/9756) of the treatment group had an MI. This is a risk reduction of 20%, with use of the angiotensin-converting enzyme (ACE) inhibitor. To calculate NNT divide 100 by this number to get 5. Therefore, we can conclude that to prevent one myocardial infarction, we need to treat five people.

The NNT can be used to help gauge the cost effectiveness of a new medication or treatment. It gives more information than relative risk because it takes into account the baseline frequency of the outcome.

The higher the NNT the less effective the treatment.

47. E 78%

$$\text{Attributable risk} = \frac{\text{incidence in exposed} - \text{incidence in unexposed}}{\text{incidence in exposed}}$$

In this example, the incidence in the exposed population = 350/1268 = 0.276. The incidence in the unexposed population = 120/1972 = 0.061.

Attributable risk = (0.276-0.061)/0.276 = 0.779 = **78%**.

48. E 97.2%

For any screening question it is advisable to create a table of the data you have been given in the question, as in **Table 3.10**.

You can then easily calculate sensitivity, specificity, false positive rates, false negative rates and the positive predictive value of the test.

Table 3.10

		Disease	
		+ve	−ve
Test	+ve	a	b
	−ve	c	d

Table 3.10 A sample table of how to lay out data provided in questions related to screening programmes.

Sensitivity = a/(a + c). This value looks at the ability of the test to identify all cases of disease.

Specificity = d/(d + b). This value looks at the ability of the test to identify those without the disease.

In the above example, data can be set out as in **Table 3.11**:

Table 3.11

		Disease		
		+ve	−ve	Total
Test	+ve	872	470	1342
	−ve	25	3633	3658
	Total	497	4103	5000

Table 3.11 Data from the breast screening programme given in question 48.

Sensitivity can then be calculated as:

True positives identified by the test/all cases of disease = 872/(872 + 25) = 0.972 = **97.2%**.

Specificity in this case would be calculated as:

True negatives identified by the case/all disease free cases = 3633/(3633 + 470) = 0.885 = **88.5%**.

49. B 28%

The data from the question can be presented as in **Table 3.12**:

Positive predictive value = $\dfrac{\text{number of true +ve identified by the screening test (a)}}{\text{total number of +ve identified by screening (a + b)}}$

= 130/(130 + 333) = 0.28 = 28%.

Table 3.12

		Disease		
		+ve	−ve	Total
Test	+ve	130	333	463
	−ve	42	495	537
	Total	172	828	1000

Table 3.12 Data from the bowel cancer screening given in question 49.

The predictive value of a screening test in dependent upon the prevalence of the condition in the population being studied.

False positive and false negative rates can also easily be calculated for the screening test

False positive rate = The likelihood of receiving a positive test if you do not have the disease
= False positive identified by the test/total number of disease free people
= $b/(b + d)$.

So, for the above example false positive rate = 333/(333 + 495) = **40%**.

False negative rate = The likelihood of receiving a negative test result even if you have the disease
= False negative result identified by the test/total number of people with the disease
= $c/(c + a)$.

So, for the example above the false negative rate = 42/(42 + 130) = **24%**.

50. A A large number of the population is affected

Wilson–Jungner criteria for identifying the validity of a screening programme are:

1. The condition being screened for should be an important health problem
2. The natural history of the condition should be well understood
3. There should be a detectable early stage
4. Treatment at an early stage should be of more benefit than at a later stage
5. A suitable test should be devised for the early stage
6. The test should be acceptable
7. Intervals for repeating the test should be determined
8. Adequate health service provision should be made for the extra clinical workload resulting from screening
9. The risks, both physical and psychological, should be less than the benefits
10. The costs should be balanced against the benefits

Therefore A is not one of the criteria – although the problem should be an important health problem, how this is decided is not specified, and does not necessarily have to affect a large number of people to warrant screening.

Wilson JMG, Jungner G. Principles and practice of screening for disease (large pdf). WHO Chronicle Geneva: World Health Organization; 1968: 22(11):473.

Chapter 4

Dermatology

1. A 32-year-old woman presented to her general practitioner with a patchy rash involving the trunk. There were small oval pinky-brown spots, some coalescing to form larger patches. Over the larger patches there was a fine white scale.

   What is the most likely causative organism?

   A *Candida albicans*
   B Herpes simplex virus
   C *Malassezia furfur*
   D *Staphylococcus aureus*
   E *Streptococcus pyogenes*

2. A 45-year-old man presented to his general practitioner with hair loss. On examination, he had patchy baldness affecting both temporal areas of the scalp. There was preservation of the hair follicle and no evidence of a rash.

   What is the most likely diagnosis?

   A Alopecia areata
   B Androgenetic alopecia
   C Discoid lupus
   D Lichen planus
   E Morphoea

3. A 32-year-old woman presented to the dermatology clinic with a hyperpigmented plaque of waxy skin on her trunk. It initially began as a 5 cm plaque of indurated mauve skin before becoming hyperpigmented with absent hair and loss of sweating.

   Which one of these conditions is not associated with this skin condition?

   A Primary biliary cirrhosis (PBC)
   B Raynaud's phenomenon
   C Systemic lupus erythematosus (SLE)
   D Type I diabetes mellitus
   E Vitiligo

4. A 75-year-old woman admitted with a chest infection was noted to have thickening, discolouration and onycholysis of her toenails. A fungal infection was suspected.

   What is the most appropriate initial diagnostic investigation?

A   Blood cultures
B   C-reactive protein (CRP)
C   Fungal culture of toe scrapings
D   Plain X-rays of both feet
E   Potassium hydroxide (KOH) test

5.   Which one of the following is not a recognised association?

A   Acquired ichthyosis and lymphoma
B   Erythema gyratum repens and bronchial carcinoma
C   Erythroderma and lymphoma
D   Necrolytic migratory erythema and insulinoma
E   Pyoderma gangrenosum and myeloproliferative tumours

6.   A 60-year-old man was admitted with a scaling, erythematous rash involving the face, trunk and limbs.

What is the most likely underlying cause?

A   Contact dermatitis
B   Eczema
C   Lichen planus
D   Mycosis fungoides
E   Psoriasis

7.   A 25-year-old man developed a pruritic linear rash on his right shin 1 week after injuring this part of his leg during a rugby match.

What is the least likely cause of the rash?

A   Keratosis follicularis
B   Lichen planus
C   Lichen sclerosus
D   Psoriasis
E   Pyoderma gangrenosum

8.   A 32-year-old woman presented to her general practitioner with hot tender red nodules on both shins that had developed over the past week. She had returned from a holiday in India 2 weeks ago. She had no past medical history and did not smoke or drink alcohol.

Investigations:

haemoglobin	120 g/L (115–165)
mean cell volume	88 fL (80–96)
white cell count	12.0×10^9/L (4.0–11.0)
platelets	276×10^9/L (150–400)

What is the most appropriate initial investigation?

A   Antistreptolysin-O titre (ASOT)
B   Chest X-ray

C   Mantoux test
D   Stool culture
E   Throat swab

9. A 34-year-old man presented to the emergency department with a blistering rash involving his arms, legs and mouth. His past medical history included asthma, for which he was taking inhalers. A few days ago, he had seen his general practitioner with a fever and sore throat, and was started on amoxicillin.

The skin lesions started in the mouth and quickly spread to his soles and palms.

He was admitted to intesive therapy unit, where the skin developed a vesicular and bullous appearance with sloughing. His temperature was 38°C, pulse 130 beats per minute and blood pressure 143/76 mmHg.

Investigations:

serum sodium	137 mmol/L (137–144)
serum potassium	3.7 mmol/L (3.5–4.9)
serum urea	9.0 mmol/L (2.5–7.0)
serum creatinine	120 µmol/L (60–110)
random serum glucose	12.0 mmol/L
serum bicarbonate	21 mmol/L (20–28)
haemoglobin	130 g/L (130–180)
white cell count	12.5×10^9/L (4.0–11.0)

Which one of the following factors is most likely to be associated with a poor prognosis?

A   Age 34
B   Bicarbonate 21 mmol/L
C   Glucose 12 mmol/L
D   Pulse 130 beats per minute
E   Urea 9 mmol/L

10. A 75-year-old man presented to the dermatology clinic with itchy, tense blisters predominantly affecting his legs and elbows. There was no mucosal involvement. He was started on oral steroids and a skin biopsy was performed to confirm the diagnosis.

What is the skin biopsy most likely to show?

A   Immunofluorescence of IgA at the dermoepidermal junction
B   Immunofluorescence of IgA in a granular pattern in the upper dermis
C   Immunofluorescence of IgG and C3 in a granular pattern in the upper dermis
D   Immunofluorescence of IgG and C3 at the dermoepidermal junction
E   Immunofluorescence of IgG directed against intercellular desmosomes

11. A 35-year-old man presented to the dermatology clinic with a widespread pruritic rash that was worse after taking a shower and at night. On examination, he had a number of erythematous lesions in the webs between his fingers.

What is the most appropriate first line treatment for this skin condition?

A   Benzoyl benzoate
B   Ivermectin
C   Lindane
D   Malathion 0.5%
E   Permethrin 5%

12. A 30-year-old woman presented to her general practitioner with a rash on her face that got worse when exposed to sunlight.

Which one of the following skin conditions is not associated with photosensitivity?

A   Dermatomyositis
B   Eczema
C   Herpes simplex infection
D   Systemic lupus erythematosus
E   Melasma

13. A 48-year-old man presented to his general practitioner with a rash affecting his face and neck that had developed over the past 3 days. He had just returned from holiday in Egypt. Whilst there he had been treated for gastroenteritis.

What is the most likely drug causing his symptoms?

A   Amoxicillin
B   Ciprofloxacin
C   Clarithromycin
D   Gentamicin
E   Metronidazole

14. A 38-year-old woman presented to her general practitioner with a rash affecting her buttocks and lower limbs. On examination, she had well-defined red plaques that were covered by white scale.

What is the most useful lifestyle change to manage her condition?

A   Increase exercise
B   Increase weight loss
C   Reduce alcohol intake
D   Reduce stress
E   Stop smoking

15. A 40-year-old man presented to his general practitioner with painless white plaques in the mouth.

On examination, they were found over both lateral borders of the tongue and on the buccal mucosa where they had a lace-like pattern. They could not be removed by scraping the tongue.

What is the most likely diagnosis?

A   Aphthous ulcer
B   Chronic candidiasis
C   Chemical burn
D   Leukoplakia
E   Lichen planus

16. An 18-year-old man presented to his general practitioner with a painful rash at the right corner of his mouth. On closer inspection, there was a cluster of small fluid-filled vesicles. Tzanck test was positive (scraping of an ulcer base and direct smear to look for multinucleated giant cells).

What is the most effective treatment?

A   Acyclovir
B   Erythromycin
C   Flucloxacillin
D   Topical fusidic acid
E   Topical mupirocin

Answers

1. C *Malassezia furfur*

This woman has the typical rash of pityriasis versicolour, which is caused by *Malassezia furfur* and, more commonly, *Malassezia globosa*.

Candida albicans tends to cause intertrigo and affect oral and genital areas.

Herpes simplex virus type 1 causes skin infection on the face and lips and type 2 in the genital areas.

Staphylococcus aureus causes folliculitis, impetigo, scalded-skin syndrome and toxic-shock syndrome.

Streptococcus pyogenes can cause cellulitis, erysipelas, impetigo, necrotising fasciitis, erythema marginatum and scarlet fever. It is also one of the most common causes of erythema nodosum and can exacerbate guttate psoriasis.

Prohic A, Ozegovic L. Malassezia species isolated from lesional and non-lesional skin in patients with pityriasis versicolor. Mycoses 2007; 50(1):58–63.

2. B Androgenetic alopecia

Alopecia can be divided into scarring (destruction of the hair follicles) or non-scarring (preservation of the hair follicles) as shown in **Table 4.1**.

Options A and B are both causes of non-scarring alopecia, but androgenetic alopecia (i.e. male pattern baldness) is the most common cause in males so option B is the

Table 4.1	
Scarring	**Non-scarring**
Hereditary – ichthyosis	Androgenetic alopecia
Bacterial – tuberculosis, syphilis	Alopecia areata
Injury – burns, radiotherapy	Endocrine – hypopituitary, hypopara-thyroidism, hyper- and hypothyroidism, pregnancy
Fungal – tinea capitis causing a kerion	
Lichen planus	Drugs – heparin, OCP, carbimazole, reti-noids, lithium, cytotoxic agents, thiouracil
Discoid lupus	
Morphoea	Nutritional – iron and zinc deficiency
Trauma	Chronic illness
	Trichotillomania
	Telogen effluvium
OCP, oral contraceptive pill.	

Table 4.1 Causes of hair loss.

most likely. It tends to cause baldness in a well-defined pattern, beginning just above both temples with thinning of the crown of the head. Alopecia areata is an autoimmune condition causing localized well-defined patches of hair loss, whose edges may contain the characteristic 'exclamation-mark' hairs (hairs that become narrower closer to the base).

Goldstein B, Goldstein A. Nonscarring hair loss. In: Basow DS (ed), UpToDate. Waltham, MA: UpToDate, 2011. http://www.uptodate.com (Last accessed 1 May 2012).

3. B Raynaud's phenomenon

This woman presents with localised scleroderma known as morphoea. It tends to occur in young adults (more in females), consists of indurated plaques of sclerotic skin that can become hypo- or hyperpigmented, and may be associated with other autoimmune conditions like primary biliary cirrhosis (PBC), systemic lupus erythematosus (SLE), type I diabetes mellitus and vitiligo. In some cases, it may improve spontaneously but topical or intralesional steroids, vitamin D analogues, immunomodulators like methotrexate or tacrolimus and UVA light therapy have been used. In its extensive form, it can be differentiated from systemic sclerosis by the lack of systemic features, non-association with Raynaud's phenomenon and lack of hand signs.

Fett N, Werth VP. Update on morphea: part I. Epidemiology, clinical presentation, and pathogenesis. J Am Acad Dermatol 2011;64(2):217–228.

4. E Potassium hydroxide (KOH) test

The potassium hydroxide test involves placing a nail sample on a slide with KOH and dissolving the skin and nail cells with gentle heating until the fungal cells are left. These can then be seen on light microscopy. 91% of positive tests are detected by this KOH (and fungal microscopy) test, which provides the most rapid diagnosis. Blood cultures should be taken if the patient spikes a temperature but yield is low. C-reactive protein is an acute phase reactant and may be elevated in any infection. X-rays of the feet will not be diagnostic. Fungal culture may be diagnostic, but can take 4–6 weeks so are less useful in the acute period. Dermatophytes, like *Trichophyton rubrum*, account for 90% of cases.

Health Protection Agency (HPA). Fungal skin & nail infections: diagnosis & laboratory investigation: quick reference guide for primary care. Health Protection Agency; 2009.

5. D Necrolytic migratory erythema and insulinoma

Necrolytic migratory erythema is a red blistering rash that spreads across the skin. Commonly affected areas are the limbs and face around the lips but can also affect the lower abdomen, buttocks, perineum and groin. It is associated with pancreatic glucagonomas (as opposed to insulinomas), chronic liver disease and intestinal malabsorption. All the other options are correctly paired.

Thiers BH, Sahn RE, Callen JP. Cutaneous manifestations of internal malignancy. CA Cancer J Clin 2009; 59(2):73–98.

6. B Eczema

This man has erythroderma, which is a confluent scaling erythematous dermatitis that involves more than 90% of a patient's skin. The most common causes of erythroderma can be remembered by the mnemonic **DESCALP**.

Drugs- arsenic, barbiturates, gold salts, mercury, penicillins
Eczema – most common
Seborrhoeic dermatitis
Contact dermatitis
Atopic dermatitis
Lichen planus/**L**eukaemia/**L**ymphoma
Psoriasis/**P**ityriasis rubra pilaris

Roujeau JC, Stern RS. Severe adverse cutaneous reactions to drugs. N Engl J Med 1994; 331(19):1272.

7. E Pyoderma gangrenosum

The appearance of this man's rash on a line of trauma suggests the Koebner phenomenon. This is seen in psoriasis, lichen planus, viral warts, vitiligo, Darier's disease (keratosis follicularis), lichen sclerosus, molluscum contagiosum and pityriasis rubra pilaris.

A similar response is pathergy, whereby minor trauma causes skin lesions or ulcers that may be resistant to healing. This cutaneous phenomenon is seen in pyoderma gangrenosum and Behçet's disease.

Sagi L, Trau H. The Koebner phenomenon. Clin Dermatol 2011; 29(2):231-236.

8. B Chest X-ray

Erythema nodosum is an inflammation of subcutaneous fat (panniculitis), which usually presents as hot tender erythematous smooth nodules on both shins (although they can be found on forearms or thighs). It can be accompanied by fever, malaise and arthralgia. Lesions tend to heal without scarring in 3–6 weeks and the most important management is to treat the underlying cause, although bed rest and non-steroidal anti-inflammatory drugs (NSAIDS) are useful.

Causes of erythema nodosum can be remembered by the mnemonic **DIPSOUT**:

Drugs – sulphonamides, omeprazole, isotretinoin, monteleukast
Infection – streptococcal infection
Pregnancy
Sarcoidosis
Oral contraceptive pill
Ulcerative colitis
Tuberculosis

Chest X-ray is the most useful investigation, in the first instance, to rule out important causes like sarcoidosis and tuberculosis. A study showed that the best predictive factors for erythema nodosum included an abnormal result on a chest radiograph, a previous history of non-streptococcal upper respiratory tract infection, and a significant change in anti-streptolysin O titre (ASOT) in 2 consecutive determinations performed in a 2–4-week interval. ASOT and throat swabs can be done to look for streptococcal throat infection, which is the most common cause, but their use is limited in the initial stages as they will take a few days to come back. A stool culture is relevant if she complained of diarrhoea to look for *Salmonella* or *Campylobacter*. A Mantoux test is useful to exclude tuberculosis.

García-Porrúa C, et al. Erythema nodosum: etiologic and predictive factors in a defined population. Arthritis Rheum 2000; 43(3):584.

9. D Pulse 130 beats per minute

The **SCORTEN** scale (**SCOR**e for **T**oxic **E**pidermal **N**ecrolysis [TEN]) is a severity of illness scale used to predict the mortality rate for a patient with TEN. There are 7 independent risk factors that each score 1, giving a maximum score of 7.

1. Age > 40 years
2. Associated malignancy
3. Heart rate > 120 beats per minute
4. Urea > 10 mmol/L
5. Involved body surface > 10%
6. Bicarbonate < 20 mmol/L
7. Glucose > 14 mmol/L

Although the score was designed for TEN, it can be used in other disorders that compromise the integrity of the skin/mucosa such as burns or Stevens–Johnson syndrome. The higher the number of risk factors, the greater the mortality rate as shown in **Table 4.2**.

Bastuji-Garin S, Fouchard N, Bertocchi M, et al. SCORTEN: a severity-of-illness score for toxic epidermal necrolysis. J Invest Dermatol 2000;149–153.

Table 4.2	
No of risk factors	**Mortality rate (%)**
0–1	3.2
2	12.1
3	35.3
4	58.3
≥ 5	90

Table 4.2 Mortality rate for toxic epidermal necrolysis.

10. D Immunofluorescence of IgG and C3 at the dermoepidermal junction

This man is suffering from bullous pemphigoid, which is an autoimmune blistering condition that is more commonly seen in elderly patients.

Table 4.3 shows the differential diagnosis of bullous eruptions.

Nousari HC, Anhalt GJ. Pemphigus and bullous pemphigoid. Lancet 1999; 21; 354(9179):667-672

Table 4.3

	Clinical features	Histology
Bullous pemphigoid	Autoimmune blistering condition, manifesting as tense blisters on the limbs, trunk and flexures (rarely affecting mucosal surfaces) that is more commonly seen in elderly patients	Immunofluorescence of IgG and C3 at the dermoepidermal junction
Pemphigus vulgaris	Autoimmune blistering condition with flaccid tender (but not usually itchy) lesions (including mucosa) that easily rupture with ulceration	Acantholysis (separation of keratinocytes) Immunofluorescence of IgG directed against intercellular desmosomes
Dermatitis herpetiformis	Autoimmune condition characterised by itchy vesicular lesions in extensor areas (commonly with coeliac disease)	Immunofluorescence of IgA in a granular pattern in the upper dermis
Epidermolysis bullosa	Group of more than 23 inherited disorders involving the formation of blisters following trivial trauma	Depends on type of epidermolysis bullosa, e.g. in epidermolysis bullosa acquisita, there are anchoring fibril structures that are located at the dermoepidermal junction

Table 4.3 Causes of bullous eruptions.

11. E Permethrin 5%

This man has scabies. It is caused by *Sarcoptes scabiei* (a mite that lays its eggs into the stratum corneum) and is spread by prolonged contact. There is a delayed type IV hypersensitivity reaction to mites/eggs which occurs about 30 days after the initial infection and this causes the intense widespread pruritus, which tends to occur along the fingers, in the interdigital webspaces and flexor aspects of the wrists. The rash tends to be worse at night and in warmth.

Management involves:

- Advice on general measures to prevent spread:
  - Avoid close physical contact until treatment complete
  - All household and close contacts should be treated at the same time even if asymptomatic
  - Launder all bedding, clothes and towels on the first day of treatment to get rid of the mites
- Drugs
  - Permethrin 5% is first line treatment and is applied to the entire skin including scalp. It is left for 12 hours and then re-applied 7 days later
  - Malathion 0.5% is second line treatment

- Ivermectin may be used orally and is the treatment of choice for crusted scabies, and is often used in combination with a topical agent
- Benzoyl benzoate and lindane are other preparations that may be useful

It is important to tell the patient that the pruritus persists for up to 4–6 weeks post eradication.

Strong M, Johnstone PW, Strong, M (Eds). Interventions for treating scabies. Cochrane Database Syst Rev 2007 (3): CD000320.

12. B Eczema

Skin conditions that are aggravated by sunlight can be remembered by the mnemonic **DR XL CHAMPS**

Dermatomyositis/**D**arier's disease/**D**rugs (see Q4.13)
Rosacea

Xeroderma pigmentosum
Lupus erythematosus

Carcinoid syndrome
Herpes simplex infection
Albinism
Melasma (dark, irregular well demarcated hyperpigmented macules to patches that occur in women during pregnancy or when they are on the oral contraceptive pill)
Pellagra/**P**olymorphic light eruption/**P**orphyrias (except acute intermittent type)
Solar urticaria

Eczema is not usually photosensitive.

Elmets C. Photosensitivity disorders (photodermatoses): Clinical manifestations, diagnosis, and treatment. In: Basow DS (ed), UpToDate. Waltham, MA: UpToDate, 2011. http://www.uptodate.com (Last accessed 1 May 2012).

13. B Ciprofloxacin

Drugs causing photosensitivity can be remembered by the mnemonic **POSTCARD:**

Psoralens/**P**iroxicam
Oral contraceptive pill
Sulphonylureas/**S**ulphonamides
Tetracycline
Ciprofloxacin
Amiodarone/**A**nti-fungals, e.g. griseofulvin/**A**ntimalarials, e.g. quinine
Retinoids
Diuretics (loop and thiazide)

Amoxicillin, clarithromycin, gentamicin and metronidazole do not usually cause photosensitivity.

Morison WL. Solar urticaria due to progesterone compounds in oral contraceptives. Photodermatol Photoimmunol Photomed 2003; 19(3):155–156.

14. E Stop smoking

Female smokers have a threefold increased risk of psoriasis and heavy smokers have more severe disease (the effect greater in women compared to men). Although alcohol and stress can also exacerbate psoriasis, the effect of smoking is greater. It is unclear whether exercise or weight loss will confer reduced risk of psoriasis severity.

Fortes C, et al. Relationship between smoking and the clinical severity of psoriasis. Arch Dermatol 2005; 141(12):1580–1584.

15. E Lichen planus

The most common presentation of oral lichen planus is the reticular form, which manifests as adherent white lace-like bands across the buccal mucosa (known as Wickham's striae) or smaller papules. The lesions are usually bilateral and asymptomatic, and may involve the gingiva, tongue, palate and lips. Candidiasis tends to be easily rubbed off. Chemical burns, e.g. phosphorous, although painless, are associated with ulceration and sloughing. Aphthous ulcers tend to be painful. Leukoplakia is a diagnosis of exclusion – it presents as painless white well-defined patches that cannot be easily rubbed off. It has been described as being precancerous so a biopsy should be carried out and is associated with smoking and alcohol consumption.

Ingafou M, et al. Oral lichen planus: a retrospective study of 690 British patients. Oral Dis 2006; 12(5):463.

16. A Acyclovir

This patient has a localised herpes simplex virus infection that should be treated with aciclovir. The Tzanck test involves scraping of an ulcer base and direct smear to look for multinucleated giant cells called Tzanck cells. These can be found in herpes simplex virus (HSV), varicella zoster virus (VZV), cytomegalovirus (CMV) and pemphigus vulgaris. The likeliest cause in this case is HSV over the others because of localisation to one site and the fact that the lesions are perioral.

The important differential of a perioral vesicular rash to consider is impetigo caused by *Staphylococcus aureus* or group A beta-haemolytic *Streptococcus*, although this tends to present in young children and the vesicles rupture forming honey-coloured crusts. Limited disease should be treated with topical fusidic acid first line and topical mupirocin second line. More extensive disease should be treated with oral flucloxacillin or erythromycin (if penicillin allergic).

Fatahzadeh M. Human herpes simplex virus infections: epidemiology, pathogenesis, symptomatology, diagnosis, and management. J Am Acad Dermatol 2007; 57(5):737–763.

Chapter 5

Endocrinology

1. A 39-year-old man was admitted to the hospital suffering with a sickle cell crisis, affecting his left leg and right arm. His pain was treated with both oral and subcutaneous analgesia. After 48 hours his pain settled, but it was noticed that he was passing large volumes of urine (500 mL/h).

   What is the most likely diagnosis?

   A   Diabetes insipidus
   B   Diuresis secondary to analgesia
   C   Obstructive uropathy
   D   Psychogenic polydipsia
   E   Syndrome of inappropriate antidiuretic hormone (ADH) secretion

2. A 45-year-old woman, with known bipolar affective disorder, presented to her general practitioner complaining of increased urinary frequency and volume.

   Investigations:

   > Urine analysis:
   > protein +
   > nitrites –
   > leucocytes –

   What is the most likely cause of her polyuria?

   A   Carbamazepine
   B   Lithium
   C   Olanzapine
   D   Psychogenic polydipsia
   E   Urinary tract infection

3. A 32-year-old woman presented to her general practitioner complaining of double vision. She was taking the oral contraceptive pill. On examination, she had mild bilateral proptosis and dysconjugate eye movements.

   What is the most likely cause of her symptoms?

   A   Cavernous sinus thrombosis
   B   Graves' disease
   C   Hyperthyroidism
   D   Orbital cellulitis
   E   Orbital meningioma

4. A 68-year-old man was referred to the endocrinology clinic by his general practitioner because of difficult-to-control blood pressure. The patient mentioned that he had noticed his rings were becoming tighter and that he had seen his dentist recently because of difficulty chewing. Visual field testing revealed no deficit.

   What is the most appropriate initial treatment?

   A   Amlodipine
   B   Bromocriptine
   C   Furosemide
   D   Octreotide
   E   Transsphenoidal surgery

5. A 45-year-old woman, with known type 2 diabetes mellitus, presented to her general practitioner for her annual diabetic review. Her drug history included metformin 500 mg twice daily, aspirin 75 mg once daily and ramipril 5 mg once daily. She was having difficulty giving up smoking. Her haemoglobin A1c was 6.1%. On examination, there was no evidence of peripheral neuropathy. Her blood pressure was 135/72 mmHg.

   What is the most appropriate next step in management?

   A   Add in gliclazide 40 mg twice daily
   B   Increase metformin to 1 g twice daily
   C   Start clopidogrel 75 mg once daily
   D   Start simvastatin 40 mg once nightly
   E   Varenicline

6. A 57-year-old man presented to his general practitioner complaining of swelling of his breasts.

   Which drug is most likely to have caused this?

   A   Amitriptyline
   B   Furosemide
   C   Methyldopa
   D   Spironolactone
   E   Verapamil

7. A 21-year-old man presented to his general practitioner complaining of short stature and poor growth of facial hair. He also mentioned that he had difficulty smelling things.

   What is the most likely diagnosis?

   A   Cushing's disease
   B   Kallmann's syndrome
   C   Klinefelter's syndrome
   D   Mumps
   E   Testicular feminisation syndrome

8. A 17-year-old girl presented to her general practitioner as she had not yet started menstruating. She had otherwise gone through puberty with no significant problems and breast development was normal.

   On examination, there were bilateral groin masses, with scanty pubic hair, but nil else of note.

   What is the most likely diagnosis?

   A   Complete androgen insensitivity syndrome
   B   Congenital adrenal hyperplasia
   C   Ovarian tumour
   D   Polycystic ovaries
   E   Turner's syndrome

9. A 29-year-old man and his wife presented to their general practitioner because she was not pregnant despite a year of trying. On examination, he was tall, with scanty pubic hair and gynaecomastia.

   What is the most likely cause of infertility?

   A   Congenital adrenal hyperplasia
   B   Cushing's syndrome
   C   Hypogonadotrophic hypogonadism
   D   Kallmann's syndrome
   E   Klinefelter's syndrome

10. A 32-year-old man presented to his general practitioner for a routine review. He was found to be hypertensive.

    Investigations:

sodium	136 mmol/L (137–144)
potassium	3.1 mmol/L (3.5–4.9)
creatinine	87 μmol/L (60–110)

    What is the most likely underlying diagnosis?

    A   Benign essential hypertension
    B   Bartter's syndrome
    C   Gittleman's syndrome
    D   Liddle's syndrome
    E   Renal tubular acidosis

11. A 36-year-old woman presented to the emergency department with a history of nausea and vomiting. She was known to suffer from hypothyroidism and was on thyroxine. On examination, her temperature was 38.2°C with blood pressure 92/47 mmHg and pulse 145 beats per minute.

    What is the most appropriate next step in management?

    A   Ciprofloxacin
    B   Hydrocortisone

    C   Prednisolone
    D   Propranolol
    E   Thyroxine

12. A 58-year-old man, a lorry driver, presented to his general practitioner complaining of polydipsia. His body mass index was 32.

Investigations:

glucose	22 mmol/L (3–6 fasting)
creatinine	95 µmol/L (60–110)
bicarbonate	23 mmol/L (20–28)
total cholesterol	7.4 mmol/L (< 5.2)
urinalysis	glucose +

What is the most appropriate management?

    A   Diet and lifestyle advice
    B   Gliclazide
    C   Insulin therapy
    D   Metformin
    E   No treatment currently and repeat blood tests in 3 weeks time

13. A 42-year-old woman presented to her general practitioner complaining of a tender neck. Two weeks ago she had been unwell with an upper respiratory tract infection. On examination, there was a palpable tender goitre.

Investigations:

thyroid-stimulating hormone (TSH)	< 0.4 mIU/L (0.4–4.5)
free T4	> 75 pmol/L (10–22)

What would be the most likely finding on radioiodine scanning?

    A   Diffuse increased uptake
    B   Diffuse reduced uptake
    C   Multiple nodules with increased uptake
    D   Normal scan
    E   Single toxic nodule

14. A 19-year-old woman presented to her general practitioner with a history of weight gain, amenorrhoea and increased growth of facial hair. Her blood pressure was 157/85 mmHg.

What is the most useful initial diagnostic test?

    A   24-hour urinary cortisol
    B   Dexamethasone suppression test
    C   Luteinising hormone (LH)/follicle stimulating hormone (FSH) ratio
    D   Pelvic ultrasound scan
    E   Petronasal sinus sampling

15. A 38-year-old woman presented to her general practitioner complaining of feeling tired all the time. Thyroid tests were performed:

Investigations:

| thyroid-stimulating hormone | < 0.4 mIU/L (0.4–4.5) |
| free T4 | 19 pmol/L (10–22) |

What would be the most likely complication if the patient were left untreated?

A Bradycardia
B Macrocytic anaemia
C Menorrhagia
D Osteoporosis
E Weight gain

16. A 35-year-old man presented to his general practitioner asking for advice on how to lose weight. He was obese with a body mass index of 34. His blood pressure was 138/72 mmHg.

Investigations:

triglyceride	1.9 mmol/L (0.45–1.69)
fasting glucose	6.6 mmol/L (3–6)
glucose 2 hours post 75 g oral glucose load	7.6 mmol/L (<7.8)

What is the most likely diagnosis?

A Benign essential hypertension
B Impaired fasting glucose
C Impaired glucose tolerance
D Type 2 diabetes mellitus
E Metabolic syndrome

17. A 16-year-old girl was brought to the emergency department as she felt dizzy and had collapsed at school. A point of care capillary blood glucose test performed by the ambulance crew showed blood glucose of 1.4 mmol/L (3–6 fasting). She had no significant past medical history. Her mother had vitiligo and her father had type 2 diabetes mellitus. On arrival at emergency department her blood tests showed:

Investigations:

plasma glucose	3.8 mmol/L (3–6 fasting)
insulin	12 mg/mL (6–10)
C-peptide	0.12 nmol/L (0.2–0.4)

What is the most likely reason for the patient's collapse?

A Hypotensive episode
B Insulin abuse
C Insulinoma
D Type 1 diabetes mellitus

    E   Type 2 diabetes mellitus

18. A 48-year-old man presented to his general practitioner complaining of new onset galactorrhoea. He had no other past medical history and did not take any regularly prescribed medications. He mentioned that he had recently had an episode of food poisoning for which he used some over the counter medications to control his symptoms, and felt that he had put on some weight over the past few months.

    His blood pressure was 128/63 mmHg. What is the most likely cause of his galactorrhoea?

    A   Acromegaly
    B   Bromocriptine
    C   Cyclizine
    D   Metoclopramide
    E   Undiagnosed hyperthyroidism

19. A 28-year-old woman presented to her general practitioner with difficulty conceiving. She had a history of polycystic ovarian syndrome (PCOS).

    What is the most appropriate initial treatment?

    A   Clomifene
    B   In vitro fertilisation (IVF)
    C   Metformin
    D   Oral contraceptive pill
    E   Weight loss

20. A 20-year-old woman presented to emergency department following sudden onset of palpitations. She also complained of headache. On examination, she was clammy to touch, pulse 110 beats per minute and blood pressure 210/108 mmHg. ECG showed a sinus tachycardia.

    What is the most useful diagnostic investigation?

    A   Dexamethasone suppression test
    B   Short synacthen test
    C   Thyroid function tests
    D   Urinary catecholamines
    E   Urinary cortisol

21. A 57-year-old man was reviewed by his general practitioner. He had been under investigation for a 6-month history of diarrhoea. He had undergone a colonoscopy, which was normal. Multiple stool samples had been sent to the laboratory for microscopy, culture and sensitivity and were all negative. He continued to open his bowels up to 20 times per day. Three months ago he was diagnosed with asthma and had been started on a salbutamol inhaler. He did not feel this was helping with his breathlessness. He also complained of facial flushing, which he thought might be due to the inhaler, as he had noticed this had started to occur at around the same time this was prescribed.

What is the most useful diagnostic investigation?

A   Allergy testing
B   Further sample for faecal microscopy, culture and sensitivity (M, C&S) and ova, cysts and parasites
C   Platelet serotonin levels
D   Urinary catecholamines
E   Urinary 5-hydroxyindoleacetic acid (5-HIAA)

22. A 34-year-old woman presented to her general practitioner with 6 months history of absent periods. She was not pregnant as confirmed by urine test. Prior to this, she had regular menses every 25–27 days.

Investigations:

thyroid-stimulating hormone	3.5 mIU/L (0.4–4.5)
free T4	19 pmol/L (10–22)
prolactin	3 ng/mL (0–10)
follicle stimulating hormone	45 IU/L (0–20)
oestradiol	18 pg/mL (30–400 premenopausal)

What is the most likely underlying cause of her amenorrhea?

A   Excessive exercise
B   Hyperprolactinaemia
C   Hyperthyroidism
D   Polycystic ovarian syndrome (PCOS)
E   Primary ovarian failure

23. A 68-year-old woman was admitted to hospital with renal colic. Her past medical history included previous transsphenoidal surgery for a pituitary tumour.

Investigations:

corrected calcium	3.2 mmol/L (2.2–2.6)
parathyroid hormone	5.9 pmol/l (0.9–5.4)
CT KUB:	renal stone in the right ureter.

What is the most likely underlying diagnosis?

A   Breast cancer
B   Dehydration
C   Multiple endocrine neoplasia (MEN) type 1
D   MEN type 2
E   Primary hyperparathyroidism

24. A 35-year-old man was newly diagnosed with type 2 diabetes. His fasting blood glucose at diagnosis was 13.7 mmol/L (3–6 fasting). He had no other past medical history, but his father had suffered a myocardial infarction at the age of 74 years. He was obese with a body mass index of 32, and had poor renal function with a creatinine of 160 μmol/L (60–110).

What is the most important factor in selecting his diabetic therapy?

A   Ability to achieve and maintain glycaemic control
B   Cardiac history
C   Fasting glucose at diagnosis
D   Patient weight
E   Renal function

25. What is the most common type of thyroid cancer?

A   Anaplastic
B   Follicular
C   Lymphoma
D   Medullary
E   Papillary

26. A 17-year-old girl was asked to attend her general practitioner as recent blood tests had shown low calcium with a parathyroid hormone (PTH) level of 9.2 pmol/L (0.9–5.4). On examination, she was noted to be quite short in stature and had shortened 4th and 5th metacarpals.

What is the underlying diagnosis?

A   Primary hyperparathyroidism
B   Primary hypoparathyroidism
C   Pseudohypoparathyroidism
D   Pseudopseudohypoparathyroidism
E   Secondary hyperparathyroidism

27. A 52-year-old man attended his general practitioner complaining of frequent muscle cramps and lethargy. Clinical examination was unremarkable and his blood pressure was 152/85 mmHg.

Investigations:

potassium	2.9 mmol/L (3.5–4.9)
pH	7.49 (7.35–7.45)
bicarbonate	34 mmol/L (20–28)
corrected calcium	2.32 mmol/L (2.2–2.6)

What is the most useful diagnostic investigation?

A   CT abdomen
B   Dexamethasone suppression test
C   Renin: aldosterone ratio
D   Short synacthen test
E   24 hour urinary cortisol

28. A 27-year-old woman attended the endocrinology clinic for monitoring of her treatment for hypothyroidism. She took thyroxine 75 µg daily. Blood tests taken on the morning of the clinic show:

Investigations:

| thyroid-stimulating hormone | 9 mU/L (0.4–5.0) |
| total T4 | 120 nmol/L (58–174) |

What is the most appropriate next step in management?

A   Decrease thyroxine to 50 µg/day
B   Education regarding her diagnosis and treatment
C   Increase thyroxine to 150 µg/day
D   No change required
E   Stop the thyroxine

29. A 17-year-old girl attended her general practitioner as she was concerned, she had not yet started menstruating. She commented that she had developed pubic and underarm hair earlier than her friends at school. On examination, she was noted to have clitoromegaly and hirsutism.

What is the most likely underlying diagnosis?

A   Congenital adrenal hyperplasia
B   Cushing's syndrome
C   Excessive exercise
D   Polycystic ovarian syndrome
E   Turner's syndrome

30. A 33-year-old woman was admitted to the emergency department with a fever and confusion. She was unable to give a history, but a packet of carbimazole is located in her handbag. She had a temperature of 38.8°C, blood pressure 175/42 mmHg and pulse 152 beats per minute. Heart sounds were normal, and there were bilateral basal crackles on auscultation of her chest. There was no skin rash.

Investigations:

chest X-ray:	cardiomegaly
urine analysis:	negative
haemoglobin	12.1 g/dL (11.5–16.5 females)
white cell count	11.3×10^9/L (4–11)
platelets	235×10^9/L (150–400)
bilirubin	27 µmol/L (1–22)
alanine aminotransferase	52 U/L (5–35)
alkaline phosphatase	62 U/L (45–105)
paracetamol level	< 10 mg/L

What is the most likely cause?

A   Anxiety disorder
B   Carbimazole side effects
C   Sepsis
D   Paracetamol overdose
E   Thyroid storm

Answers

1. A Diabetes insipidus

Patients with sickle cell disease are at risk of infarcts, particularly during a crisis. In this case, the patient most likely has developed a pituitary infarct as a result of his crisis. This results in impaired secretion of antidiuretic hormone (ADH) and an inability to concentrate urine (craniogenic diabetes insipidus). The patient therefore produces a large volume of dilute urine, and compensates by increasing his oral intake. The normal ADH pathway is outlined in **Figure 5.1**. Diagnosis is by a water deprivation test, and treatment is with desmopressin (a synthetic version of ADH).

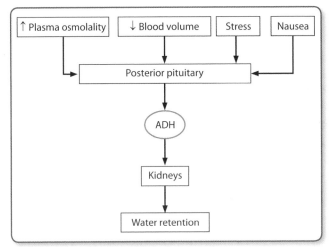

Figure 5.1 ADH pathway. In craniogenic diabetes insipidus antidiuretic hormone (ADH) is not produced by the posterior pituitary and so downstream regulation of water retention does not occur.

Syndrome of inappropriate ADH secretion (SIADH) is the opposite of diabetes insipidus, where the patient overproduces ADH, and produces concentrated urine of small volume.

Sickle cell anaemia is associated with type 1 renal tubular acidosis (distal), which can lead to abnormal build-up of calcium deposits, and therefore risk of stone formation and obstructive uropathy. For this to be the underlying cause of the polyuria, it would be expected that the patient would continue to be in pain, typically in the distribution of flank to groin.

Opiate analgesia is used to treat sickle cell crisis. This has many side effects, but does not normally cause polyuria. Urinary retention is a known side effect of opiate analgesia.

Water deprivation testing (**Table 5.1**) is used to determine the cause of polydipsia/polyuria. The patient is deprived of water and hourly urine, and plasma osmolality are measured. An injection of desmopressin acetate (DDAVP) (synthetic ADH analogue) is given when the patient has lost 3% of their body weight, and urine osmolality is re-checked.

Table 5.1				
	Initial plasma osmolality	Final urine osmolality (osmol/kg)	Urine osmolality post DDAVP (osmol/kg)	Final plasma ADH
Normal	Normal	> 600	> 600	High
Craniogenic DI	High	< 300	> 600	Low
Nephrogenic DI	High	< 300	< 300	High
Primary polydipsia	Low	300–400	400	Moderate
ADH, antidiuretic hormone; DDAVP, desmopressin acetate; DI, diabetes insipidus.				

Table 5.1 Interpretation of water deprivation testing.

2. B Lithium

This patient is suffering from nephrogenic polydipsia caused by lithium.

Diabetes insipidus can be either cranial (caused by a reduced secretion of ADH) or nephrogenic (reduced action of ADH).

Causes of cranial diabetes insipidus:

- Idiopathic
- Familial
- Craniopharyngioma
- Hypothalamic infiltration (sarcoidosis, histiocytosis X)
- Pituitary surgery
- Trauma

Causes of nephrogenic diabetes insipidus:

- Hypercalcaemia
- Hypokalaemia
- Renal disease
- Sarcoidosis
- Drugs (lithium, demeclocycline, amphotericin, glibenclamide)

3. B Graves' disease

The most likely cause of bilateral proptosis is Graves' disease. Eye signs in Graves' disease include:

- Proptosis
- Lid retraction and lid lag
- Periorbital puffiness
- Ophthalmoplegia: double vision usually maximal on upwards and outwards gaze

Graves' disease can also cause unilateral proptosis. Other causes of unilateral proptosis include:

- Wegner's granulomatosis
- Orbital tumours
- Cavernous haemangioma
- Orbital cellulitis
- Lymphoma

A patient can be hyperthyroid, hypothyroid or euthyroid when they develop eye signs in Graves' disease, and may present before any thyroid problem has been identified.

4. E Transsphenoidal surgery

This gentleman has acromegaly. Acromegaly is caused by a growth hormone-secreting pituitary tumour in the majority of cases. Rarely, it is secondary to ectopic growth hormone-releasing hormone (GHRH) secretion. Symptoms include:

- Difficult to control hypertension
- Increase in size of feet and hands
- Prognathism – the bottom jaw protrudes in front of the upper jaw
- Doughy palms
- Enlarged testes
- Carpal tunnel syndrome
- Bitemporal hemianopia
- Increased sweating

It is diagnosed by a failure of growth hormone to suppress to less than 2 mU/L at any time during a standard (75 g) oral glucose tolerance test.

Other features of acromegaly include:

- Cardiomyopathy
- Diabetes
- Raised triglycerides and phosphates
- Pseudogout
- Occurrence of colonic polyps and neoplasia

First-line treatment is transsphenoidal surgery. The cure rate is 40–70% and depends on the initial size of the tumour. Other treatments include octreotide (a somatostatin analogue) and bromocriptine (a dopamine receptor agonist).

Shlomo Melmed, MB et al. Acromegaly N Engl J Med 2006; 355:2558–2573.

5. D Start simvastatin 40 mg once nightly

Any patient over the age of 40 years with type 2 diabetes mellitus should be offered statin therapy if they have other identifiable cardiovascular risk factors such as hypertension, hyperlipidaemia or smoking.

As the patient's HbA1c implies good diabetic control there is no need to change her diabetic medications. She is already taking aspirin at the recommended dose and there is no indication that a further antiplatelet agent is required.

Varenicline is a prescription only anti-smoking agent. It binds to nicotine receptors in the brain, reducing nicotine craving. If the patient has a clear desire to stop smoking, she could be referred to a stop smoking clinic where the most appropriate treatment will be determined.

Haffner SM, et al. Mortality from coronary heart disease in subjects with type 2 diabetes and in nondiabetic subjects with or without prior myocardial infarction. N Engl J Med 1998; 339(4):229–234.

6. D Spironolactone

This man has gynaecomastia. This is an increased in male breast tissue secondary to an increase in the oestrogen:androgen ratio. Causes include:

- Physiological – in puberty
- Testicular failure
- Testicular cancer
- Liver disease
- Hyperthyroidism
- Androgen deficiency – Kallmann's and Klinefelter's syndromes
- Drugs – anabolic steroids, cannabis , cimetidine, digoxin, finasteride, gonadorelin analogues, oestrogens, spironolactone

7. B Kallmann's syndrome

Kallmann's syndrome is an inherited form of hypogonadotrophic hypogonadism. Features include:

- Poor sense of smell
- Poor facial and axially hair growth
- Short stature
- Infertility

Treatment is with hormone replacement therapy.

AACE Thyroid Task Force. AACE Hypogonadism Guidelines. Endocr Pract 2002; 8(6):441.
Styne DM, Grumbach. Puberty: Ontogeny, neuroendocrinology, physiology, and disorders (chapter 24) In: Kronenberg HM, et al (eds). Williams Textbook of Endocrinology 11th edition. Saunders Elsevier; 2008.

8. A Complete androgen insensitivity syndrome

Complete androgen insensitivity syndrome (formerly called testicular feminisation syndrome) results when a person, who is of XY genotype, is phenotypically female. It is an X-linked recessive disease, and it is caused by end organ insensitivity to androgens. Breast development results from conversion of excess testosterone into oestrogens, but development of other secondary sexual characteristics is poor. It often presents as primary amenorrhoea. The groin masses are testes present within the inguinal canal.

Treatment is with counselling and female hormone replacement, to allow the patient to be brought up as female.

Hughes IA, et al. Consensus statement on management of intersex disorders. Arch Dis Child 2006; 91(7):554.

9. E Klinefelter's syndrome

Klinefelter's syndrome occurs in approximately 1 in every 500–1000 male births. It is caused by an XXY genotype. Features include:

- Tall stature
- Small firm testes
- Infertility
- Poor secondary sexual characteristic development
- Gynaecomastia

Diagnosis is by karyotyping and testosterone treatment may be of benefit; however it is unlikely to restore fertility.

Amory JK, et al. Klinefelter's syndrome. Lancet 2000; 356(9226):333–335.

10. D Liddle's syndrome

Liddle's syndrome is an autosomal dominant inherited disorder that mimics hyperaldosteronism. It is associated with hypertension and hypokalaemia. Other causes of hypokalaemia and hypertension include:

- Cushing's syndrome/Cushing's disease
- Conn's syndrome
- 11β-Hydroxylase deficiency

Causes of hypokalaemia with a normal blood pressure include:

- Bartter's syndrome (AR – defective Na-K-2Cl co-transporter in the ascending loop of Henlé)
- Diuretic therapy
- Gittlemann's syndrome (defect in thiazide sensitive NaCl transporter in the distal convoluted tubule)
- Gastrointestinal loss
- Renal tubular acidosis types 1 and 2

11. B Hydrocortisone

This patient has presented with an addisonian crisis. Symptoms include weakness, nausea and vomiting, collapse and pyrexia. Patients typically suffer from other autoimmune conditions. Associated signs include vitiligo and hyperpigmentation, especially in sun-exposed areas and areas exposed to constant friction or pressure. Initial treatment is with intravenous hydrocortisone, as this is rapid acting.

- Primary causes:
  - Antiphospholipid syndrome
  - HIV
  - Metastatic disease
  - Tuberculosis
  - Waterhouse–Friderichsen syndrome
- Secondary causes:
  - Pituitary disorders
  - Exogenous glucocorticoid therapy

Hahner S, Allolio B. Management of adrenal insufficiency in different clinical settings. Expert Opin Pharmacother 2005; 6(14):2407–2417.

12. D Metformin

This man has type 2 diabetes. Diagnosis is either by fasting plasma glucose greater than 7.0 mmol/L, or glucose 11.1 mmol/L or greater 2 hours after a 75 g oral glucose load. In a patient with classic symptoms (polydipsia, polyuria) a diagnosis based on an elevated plasma glucose becomes more straightforward.

Metformin is a biguanide and acts by increasing insulin sensitivity and reducing hepatic gluconeogenesis. It is not associated with hypoglycaemia or weight gain, and as such is often the first line choice when treating type 2 diabetes. It is contraindicated in renal failure, and thus should be used with caution in patients with creatinine greater than 130 µmol/L. It is not recommended for use in patient with creatinine greater than 150 µmol/L. It is rarely associated with lactic acidosis.

As this man is a lorry driver, it is likely that he will not be keen to start insulin therapy (in the UK, driving regulations mean that new applicants on insulin or existing drivers are barred by law from driving heavy goods vehicles).

Gerstein HC, Haynes RB (Eds). Evidence-based diabetes care. Ontario: BC Decker, 2001.

13. B Diffuse reduced uptake

This patient has subacute thyroiditis, which typically presents as a tender goitre following a recent viral infection. Blood tests reveal hyperthyroidism, with suppressed thyroid-stimulating hormone and elevated Free T4, and there is diffuse reduced uptake on radi-iodine scanning. The disease is usually self-limiting.

14. B Dexamethasone suppression test

This patient most likely has Cushing's syndrome. Symptoms include:

- Weight gain
- Hirsutism
- Depression
- Amenorrhoea
- Hypertension
- Bruising
- Proximal weakness
- Acne

Both dexamethasone suppression testing and 24 hours urinary free cortisol are used for initial diagnosis, but a suppression test is most sensitive. Once a failure to suppress cortisol production with dexamethasone administration has been identified, adrenocorticotropic hormone (ACTH) levels can be measured to determine if the cause is adrenal (low ACTH) or pituitary/ectopic (high ACTH).

High dose dexamethasone suppression tests are used to differentiate between pituitary and ectopic ACTH production – if the source is pituitary, high-dose dexamethasone will usually suppress cortisol production. Petronasal sinus sampling may be required to differentiate between ectopic and pituitary sources.

Polycystic ovarian syndrome may also present with amenorrhoea and hirsutism, but would not cause hypertension.

15. D Osteoporosis

This patient has subclinical hyperthyroidism, identified by the low thyroid-stimulating hormone (TSH) with free T4 within the normal range. Untreated, complications associated with hyperthyroidism may occur. These include:

- Weight loss
- Amenorrhoea
- Atrial fibrillation
- Tremor
- Microcytic anaemia
- Proximal myopathy
- Osteoporosis
- Heat intolerance

16. E Metabolic syndrome

This patient meets the criteria for metabolic syndrome. The 2006 International Diabetes Federation guidelines state that a diagnosis can be made if a patient suffers with central obesity and any two of:

- Elevated triglycerides >1.7 mmol/L
- Low high-density lipoprotein (HDL) < 1.03 mmol/L in men and < 1.29 mmol/L in women
- Elevated blood pressure >130/85 mmHg
- Fasting plasma glucose >5.6 mmol/L

2006 guidelines from the World Health Organisation for fasting glucose levels state a diagnosis of diabetes can be made if fasting glucose is ≥7.0 mmol/L, or if random glucose is ≥11.1 mmol/L at 2 hours after a 75 g oral glucose tolerance test is identified.

Impaired glucose tolerance is identified when a fasting glucose is greater than or equal to 6.1 mmol/L but less than 7.0 mmol/L.

Impaired glucose tolerance can be diagnosed when fasting glucose is < 7.0 mmol/L but plasma glucose levels at 2 hours after an oral glucose tolerance test are greater than or equal to 7.8 mmol/L, but less than 11.1 mmol/L.

International Diabetes Federation: The IDF consensus worldwide definition of the metabolic syndrome. 2006. http://www.idf.org/webdata/docs/MetS_def_update2006.pdf (last accessed May 2012).

17. B Insulin abuse

Insulin abuse is identified by elevated insulin levels with a low C-peptide. The C-peptide is a by-product of insulin production. This patient has easy access to subcutaneous insulin because her father is a diabetic.

Insulinomas are pancreatic islet cell tumours that episodically secrete insulin, resulting in recurrent hypoglycaemic episodes. Diagnosis is by prolonged supervised fasting, and blood tests would show high insulin and high C-peptide levels. Treatment is surgical resection, but diazoxide and somatostatins can be used in patients who are not surgical candidates.

18. D Metoclopramide

Prolactin is secreted by the anterior pituitary. Dopamine is the main inhibitor of its release. Causes of elevated prolactin levels, and therefore galactorrhoea include:

- Prolactinoma
- Pregnancy
- Oestrogen therapy
- Stress
- Exercise
- Acromegaly
- Primary hypothyroidism
- Metoclopramide
- Domperidone
- Haloperidol
- Phenothiazines

Dopamine agonists, such as bromocriptine, can be used in the treatment of galactorrhoea. Acromegaly is unlikely to be the underlying cause in this case, as the patients blood pressure is normal.

19. E Weight loss

Polycystic ovarian syndrome (PCOS) is associated with obesity, acanthosis nigricans, oligomenorrhoea, hirsutism and subfertility. Blood tests show an elevated luteinising hormone (LH)/follicle-stimulating hormone (FSH) ratio, with insulin resistance and hyperinsulinaemia. Initial treatment for the symptoms of PCOS is weight loss. Weight loss reduces insulin and testosterone levels, and increases the chance of ovulation.

Medications used to manage PCOS include:

- Oral contraceptives: used where the patient requires contraception, and can help to establish a regular cycle.
- Metformin: used to combat insulin resistance and to promote fertility in women with PCOS; however a recent review by the Royal College of Obstetricians and Gynaecologists has suggested that metformin therapy is not first line for the management of PCOS.
- Clomiphene: a study by Legros et al. (2004) identified clomiphene as being superior to metformin in the management of infertility in women with PCOS.

Scientific Advisory Committee. Metformin Therapy for the Management of Infertility in Women with PCOS, Opinion Paper 13. Royal College of Obstetricians and Gynaecologists; 2008.
Legro RS, et al. Clomiphene, Metformin, or Both for Infertility in the Polycystic Ovary Syndrome. N Eng J Med 2007; 256:551–566.

20. D Urinary catecholamines

This patient most likely has a diagnosis of phaeochromocytoma. The triad of headache, palpitations and sweating are said to be 90% predictive.

Phaeochromocytomas are rare tumours of the adrenal medulla or ganglia of the sympathetic nervous system. They secrete adrenalin if they are located in the adrenal glands and noradrenalin/dopamine if they are extra-adrenal.

Diagnosis is by urinary catecholamine measurement, which has 87.5% sensitivity and 99.7% specificity.

The uses of the other tests are outlined in **Table 5.2**.

Table 5.2

Test	Diagnosis
Urinary catecholamines	Phaeochromocytoma
Thyroid function tests	Thyroid dysfunction
Dexamethasone suppression test	Cushing's syndrome
Urinary cortisol	Cushing's syndrome
Short synacthen test	Addison's disease

Table 5.2 Diagnostic tests.

21. E Urinary 5-hydroxyindoleacetic acid (5-HIAA)

This man has carcinoid syndrome. Carcinoid tumours arise from enterochromaffin cells of the intestinal mucosa. They secrete serotonin, which is usually metabolised by the liver, and so patients are often asymptomatic. If the tumour metastasises to the liver serotonin is secreted into the systemic circulation and carcinoid syndrome develops. This is characterised by:

- Facial flushing
- Diarrhoea
- Bronchospasm
- Tricuspid stenosis
- Pellagra
- Hypotension

Diagnosis is by urinary 5-HIAA levels (serotonin metabolite) and treatment includes surgical resection if there are no metastases. Hepatic metastases can be resected or embolised, and symptoms of the carcinoid syndrome can be controlled with somatostatin analogues such as octreotide.

Platelet serotonin levels can be measured in carcinoid, once treatment has commenced to evaluate the effect of therapy.

As multiple stool samples have already been sent to the laboratory, there is unlikely to be any benefit from sending further samples. Anaphylaxis is a differential diagnosis of carcinoid syndrome, and in patients who present with an anaphylaxis type picture, allergy testing would be important. However, in this case the symptoms have been going on for at least 6 months, so allergy testing would not be as useful a diagnostic test as urinary 5-HIAA. Urinary catecholamines are used in the diagnosis of phaeochromocytoma.

Bendelow J, et al. Carcinoid syndrome. Eur J Surg Oncol 2008;34(3):289–296.

22. E Primary ovarian failure

Causes of amenorrhoea can be primary (failure to start menses by age 16) or secondary (cessation of menses sometime after menstruation has commenced) and are outline in **Table 5.3**

Table 5.3

Primary	Secondary
Congenital adrenal hyperplasia	Hyperprolactinaemia
Congenital malformation of the genital tract	Hypothalamic amenorrhoea (stress/exercise induced)
Testicular feminisation syndrome	Premature ovarian failure
Turner's syndrome	Polycystic ovarian failure
	Thyrotoxicosis

Table 5.3 Causes of amenorrhoea.

The initial investigation that should be performed, is a pregnancy test (urinary or blood β-hCG).

In this case, the pregnancy test is negative, and the elevated follicle-stimulating hormone (FSH) level suggests that the amenorrhoea is secondary to premature ovarian failure. This is accompanied by a low oestrogen level. In a woman under the age of 40 years with secondary amenorrhea, an FSH level greater than 20 IU/L suggests ovarian failure.

A low FSH would suggest the cause was hypothalamic, and a low oestrogen level would also be expected. Prolactin levels should be measured to rule out hyperprolactinaemia. Thyroid function tests should also be checked as both hyperthyroidism and hypothyroidism can lead to amenorrhoea.

Oestrogen levels may be high in polycystic ovarian syndrome with leuteinising hormone elevated more than FSH. Testosterone levels may also be elevated in polycystic ovarian syndrome.

Kiningham RB, Apgar BS, Schwenk TL. Evaluation of amenorrhea. Am Fam Physician 1996; 53(4):1185–1194.

23. C Multiple endocrine neoplasia (MEN) type 1

Multiple endocrine neoplasias are syndromes of multiple benign endocrine neoplasms. **Table 5.4** outlines how they are classified.

Table 5.4		
Condition	**Neoplasms**	**Genetic abnormality**
MEN-1	Parathyroid Pituitary Pancreas	Menin gene on chromosome 11
MEN-2A	Parathyroid Phaeochromocytoma Medullary thyroid cancer	Ret oncogene on chromosome 10
MEN-2B	Parathyroid Phaeochromocytoma Medullary thyroid cancer Marfanoid Mucosal neuromas	Ret oncogene on chromosome 10

Table 5.4 Classification of multiple endocrine neoplasias (MEN).

Primary hyperparathyroidism usually presents asymptomatically and is identified on routine blood tests. They may present with symptoms of hypercalcaemia including thirst, renal stones, confusion, myopathy and stiff joints. In 80% of cases it is due to a solitary adenoma and technetium MIBI subtraction scans can be used to identify the hyperplastic glands. Parathyroid hormone (PTH) levels can be normal or raised. Treatment is with parathyroidectomy.

In the above case as the patient has evidence of hyperparathyroidism and previous pituitary tumour the most likely underlying diagnosis is MEN-1 rather than isolated hyperparathyroidism.

Malone JP, et al. Hyperparathyroidism and multiple endocrine neoplasia. Otolaryngol Clin North Am 2004; 37(4):715–736.

24. A Ability to achieve and maintain glycaemic control

In order to prevent the micro and macrovascular complications associated with diabetes, it is important to maintain tight glycaemic control. Microvascular complications include nephropathy, neuropathy and retinopathy. The macrovascular complications include heart disease, stroke, peripheral vascular disease and hypertension. Every percentage drop in the HbA1c is associated with a reduction in developing complications. Trial data suggests maintaining HbA1c below 7.0, but this has to be weighed against developing hypoglycaemia.

Renal function, cardiac history and patient weight may influence the decision of which agent to use. Metformin and other biguanides should be avoided in poor renal function, due to the increased risk of lactic acidosis. Metformin can be beneficial in patients who are overweight as it has a favourable effect on lipids with a reduction in total and low-density lipoprotein (LDL) cholesterol and triglycerides. Metformin, and other biguanides, can also lead to reduced absorption of the B vitamin group and folate.

Gliclazide is contraindicated in severe hepatic or renal disease and can also predispose the patient to hypoglycaemic episodes.

Glitazones are contraindicated in those with New York Heart Association grade III or IV cardiac failure.

DeFronzo RA, Goodman AM. Efficacy of metformin in patients with non-insulin-dependent diabetes mellitus. The Multicenter Metformin Study Group. N Engl J Med 1995; 333(9):541–549.
UK Prospective Diabetes Study (UKPDS) Group. Intensive blood-glucose control with sulphonylureas or insulin compared with conventional treatment and risk of complications in patients with type 2 diabetes (UKPDS 33). Lancet 1998; 352(9131):837.

25. E Papillary

There are five types of thyroid cancer. Papillary cancer is the most common (70%). It occurs most frequently in young women and is amenable to treatment with thyroidectomy and radioiodine. The next most common is follicular cancer (20%). It tends to occur in older patients and treatment is again with thyroidectomy and radioiodine.

Medullary cancer (5%) is associated with MEN-2 and arises from the C-cells of the thyroid. It secretes calcitonin, and this can be used a tumour marker.

Anaplastic cancer (1%) is highly malignant. Lymphomas are rare, and are associated with Hashimoto's thyroiditis.

26. C Pseudohypoparathyroidism

Pseudohypoparathyroidism occurs when target cells are insensitive to parathyroid hormone (PTH), leading to a low calcium, with elevated PTH levels. It is associated with specific phenotypic features, including shortened 4th and 5th metacarpals, low IQ and short stature.

Hypoparathyroidism results from a reduced secretion of PTH. Biochemistry shows a low PTH and low calcium, with elevated phosphate levels.

Pseudopseudohypoparathyroidism has the same phenotypic features as pseudohypoparathyroidism, but biochemistry is normal.

27. C Renin:aldosterone ratio

This man has presented with symptoms of hypokalaemia (weakness, muscle cramps, paraesthesia, polyuria, polydipsia), and his blood tests show a metabolic alkalosis with hypokalaemia. He is hypertensive with a normal clinical examination. This suggests a diagnosis of primary hyperaldosteronism.

Causes include:

- Conn's syndrome – aldosterone secreting adenoma
- Bilateral adrenal hyperplasia
- Unilateral adrenal hyperplasia

The initial investigation should be a renin:aldosterone ratio to identify elevated aldosterone levels in the context of low renin levels. Ideally all antihypertensives should be stopped 2–6 weeks prior to the test, as they can interfere with renin and aldosterone levels. This is not always practical.

If an elevated aldosterone level is identified a source can then be looked for, usually with imaging of the adrenals or adrenal vein sampling.

Treatment may be by surgical resection. If this is not possible spironolactone or amiloride may be used.

28. B Education regarding her diagnosis and treatment

The blood tests identify that the patient has not been taking her medication regularly (high thyroid-stimulating hormone [TSH]), but has taken it on the morning of her clinic appointment (normal T4 levels). If the patient was taking her medication regularly the TSH level should be suppressed with a normal T4 level. **Table 5.5**

Table 5.5

Condition	TFT results
Over treated hypothyroidism	Low thyroid-stimulating hormone (TSH) High t4
Undertreated hypothyroidism	Normal or high TSH Low t4
Hyperthyroidism	Low TSH High t4
Hypothyroidism	High TSH Low t4
Sub-clinical hypothyroidism	High TSH Normal t4
Sub-clinical hyperthyroidism	Low TSH Normal t4
Non-compliance with thyroxine replacement therapy	A high TSH level is expected. If the patient has taken their medication on the day of clinic T4 levels will be within the normal range. If not their T4 level will be low

Table 5.5 Interpretation of thyroid function test (TFT) results.

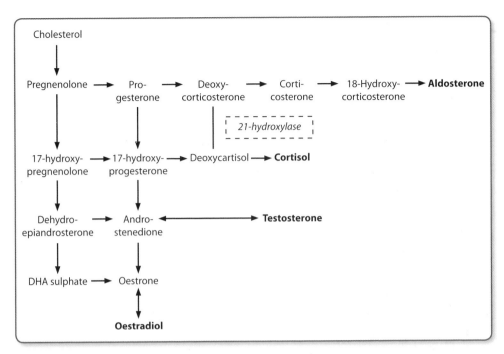

Figure 5.2 Steroid metabolism. In 21-hydroxylase deficiency the aldosterone and cortisol pathways are reduced and steroid metabolism is shifted in favour of the oestradiol and testosterone pathways, leading to excess oestradiol and testosterone production. DHA, dehydroepiandrosterone.

outlines the thyroid function test (TFT) results that would be expected with various conditions.

29. A Congenital adrenal hyperplasia

Congenital adrenal hyperplasia (CAH) results when enzyme defects lead to reduced production of cortisol, but increased production of other intermediates in steroid metabolism. It is autosomal recessive. 90% of cases are secondary to 21-hydroxlase deficiency and 5% due to 11-hydroxylase deficiency (**Figure 5.2**).

Because of the 21-hydroxylase deficiency progesterone and 17-hydroxyprogesterone cannot be metabolised onwards to produce aldosterone and cortisol. The steroid metabolism pathway is then shifted in favour of testosterone and oestradiol production. The excess of these hormones causes virilisation in females, and intersex in males.

30. E Thyroid storm

This patient is most likely suffering from a thyroid storm. This presents as:

- Fever >38.5°C

- Tachycardia
- Confusion
- Hypertension (often with a wide pulse pressure)
- Abnormal liver function tests (LFTs)

Blood tests show non-specific elevation of liver enzymes and a mild leucocytosis. Congestive cardiac failure may develop, due to the high output state.

Treatment includes symptomatic relief (e.g. paracetamol), propranolol, dexamethasone (blocks conversion of T4 to T3) and antithyroid drugs. Mortality rates are high, and the patient should be cared for in intensive care.

A thyroid storm may be precipitated by:

- Non-compliance with antithyroid therapy
- Thyroid surgery
- Radioiodine therapy
- Drugs such as salicylates and non-steroidal anti-inflammatories (NSAIDs)
- Diabetic ketoacidosis (DKA)
- Direct trauma to the thyroid gland

Although her LFTs are deranged, her paracetamol level is less than 10 mg/L, making a paracetamol overdose unlikely. In sepsis, one would expect the patient to be hypotensive, rather than hypertensive, and the clue of the carbimazole in the patients handbag, suggests she has an underlying hyperthyroidism pointing towards the diagnosis of thyroid storm.

Carbimazole side effects include nausea, mild gastrointestinal disturbances, taste disturbance, headache, fever, malaise, rash, pruritus and arthralgia. Rarely bone marrow suppression can occur, resulting in pancytopaenia and increased risk of infection. If this were the underlying cause of the symptoms in this case, a low white cell count, haemoglobin and platelet count would be expected.

Sarlis NJ, Gourgiotis L. Thyroid emergencies. Rev Endocr Metab Disord 2003; 4:129.

Chapter 6

Gastroenterology

1. A 29-year-old woman was referred to the clinic for investigation of a 6-month history of abdominal discomfort and diarrhoea.

   Which one of the following features is least consistent with a diagnosis of irritable bowel syndrome?

   A   Abdominal discomfort relieved by defecation
   B   Diarrhoea for longer than 3 months
   C   Nocturnal diarrhoea
   D   Passage of mucus mixed in with stool
   E   Sensation of abdominal bloating for longer than three months

2. A 70-year-old man attended the emergency department complaining of severe acute abdominal pain and rectal bleeding. His past medical history included ischaemic heart disease and atrial fibrillation. He was diagnosed with ischaemic colitis and underwent an urgent laparotomy.

   Which part of the large intestine is at greatest risk of bowel infarction?

   A   Anorectal junction
   B   Ascending colon
   C   Descending colon
   D   Hepatic flexure
   E   Splenic flexure

3. A 21-year-old woman was admitted to the high dependency unit after an intentional paracetamol overdose. She denied ingesting any other toxins. Her only other past medical history was depression, but she had not taken her prescribed antidepressants. She had been treated appropriately with intravenous fluids and N-acetylcysteine infusion since admission.

   Investigations 24 hours after admission:

   Arterial blood gas on air:

pH	7.28 (7.35–7.45)
pCO_2	4.0 kPa (4.7–6.0)
pO_2	14.4 kPa (11.3–12.6)
bicarbonate	14 mmol/L (21–29)
lactate	3.1 mmol/L (0.5–1.6)
oxygen saturation	98% (94–99)

Blood tests:

haemoglobin	120 g/L (115–165)
white cell count	14×10^9/L (4–11)
neutrophil count	10×10^9/L (1.5–7.0)
serum sodium	135 mmol/L (137–144)
serum potassium	4.4 mmol/L (3.5–4.9)
serum urea	11 mmol/L (2.5–7.0)
serum creatinine	201 mmol/L (60–110)
serum albumin	27 g/L (37–49)
serum total bilirubin	40 mmol/L (1–22)
serum alanine aminotransferase	8243 U/L (5–35)
serum alkaline phosphatase	240 U/L (45–105)
serum gamma glutamyl transferase	6120 U/L (4–35)
serum paracetamol	180 mg/L (<10)
prothrombin time	42 s (11.5–15.5)

Which one of the following is the single most adverse prognostic factor regarding this patient's clinical condition?

A   pH 7.28
B   prothrombin time 42 seconds
C   serum alanine aminotransferase 8243 U/L
D   serum creatinine 201 mmol/L
E   serum paracetamol 180 mg/L despite *N*-acetylcysteine

4. A 33-year-old woman underwent colonoscopy because of a 6-month history of profuse watery diarrhoea and abdominal bloating.

Investigations:

colonoscopy	brown discolouration to the colonic mucosa
histology of colonic biopsy	pigmented appearance to the macrophages of the lamina propria

What is the most appropriate next step in the management of this patient?

A   Budesonide
B   Gluten-free diet
C   Mesalazine
D   Metronidazole
E   Observation in outpatient clinic

5. A 35-year-old woman with a history of systemic sclerosis was referred to the gastroenterology clinic for investigation of a 4-month history of abdominal distension and pale, loose stools that were difficult to flush away.

Investigations:

stool cultures	no growth

What is the next most appropriate step in management?

A   Co-amoxiclav (amoxicillin-clavulanate) trial
B   Corticosteroid trial
C   Gluten-free diet
D   Lactose avoidance
E   Pancreatic enzyme supplementation

6. A 24-year-old man underwent blood tests as a routine part of a pre-employment
    medical assessment. He had been taking regular paracetamol since a knee injury
    whilst playing squash 1 week ago, but took no other regular medications. He did
    not smoke but drank approximately 21 units of alcohol per week.

    Investigations:

haemoglobin	142 g/L (130–180)
platelet count	204 × 10⁹/L (150–450)
reticulocyte count	2.3% (0.5–2.4)
prothrombin time	13.4 s (11.5–15.5)
serum total bilirubin	45 mmol/L (1–22)
serum alanine aminotransferase	33 U/L (5–35)
serum alkaline phosphatase	101 U/L (45–105)
serum gamma glutamyl transferase	29 U/L (<50)
serum albumin	39 g/L (37–49)
serum lactate dehydrogenase	104 U/L (10–250)

    What is the most likely diagnosis?

    A   Alcoholic hepatitis
    B   Gilbert's syndrome
    C   Hereditary spherocytosis
    D   Paracetamol hepatotoxicity
    E   Pyruvate kinase deficiency

7. A 55-year-old man with a background of alcoholic cirrhosis complained of a
    3-week history of dysphagia. There was no history of haematemesis or melaena. He
    had no other medical problems. He was referred for an endoscopy.

    Investigations:

gastroscopy	2 columns of medium sized oesophageal varices with no red signs

    What is the most appropriate next step in management?

    A   Band ligation of varices
    B   Isosorbide mononitrate
    C   Losartan
    D   Observe and surveillance endoscopy
    E   Propranolol

8. A 49-year-old man complained of a 6-month history of steatorrhoea and
    unintentional weight loss. He also noticed gradually progressive stiffness in his

shoulder, hips and knees. Physical examination was normal other than some cervical lymphadenopathy.

Investigations:

gastroscopy	normal oesophagus, stomach and duodenum
duodenal biopsy	macrophages stain strongly positive with periodic acid–Schiff (PAS)

What is the most likely diagnosis?

A   Coeliac disease
B   Crohn's disease
C   Giardiasis
D   Sarcoidosis
E   Whipple's disease

9. A 45-year-old woman presented with a 2-day history of jaundice and pruritis. Three weeks ago, she was diagnosed with a chest infection and was prescribed antibiotics. She had no previous medical history, family history or drug history.

Investigations:

serum total bilirubin	95 mmol/L (1–22)
serum alanine aminotransferase	88 U/L (5–35)
serum alkaline phosphatase	604 U/L (45–105)
serum gamma glutamyl transferase	168 U/L (<50)
serum albumin	42 g/L (37–49)
hepatitis serology	negative
autoantibody screen	negative
liver ultrasound	normal

Which medication is most likely to have caused her symptoms?

A   Ciprofloxacin
B   Co-amoxiclav (amoxicillin/clavulanate)
C   Phenoxymethylpenicillin (penicillin V)
D   Rifampicin
E   Tetracycline

10. A 45-year-old woman was referred by her general practitioner because of abnormal liver function tests. She complained of worsening lethargy and pruritus over the past eight months. She also had a history of hypothyroidism. She had never smoked, did not drink alcohol, and took no other medications apart from thyroxine. On examination, she was mildly icteric. She displayed xanthomata, and had excoriations on her arms and legs. The rest of the physical examination was normal.

Investigations:

serum total bilirubin	65 mmol/L (1–22)
serum alanine aminotransferase	68 U/L (5–35)

serum alkaline phosphatase	740 U/L (45–105)
serum gamma glutamyl transferase	240 U/L (<50)
serum albumin	37 g/L (37–49)
serum total protein	62 g/L (61–76)
international normalised ratio	1.1 (<1.4)
anti-neutrophil cytoplasmic antibodies	not detected
abdominal ultrasound	normal liver, gall bladder, pancreas and biliary tree

What is the most appropriate diagnostic investigation?

A   Anti-mitochondrial antibodies
B   Carbohydrate antigen (CA) 19-9
C   CT abdomen
D   Endoscopic retrograde cholangiopancreatography (ERCP)
E   Liver biopsy

11. A 49-year-old woman was suffering with watery diarrhoea. Three months ago, she had undergone laparoscopic cholecystectomy. Her bowel symptoms developed after her operation. Physical examination was normal.

What is the most appropriate next step in management?

A   Cholestyramine
B   Diphenoxylate
C   Lactose-free diet
D   Loperamide
E   Pancreatic enzyme supplementation

12. A 48-year-old man presented to the gastroenterology clinic with weight loss. He was homosexual and an ex-intravenous drug user. He no longer smoked or drank alcohol.

Investigations:

cytomegalovirus IgG	detected
cytomegalovirus IgM	not detected
hepatitis B surface antigen (HBsAg)	not detected
hepatitis B core antibody (anti-HBc)	not detected
hepatitis C IgG	detected
hepatitis C RNA	5.7 $\log_{10}$ IU/mL
HIV p24 antigen	not detected
HIV 1 & 2 antibody	not detected
liver ultrasound	small liver with coarse liver edge, no focal lesion
liver biopsy	severe fibrosis with some periportal inflammation

What is the most appropriate treatment?

A   Entecavir
B   Foscarnet

    C   Pegylated interferon-alpha and ribavirin
    D   Truvada tenofovir and emtricitabine
    E   Valganciclovir

13. A 30-year-old woman presented to the emergency department with several days of upper abdominal pain and recurrent vomiting. She was currently 36 weeks pregnant. Until now her pregnancy had been uncomplicated. This was her first pregnancy, and she had no other significant past medical history. She did not smoke or drink alcohol and took no other medications or recreational drugs. On examination, she was jaundiced, had some epigastric tenderness but no organomegaly or signs of chronic liver disease.

Investigations:

haemoglobin	116 g/L (115–165)
white cell count	14×10^9/L (4–11)
neutrophil count	11.8×10^9/L (1.5–7.0)
platelet count	88×10^9/L (150–400)
serum urea	8.4 mmol/L (2.5–7.0)
serum creatinine	166 mmol/L (60–110)
serum total bilirubin	72 mmol/L (1–22)
serum alanine aminotransferase	588 U/L (5–35)
serum aspartate aminotransferase	496 U/L (1–31)
serum alkaline phosphatase	188 U/L (45–105)
serum albumin	24 g/L (37–49)
random serum glucose	3.0 mmol/L (3.9–7.8)
serum urate	1.06 mmol/L (0.19–0.36)
international normalised ratio	1.6 (<1.4)

What is the most appropriate next step in management?

    A   Fresh frozen plasma transfusion
    B   Liaison with obstetricians regarding urgent delivery
    C   Rifaximin
    D   Ursodeoxycholic acid
    E   Vitamin K

14. A 29-year-old woman underwent screening blood tests at occupational health.

Investigations:

hepatitis B surface antigen (HBsAg)	not detected
hepatitis B surface antibody (anti-HBs)	>100 mIU/mL
hepatitis B e antigen (HBeAg)	not detected
hepatitis B e antibody (anti-HBe)	not detected
hepatitis B core antibody (anti-HBc)	not detected
hepatitis B DNA	0 IU/mL

What is the most likely explanation for these blood tests results?

    A   Acute hepatitis B infection with low infectivity
    B   Chronic hepatitis B with low infectivity

C   Cleared hepatitis B infection
D   Hepatitis B vaccination failure
E   Successful passive vaccination

15. A 35-year-old man presented with a 4-week history of worsening epigastric pain and oily stools that were difficult to flush away. He had had these symptoms intermittently for the past 2 years, and been diagnosed with peptic ulcer on two previous endoscopy procedures. His symptoms responded to high dose proton pump inhibitor therapy, but he relapsed when he stopped taking them. Recently, he had been diagnosed with primary hyperparathyroidism. He did not smoke or drink alcohol, and was not on any regular medication.

Investigations:

gastroscopy   multiple small duodenal ulcers, urease test negative

What is the most useful diagnostic investigation?

A   Abdominal ultrasound
B   Barium swallow
C   Faecal elastase
D   Fasting serum gastrin
E   Oesophageal manometry

16. A 23-year-old man presented to the emergency department with a 3-day history of vomiting and colicky abdominal pain. He had suffered from these symptoms recurrently for the past several months. He denied any change in weight or appetite. There was no past medical history, but his father had similar problems when this age and ended up requiring a laparotomy. On physical examination, he had brown-black macules on the lips and buccal mucosa. The abdomen was distended with hyperactive bowel sounds but no focal masses.

What is the most likely explanation for this man's symptoms?

A   Adhesions
B   Ileus
C   Intussusception
D   Strangulated hernia
E   Stricture

17. An 81-year-old woman was admitted to hospital with diffuse abdominal pain and a 5-day history of profuse watery diarrhoea. She took no regular medications until 4 months ago, when she had a myocardial infarction and subsequently developed atrial fibrillation.

Investigations:

stool ELISA for *Clostridium difficile* A   toxin detected

Which one of the following medications is most likely to have contributed to her current problem?

    A   Aspirin
    B   Digoxin
    C   Lansoprazole
    D   Ramipril
    E   Simvastatin

18. The pancreas secretes up to 1.5 L of alkaline fluid per day comprising proteins and electrolytes.

    Which one of the following is the only exocrine secretion?

    A   Glucagon
    B   Insulin
    C   Pancreatic polypeptide
    D   Somatostatin
    E   Trypsinogen

19. The stomach produces approximately 3 L of secretions daily.

    Which one of the following factors does not increase acid secretion?

    A   Basophilia (high basophil count)
    B   Gastrinoma
    C   Secretin
    D   Small bowel resection
    E   Systemic mastocytosis

20. Regarding iron metabolism in the body, which one of the following factors increases iron absorption?

    A   Achlorhydria
    B   Coeliac disease
    C   Crohn's disease
    D   Total gastrectomy
    E   Vitamin C

21. A 30-year-old man presented to the emergency department with severe vomiting. He had eaten a portion of reheated fried rice 5 hours ago that he had bought from the local takeaway the night before. He had no past medical history.

    What is the most likely cause for his condition?

    A   *Bacillus cereus*
    B   *Campylobacter jejuni*
    C   *Escherichia coli*
    D   *Salmonella typhi*
    E   *Staphylococcus aureus*

22. A 50-year-old woman presented to the gastroenterology clinic with an 18-month history of dysphagia for both solids and liquids. She also described occasional regurgitation of food and a night time cough. She had also lost 8 kg in weight over this time. Physical examination was normal.

Investigations:

oesophagogastroduodenoscopy (OGD)	normal
barium swallow	tapering at lower oesophageal sphincter and narrowing at the gastro-oesophageal junction

What is the most likely diagnosis?

A   Achalasia
B   Gastro-oesophageal reflux disease (GORD)
C   Oesophageal cancer
D   Oesophageal candidiasis
E   Pharyngeal pouch

23. A 56-year-old man was seen in the gastroenterology clinic with deranged liver function tests. His weight was 100 kg with a body mass index 35. He was a non-smoker and drank 6 units of alcohol per week.

Investigations:

liver ultrasound	hepatomegaly – increased echogenicity in keeping with fatty liver
liver biopsy	steatohepatitis but no fibrosis or cirrhosis
random serum glucose	9 mmol/L (3.9–7.8)

What is the most appropriate next step in management?

A   Gliclazide
B   Metformin
C   Pioglitazone
D   Simvastatin
E   Weight loss

24. A 50-year-old man presented to the emergency department with symptoms of breathlessness, lethargy and pain in both knees. He had a past medical history of cardiomyopathy and impotence. He did not drink alcohol. He had a tanned complexion and some ankle oedema. His pulse was 88 beats per minute, blood pressure 120/78 mmHg and jugular venous pressure +6 cm. There were crackles at both lung bases.

Investigations:

haemoglobin	131 g/L (130–180)
mean cell volume	98 fL (80–96)
white cell count	5.6×10^9/L (4.0–11.0)
platelets	100×10^9/L (150–400)
international normalised ratio	1.5 (<1.4)
serum sodium	139 mmol/L (137–144)
serum potassium	4.0 mmol/L (3.5–4.9)
serum urea	15 mmol/L (2.5–7.0)

serum creatinine	88 μmol/L (60–110)
random serum glucose	17 mmol/L (3.9-7.8)
serum albumin	28 g/L (37–49)
serum total bilirubin	75 μmol/L (1–22)
serum alanine aminotransferase	99 U/L (5–35)
serum alkaline phosphatase	452 U/L (45–105)
knee X-ray	chondrocalcinosis

Which is the only reversible feature of this patient's condition?

A   Arthropathy
B   Cardiomyopathy
C   Diabetes mellitus
D   Hypogonadism
E   Liver cirrhosis

25. A 50-year-old man with dyspepsia was found to be *H.pylori* positive and underwent eradication treatment. He had a breath test which showed him to still have the infection. Previously he was treated with omeprazole, amoxicillin and clarithromycin.

Which one of the following is least likely to be effective in treating *H.pylori*?

A   Isoniazid
B   Levofloxacin
C   Metronidazole
D   Rifampicin
E   Tetracycline

26. Which one of the following is not a recognised risk factor for developing adenocarcinoma of the stomach?

A   Blood group A
B   Chronic atrophic gastritis
C   Diet high in nitrites
D   Diet high in salt
E   Gastro-oesophageal reflux disease (GORD)

27. A 45-year-old woman presented to the emergency department with abdominal pain over the past year. The pain radiated to the back, occurred predominately after meals and could last for hours. She also suffered with fatty, bulky stools that were difficult to flush away. She smoked 20 cigarettes and drank a bottle of wine per day. On general observation she was cachexic, her abdomen was soft and tender in the epigastrium.

Investigations:

| random serum glucose | 15 mmol/L (3.9–7.8) |

What is the most appropriate diagnostic investigation?

A   Abdominal X-ray
B   CT abdomen
C   Endoscopic ultrasound (EUS)
D   Endoscopic retrograde cholangiopancreatography (ERCP)
E   Faecal elastase

28. A 37-year-old woman was referred by her general practitioner with jaundice, lethargy, abdominal discomfort, pruritus and arthralgia. She had been on thyroxine for 5 years for hypothyroidism. On examination, she had palmar erythema, icteric sclerae, spider naevi and 3 cm tender hepatomegaly.

Investigations:

haemoglobin	115 g/L (115–165)
mean cell volume	89 fL (80–96)
platelets	375 × 10⁹/L (150–400)
international normalised ratio	1.2 (<1.4)
serum albumin	30 g/L (37–49)
serum total bilirubin	34 µmol/L (1–22)
serum alanine aminotransferase	325 U/L (5–35)
serum alkaline phosphatase	200 U/L (45–105)
serum total protein	86 g/L (60–80)
serum immunoglobulin A	1.5 g/L (0.9–3.0)
serum immunoglobulin G	30 g/L (6–13)
serum immunoglobulin M	1.0 g/L (0.4–2.5)

What is the most appropriate treatment for this patient?

A   Azathioprine
B   Cyclophosphamide
C   Mycophenolate mofetil
D   Prednisolone
E   Ursodeoxycholic acid

29. A 28-year-old man with known left sided ulcerative colitis for the past 4 years, was seen in the gastroenterology clinic. For the past 2 weeks he complained of increased bowel frequency, some abdominal pain, but no blood in his stools. He had no recent foreign travel and had no recent infections. He was already on maximum dose oral mesalazine. On examination, his temperature was 37.2°C, pulse 88 beats per minute, and blood pressure 130/76 mmHg.

Investigations:

haemoglobin	133 g/L (130–180)
mean cell volume	80 fL (80–96)
platelets	375 × 10⁹/L (150–400)
white cell count	11.0 × 10⁹/L (4.0–11.0)
neutrophil count	7.8 × 10⁹/L (1.5–7.0)
erythrocyte sedimentation rate	20 mm/1st hour (<20)
serum C-reactive protein	15 mg/L (<10)

What is the most appropriate next step in management?

A   Azathioprine
B   Loperamide
C   Metronidazole
D   Prednisolone
E   Topical mesalazine

30. Which one of the following features is not characteristic of Crohn's disease?

A   Crypt abscesses
B   Fissuring ulcers
C   Neutrophil infiltrates
D   Non-caseating granuloma
E   Transmural inflammation

Answers

---

1. C Nocturnal diarrhoea

The diagnosis of a functional bowel disorder (such as irritable bowel syndrome) is made as a diagnosis of exclusion. However, certain features of the clinical history can suggest whether the symptoms described are more likely to have an organic basis or be functional in nature. The Rome III diagnostic criteria can be helpful in making the diagnosis of irritable bowel syndrome:

Recurrent abdominal pain or discomfort at least 3 days per month in the last 3 months, associated with two or more of the following:

- Improvement with defecation
- Onset associated with a change in frequency of stool
- Onset associated with a change in form (appearance) of stool

Gastrointestinal symptoms that should not be assumed to be functional without thorough investigation include nocturnal diarrhoea, rectal bleeding, mouth ulcers, and unintentional weight loss.

Longstreth GF, et al. Functional bowel disorders. Gastroenterol 2006; 130(5):1480–1491.

---

2. E Splenic flexure

Ischaemic colitis remains a devastating disease, with mortality rates of at least 60%. It usually occurs due to occlusion of flow in the superior mesenteric artery from causes such as thromboembolism (often from an intracardiac source), progressive atheromatous change or local thrombosis. The superior mesenteric artery is the predominant colonic arterial supply to the proximal two-thirds of the colon up to the distal transverse colon, with the inferior mesenteric artery being the major arterial source from here through to the rest of the large intestine. Because the splenic flexure is a 'watershed' area of the colon, located at the crossover between two arterial territories, and where there is scant blood flow from collateral vessels, it is particularly vulnerable to ischaemic damage if there is any disruption in its vascular supply.

Theodoropoulou A, Koutroubakis IE. Ischemic colitis: clinical practice in diagnosis and treatment. World J Gastroenterol 2008; 14(48): 7302–7308.

---

3. A pH 7.28

Several different models have been proposed for trying to estimate prognosis in acute liver failure and predict who is likely to develop fulminant disease and require consideration for liver transplantation. The most widely accepted criteria for listing for liver transplantation in the context of acute liver failure are the King's College Criteria:

For paracetamol-induced acute liver failure:

- **Either** arterial pH < 7.3 (after correction of dehydration)

- **Or ALL three of:**
  - Grade III/IV encephalopathy
  - Prothrombin time > 100 seconds (or international normalised ratio [INR] > 6.5)
  - Serum creatinine > 301 mmol/L

For acute liver failure with causes other than paracetamol:

- **Either** prothrombin time >100 s (or INR > 6.5) (regardless of the level of encephalopathy)
- **Or any three of the following** (regardless of the level of encephalopathy):
  - Age < 10 years or > 40 years
  - Aetiology – non-A, non-B hepatitis, halothane hepatitis, idiosyncratic reactions.
  - Duration of jaundice prior to onset of encephalopathy > 7 days
  - Prothrombin time > 50 s (or INR > 3.5)
  - Serum total bilirubin > 308 mmol/L

Although this woman has evidence of several markers of severity – including coagulopathy, renal failure and acidosis – it is the degree of acidosis that makes this the single worst prognostic factor.

Although paracetamol levels are crucial at the time of initial assessment in helping to decide whether the patient would benefit from treatment with *N*-acetylcysteine or not, they are not helpful as markers of severity. Very elevated alanine transaminase (ALT) levels may be found in the context of paracetamol overdose, but they also provide no prognostic information.

O'Grady J, et al. Early indicators of prognosis in fulminant hepatic failure. Gastroenterol 1989; 97 (2):439–45.

4. E Observation in outpatient clinic

The appearance of a brown discolouration to the colonic mucosa on endoscopy is known as melanosis coli. It tends to be located particularly in the region of the rectum and sigmoid colon, and may sometimes be described as having a 'tiger skin' appearance. This most often occurs as a consequence of the prolonged use of stimulant laxatives.

None of options A, B, C or D would provide any benefit. The most appropriate management is to try and minimise the patient's further use of stimulant laxatives and to follow them up in outpatient clinic.

Freeman HJ. "Melanosis" in the small and large intestine. World J Gastroenterol 2008; 14(27):4296 –4299.

5. A Co-amoxiclav (amoxicillin-clavulanate) trial

Up to 90% of patients with systemic sclerosis have an element of gastrointestinal involvement, with the common underlying pathology being abnormally slow and uncoordinated gastrointestinal tract mobility. Stasis of the small intestine provides an environment suitable for bacterial division, and therefore the risk of developing small bowel bacterial overgrowth (SBBO) (also known as 'blind loop syndrome') and consequently malabsorption. The description of steatorrhoea given here is therefore most likely to be explained by SBBO, the treatment of which is – in addition to treating any underlying cause – the use of broad-spectrum antibiotics with anaerobic cover.

Causes of SBBO may be summarised as those pathologies affecting the normal structure, function and controls on bacterial proliferation within the small bowel, namely:

- Structural – previous gastric surgery (especially Bilroth II surgery), surgical blind loops, Crohn's disease (via fistula or stricture formation), jejunal diverticulae, radiation enteritis
- Functional – autonomic neuropathy (including diabetes mellitus), systemic sclerosis
- Impaired immune function – hypogammaglobulinaemia, hypo-/achlorydia

The gold standard for diagnosis of SBBO is jejunal aspiration and culture, but this is technically difficult, invasive, and often gives false negatives, meaning it is seldom used in practice. Another, albeit less commonly used, method is the lactulose-hydrogen breath test. Lactulose is a non-absorbable disaccharide that is normally only metabolised by colonic bacteria, and releases detectable hydrogen in doing so. In the presence of bacterial overgrowth, lactulose will also be metabolised in the small bowel, with the consequence of hydrogen being detected earlier than normal.

Other causes of malabsorption include inflammatory bowel disease, coeliac disease, lactose intolerance and chronic pancreatitis, and options B, C, D and E respectively may improve symptoms in these diseases. However, they will be of no benefit to the symptoms of SBBO.

Bures J, et al. Small intestinal bacterial overgrowth syndrome. World J Gastroenterol 2010; 16(24): 2978–2990.

6. B Gilbert's syndrome

The presence of an elevated bilirubin in the presence of normal liver enzyme levels and normal markers of hepatic synthetic function (i.e. prothrombin time and albumin) makes a pre-hepatic aetiology of jaundice the most likely explanation. Options A and D can therefore be rejected.

The differentiation that then needs to be made is whether this is prehepatic jaundice because of increased bilirubin production (as is the case in haemolysis), or whether this represents an absence or inactivity of the conjugating enzymes of the liver. The presence of a normal haemoglobin level, platelet count, reticulocyte count and plasma lactate dehydrogenase make haemolysis very unlikely, and options C and E can therefore be rejected.

Gilbert's syndrome is a condition inherited in an autosomal dominant manner. It results in jaundice through the reduced activity of the hepatic glucuronyl transferase enzymes that are responsible for bilirubin conjugation and uptake by the liver. The jaundice is produced typically mild, although it may become more marked at times of stress (e.g. fasting, infection). There is no evidence of Gilbert's syndrome causing any detrimental effect to the affected person, and the only clinical finding is mild jaundice. Gilbert's syndrome is often diagnosed incidentally after the consistent finding of low grade unconjugated hyperbilirubinaemia in the absence of haemolysis.

A summary of bilirubin metabolism is given in **Figure 6.1**.

Hirschfield GM, Alexander GJ. Gilbert's syndrome: an overview for clinical biochemists. Ann Clin Biochem 2006; 43 (5):340–343.

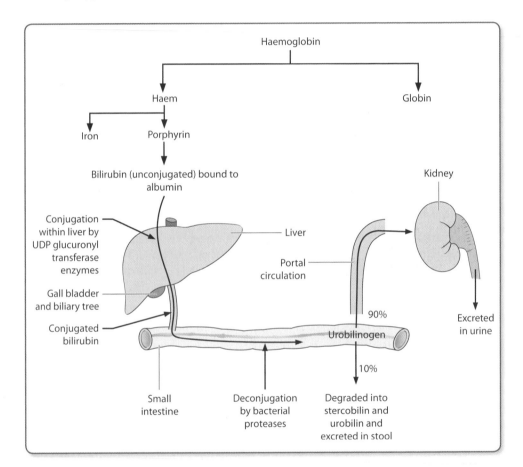

Figure 6.1 Summary of bilirubin metabolism. Patients with Gilbert's syndrome have reduced activity of uridine diphosphate (UDP) glucuronyl transferase enzymes. They therefore cannot conjugate bilirubin normally, and experience life-long unconjugated hyperbilirubinaemia.

7. E Propranolol

International guidelines describe non-selective beta-blockers (such as propranolol) and endoscopic variceal ligation as the two most effective therapies in primary prevention of variceal haemorrhage. Propranolol is the usual first treatment introduced, providing there are no contraindications to its use (such as asthma, heart block or hypotension). In patients for whom beta-blockers are inappropriate, then band ligation of varices is the appropriate next step. Nitrate-based medications appear to reduce the rate of variceal haemorrhage when given to patients who have had band ligation, but not when given alone. There is contradictory data regarding the efficacy of angiotensin II receptor antagonists (such as losartan) in reducing portal hypertension, and they are therefore not recommended by guidelines at present.

The situation is different for secondary prevention. Patients presenting with variceal haemorrhage can bleed profusely, and the immediate aim is to correct hypovolaemic shock and any accompanying coagulopathy. When safe to do so, the most appropriate definitive treatment is band ligation of the varices (**Figure 6.2**). Beta-blockers are only safe to start/restart once the patient has fully stabilised.

Garcia-Tsao G, Bosch J. Current Concepts: Management of Varices and Variceal Haemorrhage in Cirrhosis. N Engl J Med 2010; 362:823–832.
Garcia-Tsao G, et al. Prevention and Management of Gastroesophageal Varices and Variceal Hemorrhage in Cirrhosis. Hepatol 2007; 46 (3):922–938.

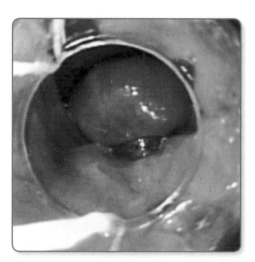

Figure 6.2 Banded oesophageal varix. There is an oesophageal varix which has had an elastic band deployed at the base of the varix. Within 2–5 days the band will fall off to leave a ulcer that will heal within 2–3 weeks before possible re-banding of the varix.

8. E Whipple's disease

Whipple's disease is a rare condition, caused by infection with the gram-positive bacillus *Tropheryma whipplei*, a bacterium resident within the macrophages of the small intestinal mucosa. The major pathogenic effect is the infiltration of the small intestinal mucosa by 'foamy', lipid-rich macrophages that stain positive with periodic acid–Schiff (PAS) reagent. As such, endoscopy and biopsy is the major route by which the diagnosis of Whipple's disease is confirmed. All of the options offered may present with malabsorption, but Whipple's disease is the only one of the options that typically gives these duodenal biopsy findings.

Whipple's disease is often thought of as a great mimic, not least because its symptoms and signs are so diverse. These include:

- Gastrointestinal – the most frequently found category, including steatorrhoea, weight loss, and hepatosplenomegaly
- Rheumatological – seronegative migratory large joint polyarthritis
- Cardiac – myocarditis, pericarditis, or an endocarditis-like disorder
- Neurological – cognitive impairment, sterile meningitis, or involuntary movements
- Others – fever, lymphadenopathy, pigmentation

The most commonly used treatment regimen is with 2 weeks of intravenous ceftriaxone, followed by 1 year of oral trimethoprim–sulphamethoxazole. The prognosis is usually good.

Afshar P, Redfield DC, Higginbottom PA. Whipple's disease: a rare disease revisited. Curr Gastroenterol Rep 2010; 12(4):263–269.

9. B Co-amoxiclav (amoxicillin-clavulanate)

The spectrum of drug-induced liver injury (DILI) can range from the mild and self-limiting (as in the majority of cases) up to fulminant liver failure. Co-amoxiclav is one of the drugs most frequently implicated in drug-induced liver injury worldwide, characteristically causing a cholestatic pattern of liver function tests; options D and E are associated with hepatocellular injury rather than cholestasis, whilst options A and C have very little association with DILI. Some of the drugs most commonly associated with DILI, and the pattern of injury they cause are shown in **Table 6.1.**

Chang CY, Schiano TD. Review article: drug hepatotoxicity. Aliment Pharmacol Ther 2007; 25(10): 1135–1151.

Table 6.1

Hepatocellular	Cholestatic	Mixed
Isoniazid	Co-amoxiclav	Carbamazepine
Rifampicin	Flucloxacillin	Phenytoin
Tetracycline	Erythromycin	Phenobarbitone
Diclofenac	Oestrogens	Nitrofurantoin
Paracetamol	Anabolic steroids	Clindamycin
Sulphonylureas	Chlorpromazine	Ibuprofen
Statins	Ethanol	Verapamil
Sodium valproate	Terbinafine	
Halothane		
Ketoconazole		

Hepatocellular defined as alanine transaminase (ALT) > 3 × upper limit of normal; cholestasis defined as alkaline phosphate (ALP) > 2 × upper limit of normal; mixed where elements of both present.

Table 6.1 Typical causes of drug-induced liver injury.

10. A Anti-mitochondrial antibodies

The differential diagnosis for this scenario includes primary biliary cirrhosis (PBC), autoimmune hepatitis, primary sclerosing cholangitis (PSC), drug-induced liver injury, and malignancy (e.g. pancreatic head adenocarcinoma). Cholestatic rather than hepatitic liver function tests (LFTs) make autoimmune hepatitis improbable. PSC seems unlikely given the apparent lack of bowel symptoms and negative anti-neutrophil cytoplasmic antibodies (ANCAs) (p-ANCA is positive in up to 80% of cases). A normal ultrasound makes malignancy unlikely. PBC is therefore the most likely diagnosis.

Primary biliary cirrhosis is an autoimmune disease of uncertain aetiology characterised by chronic, progressive intra-hepatic cholestasis. The typical first presentation of PBC is with progressive lethargy and pruritus, but the diagnosis may also be made in patients who are asymptomatic and undergoing investigations for abnormal LFTs. Up to 80% of patients with PBC have other autoimmune diseases, including thyroid disease, keratoconjunctivitis sicca, pernicious anaemia and rheumatoid arthritis. Xanthomata and other features of dyslipidaemia are other common associations.

Anti-mitochondrial antibodies are detectable in the serum of at least 95% of patients with PBC. Given that this is such a sensitive and specific test for the condition, liver biopsy is not required additionally to make the diagnosis unless clinical and serological features are equivocal. As such, option A is preferable to option E.

CA 19-9 is a tumour marker that is useful in some circumstances as part of investigations for possible cholangiocarcinoma, but has no utility in making the diagnosis of PBC. Neither CT abdomen nor endoscopic retrograde cholangiopancreatography (ERCP) will help in diagnosing PBC either – PBC is a disorder of the intra-hepatic biliary tree, whilst these investigations are most of use in looking for disease of the extra-hepatic tree (e.g. malignancy, PSC).

Poupon R. Primary biliary cirrhosis: a 2010 update. J Hepatol 2010; 52(5):745–758.

11. A Cholestyramine

Approximately 10% of patients who have undergone cholecystectomy will experience problems with diarrhoea afterwards due to bile acid malabsorption. Without the gall bladder present to act as a reservoir for bile, bile salts drain at a high rate straight into the small bowel, and potentially at a rate that exceeds the reabsorptive ability of the terminal ileum. Free bile salts in the colon stimulate water and electrolyte secretion, hence chronic diarrhoea may be generated. Most patients respond to the use of bile salt binding resins, such as cholestyramine.

Options C and E are the first-line treatments for lactose intolerance and pancreatic exocrine insufficiency respectively, but would not be of any benefit here. Options B and D are symptomatic treatments for diarrhoea.

Walters JR, Pattni SS. Managing bile acid diarrhoea. Ther Adv Gastroenterol 2010; 3(6):349–357.

12. C Pegylated interferon-alpha and ribavarin

The presence of IgG but not IgM antibodies to cytomegalovirus implies that this man has been exposed to this infection in the past rather than recently. Foscarnet and valganciclovir are licensed for use in active cytomegalovirus (CMV) disease (with particular use being in immunocompromised patients), but there is no indication for their use here. The hepatitis B and HIV serology results imply that this man has not been exposed to either virus previously. However, the blood results confirm that this man is hepatitis C positive.

This patient has severe fibrosis/cirrhosis and so will need treatment regardless of viral load, alanine transferase (ALT) or hepatitis C genotype. The genotype determines the likelihood of eradication with drug therapy and the duration of treatment that is used. The current standard of care is pegylated interferon-alpha given subcutaneously weekly and daily ribavirin for between 24 and 48 weeks. Although active drinking of alcohol is not a contraindication to starting treatment, it certainly decreases the chances of sustained virological response significantly and so patients are encouraged to abstain from alcohol before treatment commences.

Rosen HR. Chronic Hepatitis C Infection. N Engl J Medicine 2011; 364:2429–2438.

13. B Liaison with obstetricians regarding urgent delivery

The most likely diagnosis is acute fatty liver of pregnancy which usually presents in the last trimester of pregnancy. It presents initially with abdominal pain and nausea, but may progress to jaundice, coagulopathy, elevated liver enzymes, hypoglycaemia, encephalopathy and eventual multi-organ failure. The condition appears to be caused by a defect in beta-oxidation of fatty acids within mitochondria. The presence of microvesicular fatty infiltration of hepatocytes on liver biopsy is the diagnostic gold standard, although practically the diagnosis is usually made clinically. If left untreated, maternal mortality can be up to 3%, with fetal mortality up to 45%. However, following delivery, the condition begins to quickly resolve and usually leaves no long term adverse effects. As such, urgent delivery is the most definitive treatment in management of this patient. Although correcting coagulopathy (options A and E) and treating encephalopathy (option C) may be important parts of supportive management for the condition, the key to successful management is in arranging delivery once safe to do so.

The HELLP (haemolysis, elevated liver enzymes and low platelets) syndrome is a condition most often found in multiparous women in late pregnancy, particularly those with previous pre-eclampsia. It has considerable overlap with the features of acute fatty liver of pregnancy, but is additionally characterised by microangiopathic haemolytic anaemia, coagulopathy and placental abruption. Again, urgent delivery is the definitive management. Intrahepatic cholestasis of pregnancy most often occurs in the third trimester, and is characterised by pruritus in association with elevated serum bile acids; ursodeoxycholic acid – a hydrophilic bile acid is the mainstay of treatment.

Joshi D, et al. Liver disease in pregnancy. Lancet 2010; 375:594–605.

14. E Successful passive vaccination

The serology findings at different stages of hepatitis B infection/in response to vaccination against the virus are summarised in **Table 6.2**.

Chronic hepatitis is by definition the persistence of HBsAg in the serum for greater than six months, helping to make the distinction between an acute and chronic infection. The presence of anti-HBs indicates either complete elimination of the virus by the immune system following infection, or prior passive vaccination. Anti-HBc antibodies appear in the serum weeks after infection, and are usually detectable for life; however, they are not detectable in the case of passive vaccination. This helps to differentiate a successfully cleared infection from passive vaccination. The presence of anti-HBs but not anti-HBc in this patient's serum means the answer is either option D or E.

Following vaccination against hepatitis B, levels of anti-HBs are measured as a means of establishing whether vaccination has been successful or not. Levels of anti-HBs > 10 mIU/mL are widely-accepted as indicating a good level of immunity. Those with lower levels are often given a booster vaccine in the first instance. The high anti-HBs level detected here makes option E the correct answer.

HBeAg appears in the serum soon after viral infection and is a marker of ongoing viral replication within the liver, a good surrogate marker of infectivity. The decline of HBeAg levels in the serum and appearance of anti-HBe are signs of reduced infectivity. However, there are also recognised mutant forms of the hepatitis B virus that fail to express the e antigen but are as infective as forms of the virus that do. As such, assays for hepatitis B DNA should be performed in addition to serology in helping to establish the degree of infectivity.

Centers for Disease Control and Prevention (CDC) Hepatitis B information: http://www.cdc.gov/hepatitis/hbv/hbvfaq.htm (Last accessed May 2012).

Table 6.2

Stage of disease	Serological marker		
	HBsAg	Anti-HBs	Anti-HBc
Acute hepatitis B	+	−	+ for IgM at first and then + for IgG later
Chronic hepatitis B	+	−	+
Cleared infection	−	+	+
Passive vaccination	−	+	−

Table 6.2 Serological findings in hepatitis B.

15. D Fasting serum gastrin

The presence of recurrent peptic ulcers (in the absence of any other obvious cause, such as *Helicobacter pylori* or non-steroidal anti-inflammatory drugs [NSAIDs]) and steatorrhoea is very characteristic of Zollinger–Ellison syndrome, reflecting an underlying gastrinoma. Fasting plasma gastrin is the usual first-line test where this diagnosis is being considered; subsequent investigations include tumour staging, either with CT scan, MRI or endoscopic ultrasound. Symptoms may be managed medically with proton pump inhibitors or H2-antagonists, but surgical resection remains the definitive management.

Gastro-intestinal neuro endocrine tumours are rare in clinical practice but may present with very characteristic clinical syndromes. Syndromes that may be seen include:

- Glucagonoma – hyperglycaemia/diabetes mellitus, necrolytic migratory erythema, stomatitis, flushing, weight loss.
- Insulinoma – recurrent hypoglycaemia.
- Somatostatinoma – hyperglycaemia/diabetes mellitus, gallstones, steatorrhoea.
- VIPoma – profuse watery diarrhoea, hypokalaemia.

Note that up to 20% of cases of gastro intestinal neuro endocrine tumours – particularly those situated in the pancreas - occur as part of the multiple endocrine neoplasia 1 syndrome. The past medical history in this patient of parathyroid disease makes it possible that this is the case here.

Öberg KE. Gastrointestinal neuroendocrine tumours. Ann Oncology 2010; 21:vii72–80.

16. C Intussusception

Peutz–Jeghers syndrome is a rare autosomal dominant disorder associated with mutation of the gene encoding serine threonine kinase (STK11) on chromosome 19. There are two major categories of clinical features:

1. Pigmented macules – these may affect the hands, feet, lips and buccal mucosa, but spare the tongue. The description of such macules in the patient in this scenario along with the suggestion of a family history of disease is very suggestive that this is the underlying diagnosis here.
2. Gastrointestinal hamartomatous polyps – these may begin to develop anywhere within the gastrointestinal tract within the first decade of life, and tend to become symptomatic between the ages of 10 and 30 years. They are most often found in the small intestine, with the large intestine and stomach the second and third most prevalent sites, respectively.

The usual means by which these polyps first present is through intestinal obstruction. This either occurs through polyps acting as an anchor site for intussusception, or else through large polyps occluding the intestinal lumen. Although intussusception accounts for only approximately 5% of cases of small bowel obstruction in the total adult population, it is the most common cause in those with Peutz–Jeghers syndrome, with the majority of sufferers affected at some point. In the absence of any other obvious risk factor for intestinal obstruction within the scenario (such as prior surgery predisposing to adhesions, or a hernia on clinical examination), option D is the correct answer. Other means by which the polyps may be first detected are through investigations for rectal bleeding or iron-deficiency anaemia.

Peutz–Jeghers syndrome is also notable for its association with malignancy, increasing an individual's lifetime risk of developing cancer approximately ten-fold.

This risk is both for gastrointestinal cancers and for those at other sites (especially breast, ovarian, uterine and testicular). Appropriate screening should be started at an early age.

van Lier MG, et al. High cumulative risk of intussusception in patients with peutz-jeghers syndrome: time to update surveillance guidelines? Am J Gastroenterol 2011; 106:940–945.

17. C Lansoprazole

Almost all medications may be associated with gastrointestinal disturbance as a side effect, but at least three of this woman's regular medications (digoxin, statin and proton pump inhibitor) have a particularly strong association with the development of loose stool. However, of the medications listed, only lansoprazole has any significant association with the development of *C. difficile* infection. The risk factors for *C. difficile* infection are summarised in **Table 6.3**.

Table 6.3	
Risk factor	**Details**
Antibiotics	Antibiotics disrupt the balance of the normal colonic flora, allowing *C. difficile* multiplication and toxin release. The most frequently implicated antibiotics are fluoroquinolones and cephalosporins.
Gastric acid inhibition	Gastric acid appears to have a role in destroying *C. difficile* spores. There is an epidemiological association between the use of proton pump inhibitors/ H2-antagonists and the develop of *C. difficile* infection
Age	Increasing age is associated with a diminished immune response to spore exposure, and an increased risk of polypharmacy (and hence a greater likelihood of exposure to medications associated with infection).

Table 6.3 Risk factors for *Clostridium difficile* infection.

Diagnosis is made through the use of ELISA to detect one or both of the *C. difficile* toxins. First-line management is oral metronidazole; if the diarrhoea fails to resolve, then oral vancomycin and/or intravenous metronidazole are generally used next. Colonic resection may be required in the most severe cases.

Linsky A, et al. Proton pump inhibitors and risk for recurrent Clostridium difficile infection. Arch Intern Med 2010; 170:772–778.
Howell, MD et al. Iatrogenic gastric acid suppression and the risk of nosocomial Clostridium difficile infection. Arch Intern Med 2010; 170:784–790.

18. E Trypsinogen

The pancreas is innervated by the coeliac plexus and is made up of exocrine acini of epithelial cells (98%) and endocrine islet cells of Langerhans (2%). **Table 6.4** illustrates the different pancreatic secretions.

Chandra R, Liddle RA. Recent advances in pancreatic endocrine and exocrine secretion. Curr Opin Gastroenterol 2011; 27(5):439–443.

Table 6.4

Endocrine	Exocrine
Glucagon from α cells	Chymotrypsinogen
Insulin from β cells	Lipase
Pancreatic polypeptide	Pancreatic amylase
Somatostatin from δ cells	Trypsinogen

Table 6.4 Endocrine and exocrine pancreatic secretions.

19. C Secretin

Gastric acid secretion is mediated by gastrin, histamine and vagal stimulation. **Figure 6.3** shows how these three factors act on the parietal cell to produce gastric acid.

Table 6.5 Illustrates the factors affecting gastric acid secretion.

Soll A. Physiology of gastric acid secretion. In: Basow DS (ed), UpToDate. Waltham, MA: UpToDate, 2010. http://www.uptodate.com (Last accessed 1 May 2012).

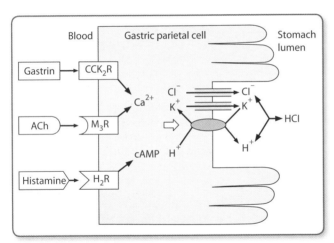

Figure 6.3 Gastric acid secretion from the parietal cell. ACh, acetylcholine; cAMP, cyclic adenosine monophosphate; CCK_2R, cholecystokinin receptor; H_2R, histamine receptor; M_3R, muscarinic receptor.

Table 6.5

Increase acid secretion	Decrease acid secretion
Basophilia – basophils produce histamine	Drugs – histamine-2 antagonists, proton pump inhibitors
Gastrinoma	
Small bowel resection	Hormones – cholecystokinin-pancreozymin (CCK-PZ), gastric inhibitory peptide (GIP), secretin, vasoactive intestinal peptide (VIP)
Systemic mastocytosis (increases histamine)	
	Low pH

Table 6.5 Factors affecting gastric acid secretion

20. E Vitamin C

Iron is absorbed in the duodenum by enterocytes of the duodenal lining and a well-nourished person will have between 4 and 5 g in their body. Most iron intake, be that from supplements or food, is in the Fe^{3+} form and only around 10% of that consumed is absorbed (more is absorbed from foods of animal origin compared to plant origin). **Table 6.6** illustrates the factors affecting iron absorption.

Hallberg L, Hulthén L. Perspectives on iron absorption. Blood Cells Mol Dis 2002; 29(3):562–573.

Table 6.6	
Increase iron absorption	**Decrease iron absorption**
Gastric acid	Achlorhydria
Gastrointestinal blood loss	Coeliac disease
Increased erythropoiesis, e.g. pregnancy	Crohn's disease
Vitamin C	Drugs, e.g. desferrioxamine
	Partial/total gastrectomy

Table 6.6 Factors affecting iron absorption.

21. A *Bacillus cereus*

This is a case of gastroenteritis, which can be predominantly 'vomiting' or predominantly 'diarrhoea'. Options B, C and D are causes of diarrhoeal illness, which can also be bloody. This leaves option A and E as possible answers. Both *Bacillus cereus* and *Staphylococcus aureus* cause acute food poisoning, which manifests as severe vomiting, within 1–6 hours of ingestion of the offending food. What differentiates them is that with *Bacillus*, there are two types of illness:

- Vomiting within 1–6 hours, where the offending food is usually rice or noodles
- Diarrhoea with an incubation period of 6–14 hours

Table 6.7 shows the different bacterial causes of acute food poisoning, how they present and their incubation periods.

Most cases of food poisoning settle with rest and adequate hydration, and antibiotics tend not to be needed.

Acheson D. Differential diagnosis of microbial foodborne disease. In: Basow DS (ed), UpToDate. Waltham, MA: UpToDate, 2010. http://www.uptodate.com (Last accessed 1 May 2012).

22. A Achalasia

Dysphagia for both solids and liquids is the hallmark feature of achalasia. Other symptoms include heartburn and regurgitation of food (which can lead to coughing which is worse at night when lying supine and aspiration pneumonia) and weight loss. The typical 'bird's beak' appearance of the barium swallow seen in achalasia is described in the question.

Table 6.7

Cause	Clinical features	Incubation period (hours)
Bacillus cereus	Two types:	
	Vomiting (usually due to rice or noodles)	1–6
	Diarrhoea	6–14
Campylobacter jejuni	Flu like prodrome which is then followed by fever, abdominal cramps and diarrhoea (may be bloody)	48–72
Clostridium perfringens	Abdominal cramps and diarrhoea (usually after eating inadequately cooked meat)	6–24
Escherichia coli	Abdominal cramps, nausea, watery diarrhoea	12–48
Salmonella	Diarrhoea (usually after eating eggs or inadequately cooked poultry)	12–48
Shigella	Abdominal pain, bloody diarrhoea, vomiting	48–72
Staphylococcus aureus	Severe vomiting	1–6

Table 6.7 Causes of food poisoning.

With oesophageal cancer, there would be symptoms of weight loss, anorexia, vomiting during eating and a history of gastro-oesophageal reflux disease (GORD), Barrett's oesophagus, smoking or alcohol. The duration of symptoms also goes against this option.

Oesophageal candidiasis is associated with any form of immunosuppression, e.g. retroviral disease or steroid inhaler use, and the cardinal symptom is odynophagia.

Oesophagitis may present with heartburn and/or odynophagia (usually without weight loss).

Like achalasia, a pharyngeal pouch can present with dysphagia, heartburn, food regurgitation, aspiration and chronic cough so it can be difficult to differentiate the two. However, patients with a pharyngeal pouch often complain of food getting stuck high up in the throat and there may be halitosis and (if large) a midline neck lump that gurgles on palpation and drinking is seen.

Fass R. Evaluation of dysphagia in adults. In: Basow DS (ed), UpToDate. Waltham, MA: UpToDate, 2010. http://www.uptodate.com (Last accessed 1 May 2012).

23. E Weight loss

This patient has non-alcoholic steatohepatitis (NASH). It can vary from non-alcoholic fatty liver disease (NAFLD) at one end of the spectrum to cirrhosis at the other end. This patient has fatty inflammation of the liver (steatohepatitis) but no more significant liver damage (as characterised by fibrosis). There is currently no cure for

NASH and management involves controlling conditions associated with NASH such as obesity, hyperlipidaemia and diabetes mellitus:

- Lifestyle changes, like smoking cessation and particularly weight loss, improved histological disease activity
- Treatment of insulin resistance – thiazolidinediones like pioglitazone improved steatosis and inflammation but caused significant weight gain
- Polyunsaturated fatty acids (PUFA) ameliorate biochemical and radiological markers of NASH

There is ongoing debate as to whether weight-loss surgery like gastric banding has a role in the improvement of NASH.

Musso G, et al. A meta-analysis of randomized trials for the treatment of nonalcoholic fatty liver disease. Hepatol 2010; 52(1):79.

24. B Cardiomyopathy

This patient has haemochromatosis as evidenced by arthralgia, impotence (secondary to hypogonadism), heart failure (secondary to cardiomyopathy), arthropathy (secondary to crystal deposition), diabetes and cirrhosis (thrombocytopaenia, macrocytosis, deranged liver function tests and elevated international normalised ratio [INR]).

Table 6.8 shows the reversibility of the features of haemochromatosis.

Niederau C, et al. Long-term survival in patients with hereditary hemochromatosis. Gastroenterol 1996; 110(4):1107–1119.

Table 6.8	
Reversible (on venesection)	**Irreversible**
Cardiomyopathy	Liver cirrhosis
Skin pigmentation	Diabetes mellitus
Hepatomegaly	Hypogonadotrophic hypogonadism
	Arthropathy

Table 6.8 Reversibility of the features of haemochromatosis.

25. A Isoniazid

Helicobacter pylori is a gram-negative spiral bacillus associated with:

- Atrophic gastritis
- B-cell lymphoma of mucosa-associated lymphoid tissue (MALT) tissue
- Gastric adenocarcinoma
- Peptic ulcer disease (found in >90% of patients with duodenal ulcer, >70% with gastric ulcer)

There is currently no agreed treatment regimen. Amoxicillin seems to be the most important antibiotic and most resistance is to clarithromycin. Re-treatment should probably involve quadruple treatment: protein pump inhibitor + bismuth + amoxicillin + another antibiotic, e.g. metronidazole, tetracycline or rifampicin.

Ahuja V, et al. Efficacy and tolerability of rifampicin-based rescue therapy for *Helicobacter pylori* eradication failure in peptic ulcer disease. Dig Dis Sci 2005; 50:630–663.
Malfertheiner P, et al. *Helicobacter pylori* eradication with a capsule containing bismuth subcitrate potassium, metronidazole, and tetracycline given with omeprazole versus clarithromycin-based triple therapy: a randomised, open-label, non-inferiority, phase 3 trial. Lancet 2011; 377(9769):905–913.
Mirbagheri SA, et al. Triple, standard quadruple and ampicillin-sulbactam-based quadruple therapies for *H. pylori* eradication: A comparative three-armed randomized clinical trial. World J Gastroenterol 2006; 12 (30):4888–4891.

26. E Gastro-oesophageal reflux disease (GORD)

GORD is a risk factor for oesophageal carcinoma but not gastric carcinoma. Gastric carcinoma remains one of the commonest causes of cancer deaths despite the incidence in the Western world decreasing. This is because most patients have local spread of the disease at time of diagnosis, thus making curative resection unfeasible. The commonest site for cancer is in the pylorus but the incidence of tumours in the cardia is rising.

Risk factors include:

- Blood group A
- Hypo- and/or achlorhydria (chronic atrophic gastritis, hypertrophic gastritis, partial gastrectomy, pernicious anaemia)
- Diets high in salt or nitrites
- Family history of gastric carcinoma
- Gastric polyps
- *Helicobacter pylori* infection
- Japanese/Chinese ethnicity
- Smoking

Peleteiro B, et al. Salt intake and gastric cancer risk according to *Helicobacter pylori* infection, smoking, tumour site and histological type. Br J Cancer 2011; 104:198.
González CA, et al. Smoking and the risk of gastric cancer in the European Prospective Investigation Into Cancer and Nutrition (EPIC). Int J Cancer 2003; 107:629.

27. B CT abdomen

This is a case of chronic pancreatitis as characterised by the abdominal pain (radiating to the back and after meals), cachexia (malabsorption), steatorrhoea and diabetes mellitus. It is a chronic inflammatory condition that irreversibly affects the exocrine, and later the endocrine, function of the pancreas. The commonest cause is alcohol (80% of cases) and may occasionally be due to cystic fibrosis.

All of the options may be useful in making a diagnosis of chronic pancreatitis but CT is the most sensitive for detection of pancreatic calcification, which is highly suggestive of the disease. CT would also be useful to exclude pancreatic carcinoma in a patient with abdominal pain and losing weight. Plain X-ray is a useful initial investigation that may show speckled pancreatic calcification in 30–60% of patients. Endoscopic retrograde cholangiopancreatography (ERCP) and magnetic resonance cholangiopancreatography (MRCP) can show irregular dilatation and stricturing of the pancreatic ducts and look for stones in the ducts with a view to performing therapeutic procedures like pancreatic duct stent insertion in the former. Endoscopic ultrasound (EUS) is another investigation that is sensitive in diagnosing early and late changes of chronic pancreatitis but, like ERCP, is invasive. The faecal elastase test uses an enzyme-linked immunosorbent assay to measure the concentration of the elastase-3B enzyme found in faecal matter. Faecal elastase <200 μg/g of stool indicates exocrine insufficiency.

Shams J, Stein A, Cooperman AM. Computed tomography for pancreatic diseases. Surg Clin North Am 2001; 81(2):283–306.

28. D Prednisolone

The hepatocellular picture in the derangement of liver function tests, association with other autoimmune disorders (i.e. hypothyroidism) and hypergammaglobulinaemia point to a diagnosis of autoimmune hepatitis (AIH). The patient has an elevated globulin (protein minus albumin) which is also in keeping with AIH and useful for monitoring response to treatment.

There are three types of autoimmune hepatitis:

- Type 1 affecting adults and children – anti-nuclear antibody (ANA) and/or anti-smooth muscle antibody (SMA)
- Type 2 affecting children only – anti-liver kidney microsomal 1 (LKM) antibody
- Type 3 affecting middle-aged adults – anti-soluble liver/kidney antigen

Indications for therapy are shown in **Table 6.9**.

The mainstay of treatment is immunosuppressants either with steroids (prednisolone or budesonide) alone or in combination with azathioprine. Azathioprine takes about 3 months to exert its effects and can be used to maintain remission but cannot be used as monotherapy to induce remission.

Manns MP, et al. Diagnosis and management of autoimmune hepatitis. Hepatol 2010; 51(6):2193–2213.

Table 6.9

Absolute	Relative
ALT/AST >10 ULN	Symptoms (e.g. fatigue, arthralgia, jaundice)
ALT/AST >5 ULN and gamma globulin >2 ULN	ALT/AST <5 ULN and gamma globulin <2 ULN
Bridging or multi-acinar necrosis on biopsy	Interface hepatitis on biopsy
ALT, alanine transaminase; AST, aspartate transaminase; ULN, upper limit of normal.	

Table 6.9 Indications for therapy in autoimmune hepatitis, from the American Association for the Study of Liver Diseases.

29. E Topical mesalazine

This man appears to be having a mild flare up of his ulcerative colitis . He is already on oral mesalazine so the next most appropriate option would be rectal 5-ASA (aminosalicylic acid) or topical steroids. If this fails then one should consider oral steroids. As the patient does not complain of bloody diarrhoea, oral steroids do not need to be started right now. In patients who have recurrent flare ups, azathioprine can be used as a steroid-sparing agent to maintain remission; it does not induce remission. Metronidazole is of benefit in patients with Crohn's disease. Loperamide should not be given to patients with colitis because of the risk of developing toxic megacolon.

Faecal calprotectin is a useful test in this situation as an elevated result would be consistent with a flare up and could spare the patient from being subjected to a flexible sigmoidoscopy.

Marshall JK, Irvine EJ. Rectal aminosalicylate therapy for distal ulcerative colitis: a meta-analysis. Aliment Pharmacol Ther 1995; 9(3):293.

30. A Crypt abscesses

Table 6.10 illustrates the differences between Crohn's disease and ulcerative colitis.

Abraham C, Cho J. Inflammatory bowel disease. N Engl J Med 2009; 361:2066–220.

Table 6.10		
	Crohn's disease	**Ulcerative colitis**
Mucosal involvement	Transmural inflammation	Inflammation confined to the mucosa and submucosa
Inflammatory infiltrate	Neutrophil infiltrates	Inflammatory cell infiltrate in lamina propria
Architecture	Fissuring ulcers ('rose-thorn ulcers')	Crypt abscesses
Imaging	'Cobblestoning', skip lesions	'Pseudopolyps'
Presence of granuloma	Non-caseating granuloma	Rare

Table 6.10 Differences between Crohn's disease and ulcerative colitis.

Chapter 7

Haematology and oncology

1. A 55-year-old Caucasian woman presented to her general practitioner with tiredness and shortness of breath on exertion, worsening over the past 6 months. On examination, she had conjunctival pallor, but chest, cardiovascular and abdominal examinations were otherwise unremarkable.

   Investigations:

haemoglobin	90 g/L (115–165)
mean cell volume	110 fL (80–96)
white cell count	6.8×10^9/L (4.0–11.0)
platelet count	340×10^9/L (150–400)

   What is the least likely cause of this presentation?

   A B_{12} deficiency
   B Folate deficiency
   C Iron deficiency
   D Myelodysplasia
   E Myxoedema

2. Which one of the following features on a blood film is most consistent with iron deficiency anaemia?

   A Bite cell
   B Helmet cell
   C Oval cell
   D Pencil cell
   E Teardrop cell

3. Which one of the following is considered to be a good prognostic indicator in acute myeloid leukaemia (AML)?

   A Age > 60 years
   B Deletions of chromosome 5 or 7
   C History of myelodysplasia or other preleukaemic condition
   D Translocation (8;21)
   E Translocation (9;22)

4. A 25-year-old man presented to the emergency department with fever and shortness of breath. He described a 4-week history of general weakness, epistaxis and easy fatiguability. He had no significant past medical history and no history of recent travel. On examination, he had evidence of gingival bleeding, pallor and had multiple ecchymoses on his trunk and limbs. His temperature was 39.0°C, pulse 130 beats per minute, blood pressure 90/50 mmHg, respiratory rate 35 breaths per minute and oxygen saturation 94% on 5 L/minute of oxygen. He had bilateral coarse crackles on chest examination.

Investigations:

haemoglobin	78 g/L (130–180)
mean cell volume	89 fL (80–96)
white cell count	2.1×10^9/L (4.0–11.0)
neutrophil count	0.8×10^9/L (1.5–7.0)
platelets	40×10^9/L (150–400)
international normalised ratio	1.6 (<1.4)
D-dimer	2.0 mg/L (<0.5)
fibrinogen	1.2 g/L (1.8–5.4)
blood film	multiple helmet cells
bone marrow aspirate	auer rods and faggot cells

What is the most appropriate treatment for this patient?

A   All-trans retinoic acid (ATRA)
B   Arsenic trioxide
C   Chlorambucil
D   Imatinib
E   Methylprednisolone

5. An 18-year-old man presented to the emergency department with a large haemarthrosis in the left knee that developed after he was tripped playing football.

Investigations:

haemoglobin	131 g/L (130–180)
international normalised ratio	1.0 (<1.4)
prothrombin time	12 s (11.5–15.5)
activated partial thromboplastin time	65 s (30–40)
bleeding time	7 min (3–8)
factor VIIIc activity	normal

What is the most likely diagnosis?

A   Antiphospholipid syndrome
B   Factor VII deficiency
C   Haemophilia A
D   Haemophilia B
E   von Willebrand's disease

6. Which one of the following investigations is the most useful marker of prognosis in myeloma?

   A   Albumin
   B   Alkaline phosphatase (ALP)
   C β_2-microglobulin
   D   C-reactive protein (CRP)
   E   Lactate dehydrogenase (LDH)

7. Which one of the following types of Hodgkin's lymphoma (HL) is associated with the best prognosis?

   A   Lymphocyte depleted classical HL
   B   Lymphocyte rich classical HL
   C   Mixed cellularity classical HL
   D   Nodular lymphocyte predominant HL
   E   Nodular sclerosis classical HL

8. Which one of the following conditions is least likely to cause a warm autoimmune haemolytic anaemia?

   A   Chronic lymphocytic leukaemia
   B   *Mycoplasma* infection
   C   Non-Hodgkin's lymphoma
   D   Penicillin therapy
   E   Systemic lupus erythematosus (SLE)

9. A 20-year-old woman presented with one week of recurrent nose bleeds. She had no past medical history of note, and took no regular medications. Examination revealed normal physical observations, some scattered petechiae over her arms and legs, but no evidence of lymphadenopathy or hepatosplenomegaly.

   Investigations:

haemoglobin	129 g/L (115–165)
mean cell volume	89 fL (80–96)
white cell count	6.2×10^9/L (4.0–11.0)
platelet count	8×10^9/L (150–400)
international normalised ratio	1.0 (<1.4)
blood film	isolated thrombocytopenia, no evidence of platelet clumping
HIV serology	negative
hepatitis C serology	negative
autoantibody screen	negative

   What is the most appropriate treatment?

   A   Azathioprine
   B   Intravenous immunoglobulin (IVIG)

    C   Prednisolone

    D   Recombinant human factor VIIa

    E   Splenectomy

10. A 78-year-old man underwent investigation after experiencing worsening lethargy for several months. He had no past medical history of note and took no regular medications. Examination revealed widespread lymphadenopathy and splenomegaly.

Investigations:

haemoglobin	134 g/L (130 – 180)
white cell count	27×10^9/L (4–11)
lymphocyte count	26×10^9/L (1.5–4.0)
platelet count	172×10^9/L (150–400)
blood film	smudge cells

What is the most appropriate next investigation?

    A   Abdominal ultrasound

    B   Bone marrow aspiration

    C   Immunophenotyping

    D   Mutational analysis for immunoglobulin V_H gene (IgV_H)

    E   Serum β_2-microglobulin

11. Which virus is most closely associated with Burkitt's lymphoma?

    A   Cytomegalovirus

    B   Epstein–Barr virus

    C   Herpes simplex virus

    D   Human herpes virus 8

    E   Varicella zoster virus

12. A 78-year-old woman attended a routine anti-coagulation clinic appointment. She had received warfarin therapy for several years because of recurrent pulmonary emboli. Her other past medical history was of hypertension. Examination did not reveal any evidence of bleeding.

Investigations:

haemoglobin	141 g/L (115–165)
platelet count	392×10^9/L (150–450)
white cell count	6.8×10^9/L (4–11)
international normalised ratio	9.1 (<1.4)
serum albumin	42 g/L (37–49)

In addition to temporarily withholding warfarin, what is the most appropriate next step in management?

    A   Fresh frozen plasma

    B   Oral vitamin K

    C   Protamine

D   Prothrombin complex concentrate
E   Subcutaneous vitamin K

13. A 53-year-old man underwent investigation for 6 months of weight loss, sweating and abdominal pain. Examination revealed pallor and very marked splenomegaly.

Investigations:

haemoglobin	91 g/L (130–180)
mean cell volume	91 fL (80–96)
platelet count	588×10^9/L (150–450)
white cell count	104×10^9/L (4–11)

Blood film and differential:

lymphocytes	8% (20–40)
neutrophils	44% (40–60)
bands	13% (<3)
metamyelocytes	7% (<1)
myelocytes	15% (<1)
basophils	2.0% (0.5–1.0)
monocytes	10% (2–8)
eosinophils	1.0% (1.0–4.0)
bone marrow aspirate	hypercellular marrow with granulocytic predominance. All levels of granulocytic maturation noted

What is the most likely finding on genetic testing?

A   del(5q)
B   del(13q)
C   inv(16)
D   t(9; 22)
E   t(15; 17)

14. Which electrolyte abnormality is most commonly associated with massive blood transfusion?

A   Hypocalcaemia
B   Hypokalaemia
C   Hypomagnesaemia
D   Hyponatraemia
E   Hypophosphataemia

15. A 29-year-old woman underwent investigation for recurrent headache and was diagnosed with sagittal sinus thrombosis. She had a past medical history of deep vein thrombosis of her left leg 2 years ago, for which she was treated with anticoagulation for several months. Her mother had suffered from recurrent deep vein thromboses. She did not smoke, drink alcohol or use the oral contraceptive pill. Examination was normal.

Which of the following disorders is she least likely to be suffering from?

A Antithrombin III deficiency
B Factor V Leiden
C Protein C deficiency
D Protein S deficiency
E Prothrombin deficiency

16. A 23-year-old woman presented with several months of lethargy. She denied any gastrointestinal symptoms or menorrhagia. There was no past medical history of note, and she took no regular medications. Examination was normal.

Investigations:

haemoglobin	98 g/L (115–165)
mean cell volume	63 fL (80–96)
platelet count	284 × 10⁹/L (150–450)
white cell count	8.2 × 10⁹/L (4–11)
serum iron	14 mmol/L (12–30)
serum iron-binding capacity	50 mmol/L (45–75)
serum ferritin	47 mg/L (15–300)
blood film	hypochromic microcytic anaemia, occasional target cells

What is the most likely diagnosis?

A β-thalassaemia minor
B Congenital sideroblastic anaemia
C Copper deficiency
D Iron-deficiency anaemia
E Underlying chronic disease

17. A 59-year-old man underwent investigation for several months of pruritus. He described the pruritus as particularly marked when he had a bath. He had no past medical history of note, had never smoked, and felt otherwise well. Examination revealed a plethoric man with oxygen saturations of 99% on room air. He had splenomegaly.

Investigations:

haemoglobin	193 g/L (130–180)
haematocrit	0.59 (0.40–0.52)
platelet count	396 × 10⁹/L (150–450)
white cell count	10.4 × 10⁹/L (4–11)
neutrophil count	9.4 × 10⁹/L (1.5–7.0)
erythrocyte sedimentation rate	4 mm/1st hour (<20)
serum sodium	137 mmol/L (137–144)
serum potassium	4.3 mmol/L (3.5–4.9)
serum urea	5.3 mmol/L (2.5–7.0)
serum creatinine	88 mmol/L (60–110)
serum C-reactive protein	<5 mg/L (<10)

What is the most appropriate next investigation?

A   Abdominal ultrasound
B   Arterial blood gas
C   Bone marrow aspirate and trephine
D   Genetic screening for *JAK2* mutation
E   Serum erythropoietin level

18. A 31-year-old woman had recently undergone investigations for menorrhagia and had been diagnosed with von Willebrand's disease. Aside from the menorrhagia, she had no history of excessive bleeding. She was due to visit her dentist in 4 days time for a tooth extraction.

What would be the most appropriate bleeding prophylaxis for her extraction?

A   Desmopressin
B   Factor VIII concentrate
C   Protamine
D   Prothrombin complex concentrate
E   Vitamin K

19. An 80-year-old woman was referred for knee arthroscopy. She had no significant past medical history and felt completely well aside from knee problems. She underwent blood tests as part of routine pre-operative assessment.

Investigations:

haemoglobin	121 g/L (115–165)
platelet count	190 × 10⁹/L (150–450)
white cell count	28.0 × 10⁹/L (4–11)
lymphocyte count	27.1 × 10⁹/L (1.5–4.0)
blood film	smudge cells

Further investigations confirmed the diagnosis of chronic lymphocytic leukaemia

What is the most appropriate next step in management?

A   Alemtuzumab
B   Bone marrow transplantation
C   Chlorambucil
D   Continue with surgery, for regular follow-up in haematology clinic afterwards
E   Splenectomy

20. A 21-year-old man presented with several days of worsening nausea and rash. He was normally fit and well, although he described several days of blood-stained diarrhoea whilst backpacking in India 1 week earlier. On examination, he was afebrile and had a widespread petechial rash. His blood pressure was 192/102 mmHg.

Investigations:

haemoglobin	84 g/L (130–180)
white cell count	14.4 × 10⁹/L (4–11)
platelet count	46 × 10⁹/L (150–450)

reticulocyte count	280×10^9/L (25–85)
international normalised ratio	1.0 (<1.4)
blood film	multiple schistocytes
serum sodium	139 mmol/L (137–144)
serum potassium	5.4 mmol/L (3.5–4.9)
serum urea	13.4 mmol/L (2.5–7.0)
serum creatinine	222 mmol/L (106 mmol/L one year earlier) (60–110)
serum C-reactive protein	<5 mg/L (<10)
antineutrophil cytoplasmic antibodies	negative
anti nuclear antibodies	negative

What is the most likely diagnosis?

A   Antiphospholipid syndrome
B   Disseminated intravascular coagulopathy
C   Haemolytic–uraemic syndrome
D   Scleroderma renal crisis
E   Thrombotic thrombocytopenic purpura

21. A 74-year-old woman underwent investigation because of 3 months history of worsening lethargy, night sweats and abdominal pain. She had no past medical history of note and took no regular medications. Examination revealed pallor, hepatomegaly and massive splenomegaly.

Investigations:

haemoglobin	101 g/L (115–165)
white cell count	14.9×10^9/L (4–11)
platelet count	310×10^9/L (150–450)
blood film	leukoerythroblastic film with tear-drop poikilocytes

What is the most likely diagnosis?

A   Bacterial sepsis
B   β-thalassaemia major
C   Chronic lymphocytic leukaemia
D   Myelodysplastic syndrome
E   Myelofibrosis

22. Which one of the following is not a cause for Howell–Jolly bodies on a blood film?

A   Chronic myeloid leukaemia
B   Coeliac disease
C   Multiple myeloma
D   Sickle cell anaemia
E   Splenectomy

23. A 77-year-old man was admitted to hospital with a swollen leg, and diagnosed with a deep vein thrombosis. He reported feeling unwell for several months, with

symptoms including weight loss, night sweats and lethargy. He had no other past medical history of note and took no regular medications. Examination revealed generalised lymphadenopathy.

Investigations:

haemoglobin	103 g/L (130–180)
white cell count	5.6 × 10⁹/L (4–11)
platelet count	180 × 10⁹/L (150–450)
serum sodium	139 mmol/L (137–144)
serum potassium	4.1 mmol/L (3.5–4.9)
serum urea	4.7 mmol/L (2.5–7.0)
serum creatinine	102 mmol/L (60–110)
serum corrected calcium	2.5 mmol/L (2.2–2.6)
serum immunoglobulin G	8.0 g/L (6–13)
serum immunoglobulin A	2.1 g/L (0.8–3.0)
serum immunoglobulin M	11.8 g/L (0.4–2.5)
serum electrophoresis	monoclonal immunoglobulin M protein

What is the most likely diagnosis?

A   Chronic lymphocytic leukaemia
B   Chronic myeloid leukaemia
C   Monoclonal gammopathy of uncertain significance
D   Multiple myeloma
E   Waldenström's macroglobulinaemia

24. A 18-year-old man presented with several days of worsening abdominal pain. He was known to have sickle cell anaemia. Examination revealed pallor, marked splenomegaly and tenderness in the left upper quadrant of the abdomen.

Investigations:

haemoglobin	92 g/L (130–180)
mean cell volume	104 fL (80–96)
white cell count	4.8 × 10⁹/L (4–11)
platelet count	164 × 10⁹/L (150–450)
reticulocyte count	134 × 10⁹/L (25–85)

What is the most likely diagnosis?

A   Aplastic crisis
B   Gastritis
C   Papillary necrosis
D   Sequestration crisis
E   Vaso-occlusive crisis

25. A 30-year-old woman was 32 weeks pregnant with her second child. She attended antenatal clinic and underwent routine tests. Her pregnancy had been uncomplicated to date and she felt completely well. The only past medical history she gave was of thrombocytopenia during her first pregnancy, which resolved fully

after delivery of the child. She had no family history of note and took no regular medications. Her last child had a full blood count performed shortly after birth, which was normal. Examination revealed normal blood pressure and no evidence of bruising.

Investigations:

haemoglobin	115 g/L (115–165)
mean cell volume	95 fL (80–96)
white cell count	9.9×10^9/L (4–11)
platelet count	79×10^9/L (180×10^9/L one year earlier) (150–450)
reticulocyte count	82×10^9/L (25–85)
international normalised ratio	1.0 (<1.4)
blood film	isolated thrombocytopenia, no platelet clumping
serum urea	5.4 mmol/L (2.5–7.0)
serum creatinine	80 mmol/L (60–110)
serum alanine aminotransferase	31 U/L (5–35)
serum alkaline phosphatase	104 U/L (45–105)
urine dipstick	negative

What is the most likely diagnosis?

A Disseminated intravascular coagulopathy
B Gestational thrombocytopenia
C HELLP syndrome
D Pre-eclampsia
E Thrombotic thrombocytopenic purpura

26. A 51-year-old woman presented with 3 months of progressive dyspnoea. She had a past medical history of Hodgkin's lymphoma, which had been successfully treated with chemotherapy and radiotherapy 30 years earlier. She had never smoked. Examination revealed radiotherapy changes to the skin, and signs consistent with a right sided pleural effusion.

Investigations:

chest X-ray	moderate right sided pleural effusion
pleural fluid cytology	multiple lymphocytes, adenocarcinoma cells

Which one of the following is the most likely cause of the pleural effusion?

A Carcinoma of the breast
B Carcinoma of the oesophagus
C Carcinoma of the thyroid
D Meig's syndrome
E Recurrent lymphoma

27. A 27-year-old man presented to the emergency department with several hours of fevers and chills. He had recently been diagnosed with acute myeloid leukaemia, and completed his first course of chemotherapy 10 days earlier. He had no other past medical history of note. Examination revealed a temperature of 38.6°C, pulse 104 beats per minute and blood pressure 104/82 mmHg. The patient was pale and had scattered purpura on his arms, but the rest of the general examination was normal. Ten days earlier his neutrophil count was 1.5×10^9/L (1.5–7.0). Blood tests including cultures had just been taken.

What is the most appropriate next step in management?

A   Immediate intravenous aciclovir
B   Immediate intravenous amphotericin
C   Immediate intravenous filgrastim
D   Immediate intravenous piperacillin–tazobactam and amikacin
E   Regular paracetamol pending neutrophil count result

28. A 32-year-old man was recovering on the ward after resection of a testicular mass one day earlier.

Investigations:

histology of frozen section from mass	teratoma

Which one of the blood test combinations should be checked during the patient's recovery?

A   α-fetoprotein and β-human chorionic gonadotropin
B   α-fetoprotein and β_2-microglobulin
C   α-fetoprotein and carbohydrate antigen (CA)125
D   β-human chorionic gonadotropin and β_2-microglobulin
E β_2-microglobulin and CA125

29. A 23-year-old man presented with several hours of vomiting and severe generalised muscular pain. He had recently been diagnosed with acute lymphoblastic leukaemia, and undergone the first course of chemotherapy with cyclophosphamide, vincristine, doxorubicin and dexamethasone one day earlier. Examination revealed diffuse muscular tenderness, but there was no evidence of synovitis or arthritis.

Investigations:

	Now	One day earlier
serum sodium	137 mmol/L	138 mmol/L (137–144)
serum potassium	5.7 mmol/L	4.3 mmol/L (3.5–4.9)
serum urea	12.3 mmol/L	5.4 mmol/L (2.5–7.0)
serum creatinine	178 mmol/L	104 mmol/L (60–110)
serum corrected calcium	2.0 mmol/L	2.4 mmol/L (2.2–2.6)
serum phosphate	1.9 mmol/L	1.1 mmol/L (0.8–1.4)
serum urate	0.64 mmol/L	0.34 mmol/L (0.23–0.46)
serum creatine kinase	190 U/L	88 U/L (24–195)

| urine dipstick | blood +1, protein +1 |
| urine microscopy | uric acid crystals |

What is the most likely diagnosis?

A   Dexamethasone-related rhabdomyolysis
B   Gout
C   Polymyositis
D   Tumour lysis syndrome
E   Vincristine toxicity

30. A 62-year-old woman complained of nausea and vomiting for the past 2 days. She had recently been diagnosed with carcinoma of the bladder, and had undergone her first cycle of cisplatin-based chemotherapy 3 days earlier. Despite taking regular ondansetron since the day of her chemotherapy, she had not noticed any improvement of her symptoms. Examination of her gastrointestinal system was normal.

What is the most appropriate next step in her management?

A   Cyclizine
B   Dexamethasone
C   Metoclopramide
D   Olanzapine
E   Prochlorperazine

Answers

1. C Iron deficiency

This patient has a macrocytic anaemia. **Table 7.1** shows the different causes of macrocytic anaemia divided into whether they involve megaloblastic or normoblastic bone marrow or specific haematological diseases.

Hoffbrand V, Provan D. ABC of clinical haematology. Macrocytic anaemias. BMJ 1997; 314(7078):430
Colon-Otero G, et al. A practical approach to the differential diagnosis and evaluation of the adult patient with macrocytic anemia. Med Clin North Am 1992; 76(3):581.

Table 7.1		
Megaloblastic	**Normoblastic**	**Haematological disease**
B_{12} deficiency	Alcohol	Aplastic anaemia
Folate deficiency	Liver disease	Myelodysplasia
Drugs – 'MACH'	Myxoedema	Myeloma
Methotrexate	Pregnancy	Myeloproliferative disorders
Azathioprine	Reticulocytosis	
Cytosine		
Hydroxycarbamide		

Table 7.1 Causes of macrocytic anaemia.

2. D Pencil cells

Red blood cells should appear essentially round and have a smooth contour. Abnormalities in red cell shape are called poikilocytosis and this can signify pathology, as shown in **Table 7.2**.

Rosenthal D. Evaluation of the peripheral blood smear. In: Basow DS (ed), UpToDate. Waltham, MA: UpToDate, 2011. http://www.uptodate.com (Last accessed 1 May 2012).
Bain BJ. Diagnosis from the blood smear. N Engl J Med 2005; 353(5):498.

3. D Translocation (8;21)

Prognostic indicators for acute myeloid leukaemia are summarised in **Table 7.3**.

Appelbaum FR, et al. The clinical spectrum of adult acute myeloid leukaemia associated with core binding factor translocations. Br J Haematol 2006; 135(2):165.
Schiffer C. Prognosis of acute myeloid leukaemia. In: Basow DS (ed), UpToDate. Waltham, MA: UpToDate, 2012. http://www.uptodate.com (Last accessed 1 May 2012).

Table 7.2

Shape of cell	Associated condition(s)
Bite cell	G6PD deficiency
Burr cell	Uraemia
Elliptocyte	Hereditary elliptocytosis
Helmet cell	Microangiopathic haemolytic anaemia, e.g. DIC, HUS, TTP
Oval cell	Megaloblastic anaemia
Pencil cell	Iron deficiency anaemia
Sickle cell	Sickle cell anaemia
Spur cell	Liver disease
Target cell	Iron deficiency anaemia, liver disease, post-splenectomy, thalassaemia and haemoglobinopathies

DIC, disseminated intravascular coagulation; G6PD, glucose-6-phosphate dehydrogenase; HUS, haemolytic uraemic syndrome; TTP, thrombotic thrombocytopaenic purpura.

Table 7.2 Poikilocytosis and their disease associations.

Table 7.3

Type of indicator	GOOD	BAD
Age	< 50	> 60
Cytogenetics	Hyperdiploidy, inv (16) (AML M4), t(8;21) (AML M2)	deletions of chromosome 5 or 7, Philadelphia translocation (9;22)
Tumour characteristics	MDR-1 phenotype negative	MDR-1 phenotype positive
Gene mutations	*NPM1* *CEBPA*	*FLT3/ITD* *IDH1* and/or *IDH2* *MLL* partial tandem duplication *BAALC* overexpression
Response to chemotherapy		> 20% blasts after first course of chemotherapy
Performance status- Karnofsky score (%)	> 60	< 60
History of prior preleu- kaemic condition	No	Yes
History of prior chemo- or radiotherapy	No	Yes

BAALC, brain and acute leukaemia, cytoplasmic; CEBPA, CCAAT enhancer binding protein alpha; FLT, FMS-like tyrosine kinase receptor; IDH, isocitrate dehydrogenase; ITD, internal tandem duplication; MDR, multi drug resistant; MLL, myeloid/lymphoid; NPM, nucleophosmin.

Table 7.3 Prognostic indicators for acute myeloid leukaemia (AML).

4. A All-trans retinoic acid (ATRA)

This man has acute promyelocytic leukaemia (APL), which is the M3 subtype in the French–American–British (FAB) classification of acute leukaemia. It tends to present earlier than other types of acute myloid leukaemia (average age 25) and often includes disseminated intravascular coagulation or thrombocytopenia at first presentation.

Figure 7.1 shows the appearance of Auer rods on a blood film.

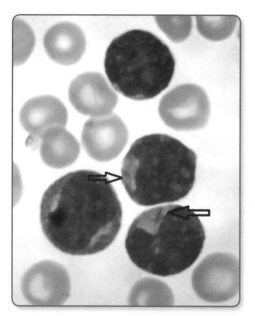

Figure 7.1 Auer rods on a blood film. These are collections of granular material that clump together in the shape of a needle and are found in the cytoplasm of leukaemic blast cells of acute myeloid leukaemia.

95% of APL cases are associated with a chromosomal translocation, i.e. t(15;17), involving the retinoic acid receptor-alpha (RARα) gene on chromosome 17. Most of the leukaemic cells are abnormal hypergranular promyelocytes.

Diagnosis is made from cytogenetic analysis of peripheral blood or bone marrow looking for the *PML/RARα* fusion gene. It is important to recognise the diagnosis early because the prognosis is good if correctly managed. ATRA should be started without delay to induce remission as soon as acute promyelocytic leukaemia is suspected even before cytogenetic confirmation of the diagnosis because there is a high-risk of mortality from haemorrhage due to the coagulopathy. Arsenic trioxide is currently being studied in combination with ATRA for treatment in relapsed/refractory disease.

Tallman MS, Altman JK. How I treat acute promyelocytic leukemia. Blood 2009; 114(25):5126.

5. D Haemophilia B

Table 7.4 shows the different coagulation profiles expected for each of the above diseases:

Hoots WK, Shapiro AD. Clinical manifestations and diagnosis of hemophilia. In: Basow DS (ed), UpToDate. Waltham, MA: UpToDate, 2011. http://www.uptodate.com (Last accessed 1 May 2012).

Table 7.4

Disease	PT*	BT	APTT*	Factor VIIIc activity
Antiphospholipid syndrome	Normal	Normal	High	Normal
Factor VII deficiency	High	Normal	Normal	Normal
Haemophilia A (Factor VIII deficiency)	Normal	Normal	High	Low
Haemophilia B (Factor IX deficiency)	Normal	Normal	High	Normal
von Willebrand's disease	Normal	High	High/Normal	Low/Normal

PT, prothrombin time; BT, bleeding time; APTT, activated partial thromboplastin time.
* When an abnormality is detected in the PT or APTT the tests are repeated with a 50:50 mix of test and normal plasma: straightforward factor deficiencies will correct with mixing, but inhibitors (e.g. lupus anticoagulant in antiphospholipid syndrome) do not correct.

Table 7.4 Coagulation profiles for the different blood disorders.

6. C β_2-microglobulin

Table 7.5 shows the variables included in the international staging system for multiple myeloma, which can be used to predict survival.

Greipp PR, et al. International Staging System for multiple myeloma. J Clin Oncol 2005; 23(15):3412–3420.

Table 7.5

Stage	Criteria	Median survival (months)
I	β_2-microglobulin < 3.5 mg/L + albumin > 35 g/L	62
II	$3.5 \leq \beta_2$-microglobulin ≤ 5.5 mg/L	44
III	β_2-microglobulin > 5.5 mg/L	29

Table 7.5 International staging system for multiple myeloma.

7. B Lymphocyte rich classical HL

Table 7.6 shows the differences between the four types of classical Hodgkin's lymphoma (HL) and the other major sub-group of HL (nodular lymphocyte predominant HL).

Swerdlow SH, et al. WHO classification of Tumors of Haematopoietic and Lymphoid Tissues. Lyon: IARC Press, 2008.
Aster JC. Epidemiology, pathologic features, and diagnosis of classical Hodgkin lymphoma. In: Basow DS (ed), UpToDate. Waltham, MA: UpToDate, 2011. http://www.uptodate.com (Last accessed 1 May 2012).

Table 7.6

WHO classification type	How common	Prognosis
Lymphocyte depleted classical HL	<1%	Worst
Lymphocyte rich classical HL	5%	Best
Mixed cellularity classical HL	20%	Good
Nodular sclerosis classical HL	70%	Good
Nodular lymphocyte predominant HL	5%	Good

Table 7.6 Different types of Hodgkin's lymphoma (HL).

8. B *Mycoplasma* infection

Autoimmune haemolytic anaemia can be described as warm or cold depending on the temperature that the antibodies cause haemolysis. **Table 7.7** shows the different causes:

Johnson ST, et al. One center's experience: the serology and drugs associated with drug-induced immune hemolytic anemia – a new paradigm. Transfusion 2007; 47(4):697.
Horwitz CA, et al. Cold agglutinins in infectious mononucleosis and heterophil-antibody-negative mononucleosis-like syndromes. Blood 1977; 50(2):195.

Table 7.7

	Warm	Cold
Temperature at which antibodies cause haemolysis	Body temperature	4°C
Antibody	IgG	IgM
Where haemolysis occurs	Extravascular	Intravascular
Causes	Autoimmune disease, e.g. SLE Drugs – penicillin/penicillin derivatives, cephalosporins, interferon, levodopa, methyldopa, quinine/quinidine and some NSAIDs Immune deficiency syndromes, e.g common variable immunodeficiency Neoplasia, e.g. CLL, NHL	Infections – EBV, mycoplasma Haematological disease, e.g. Waldenström's macroglobulinaemia Neoplasia, e.g. lymphoma

CLL, chronic lymphocytic leukaemia; EBV, Epstein–Barr virus; NHL, non-Hodgkin's lymphoma; NSAIDs, non-steroidal anti-inflammatory drugs; SLE, systemic lupus erythematosus.

Table 7.7 Differences between warm and cold autoimmune haemolytic anaemia.

9. C Prednisolone

Immune (idiopathic) thrombocytopaenia (also known as immune [idiopathic] thrombocytopaenic purpura [ITP]) is a condition characterised by an isolated thrombocytopaenia in the absence of any identifiable precipitant. The exact pathogenesis is unclear, although it is understood to be an autoimmune condition. The onset of disease may be triggered by exposure to certain drugs or viruses that generate the production of the causative autoantibodies. ITP is a diagnosis of exclusion, with the diagnosis only made after other causes of isolated thrombocytopaenia have been excluded. This includes excluding leukaemia and myelodysplastic disease (through the full blood count and blood film), viral causes (especially HIV and hepatitis C) and autoimmune causes (e.g. SLE).

Although there is some debate as to which patients require treatment, most haematologists would recommend treating patients with a platelet count $< 30 \times 10^9$/L and/or recurrent mucosal bleeding. Guidelines recommend that corticosteroids are the most effective first-line therapy in this scenario, and hence option C is the correct answer here. Intravenous immunoglobulin would be the appropriate choice if the patient failed to respond to corticosteroids or if the patient was haemodynamically unstable because of bleeding attributed to ITP, but the normal physical observations and haemoglobin count go against this being a very significant bleed.

Other treatment options available in the scenario where patients have significant bleeding attributable to ITP include recombinant human factor VIIa and platelet transfusions. However, platelet transfusions must be administered with care, due to the risk of platelet haemolysis by the autoantibodies that cause the disease. Where ITP remains refractory to first-line therapies, other treatments that may be tried include immunosuppressants (including azathioprine and rituximab) and splenectomy.

Neunert C, et al. The American Society of Haematology 2011 evidence-based practice guideline for immune thrombocytopenia. Blood 2011; 117:4190–4207.

10. C Immunophenotyping

The combination of lymphadenopathy, splenomegaly, lymphocytosis and smudge cells on a blood film (**Figure 7.2**) is highly suggestive of chronic lymphocytic leukaemia (CLL). The most appropriate means of confirming the diagnosis is through immunophenotyping of lymphocytes in peripheral blood. Lymphocytic leukaemia cells characteristically co-express the T cell antigens CD5 and B cell antigens CD19, CD20 and CD23. Expression of CD38 is variable, and appears to have some prognostic influence.

Many patients with CLL do not require treatment, as the risks of treatment side effects may outweigh the possible benefits that may be derived. Bone marrow examination can give useful prognostic information, but is an invasive procedure with considerable associated morbidity. As such, most haematologists would now only perform a bone marrow aspirate if treatment was being imminently planned (to give information regarding prognosis), or if the patient presented with co-existing thrombocytopenia or anaemia (to help clarify whether this represented leukaemic progression into bone marrow or was autoimmune in nature). Other prognostic factors can be derived from

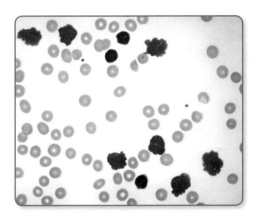

Figure 7.2 Smudge cells. These are lymphocytes whose cell membranes have broken in preparation of the blood film. They are most commonly associated with chronic lymphocytic anaemia.

molecular cytogenetics, mutational analysis (e.g. of the immunoglobulin V_H gene) and measurement of serum markers (e.g. β_2-microglobulin); however, these tests are only indicated as part of a pre-treatment work up, not as a means of establishing the diagnosis of CLL. Abdominal ultrasound would confirm the presence of splenomegaly, but would not help in making the diagnosis.

Gribben JC. How I treat CLL up front. Blood 2010; 115:187–197.
Hallek M, et al. Guidelines for the diagnosis and treatment of chronic lymphocytic leukaemia: a report from the International Workshop on Chronic Lymphocytic Leukaemia updating the National Cancer Institute-Working Group 1996 guidelines. Blood 2008; 111:5446–5456.

11. B Epstein–Barr virus

Burkitt's lymphoma is a group of very aggressive B-cell lymphomas. At the molecular level, these tumours appear to develop as a consequence of overexpression of the transcription factor c-myc. Epstein–Barr virus (EBV) is detectable in almost all African patients with Burkitt's lymphoma; the exact role for EBV in pathogenesis of Burkitt's lymphoma is not fully defined, but there is some evidence for EBV causing B cell expansion, chromosomal translocation, and consequently c-myc overexpression.

A number of viruses have been associated with haematological malignancies, particularly in immunosuppressed patients. These are summarised in the **Table 7.8**.

Klapproth K, Wirth T. Advances in the understanding of MYC-induced lymphomagenesis. Brit J Haematol 2010; 149 (4):484–497.

12. B Oral vitamin K

If no action is taken to correct this patient's excessive anticoagulation, then she is at significantly increased risk of the bleeding complications associated with warfarin. However, it is also recognised that overaggressive treatment to restore a raised INR back to normal can leave patients resistant to the effects of warfarin for between up to several weeks; this could risk the possibility of further pulmonary emboli.

Trials of using vitamin K in warfarinised patients with raised international normalised ratio (INR) but no bleeding have demonstrated that oral and intravenous vitamin K appear to be equally as effective as each other. Subcutaneous vitamin K produces

Table 7.8

Virus	Malignancy
Epstein–Barr (EBV)	Burkitt's lymphoma
	Nasopharyngeal carcinoma
	Non-Hodgkin's lymphoma
Human herpes virus 8 (HHV8)	Primary effusion (B-cell) lymphoma
	Castleman's disease
HIV	Non-Hodgkin's lymphoma
	Increased risk of EBV and HHV8 associated cancers
Human T-lymphotrophic virus 1 (HTLV1)	Adult T-cell leukaemia-lymphoma

Table 7.8 Viruses associated with haematological malignancies.

inconsistent degrees of correction of anticoagulation, and can result in haematoma formation, so it is not the preferred option. From the options given, oral vitamin K is the most appropriate choice.

Protamine is used in reversing the effect of heparin, but is not an antidote for warfarin.

A summary of the means by which raised INR and/or bleeding occurring in association with overtreatment of warfarin may be treated is provided in **Figure 7.3**.

Ansell J, et al. Pharmacology and management of the vitamin K antagonists: American College of Chest Physicians Evidence-Based Clinical Practice Guidelines, 8th Edition. Chest 2008; 133:160S– 198S.

13. D t(9;22)

Chronic myeloid leukaemia (CML) is a myeloproliferative disease characterised by huge proliferation of cells in the granulocytic series. The typical presentation is with constitutional symptoms (including weight loss, sweating and fever), although some cases may be detected incidentally during blood tests for other reasons. Characteristic examination findings include huge splenomegaly, along with signs related to bone marrow failure (such as clinical anaemia, purpura as a result of thrombocytopaenia, etc). Less commonly, patients may present with features relating to hyperuricaemia (e.g. gout) or leucostasis (e.g. visual difficulties). The full blood count typically shows a profound leucocytosis (often in excess of 100 x 10^9 cells/L), with the full range of granulocytic cells being detectable; this is often accompanied by a normocytic anaemia and a raised platelet count, although thrombocytopaenia may also occur in some cases. Bone marrow findings are as described in the question.

One distinctive feature of CML is the very consistent chromosomal abnormality associated with it. The key event in the pathogenesis of the disease in at least 95% of cases appears to be a reciprocal chromosomal translocation between chromosomes 9 and 22 in a haematopoietic stem cell, the so-called 'Philadelphia chromosome'. The break on chromosome 22 occurs in the breakpoint cluster region

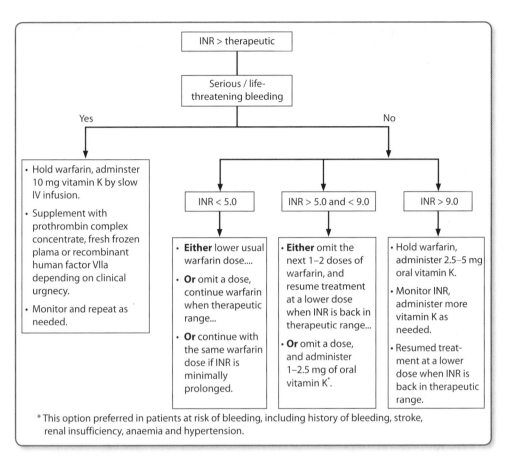

Figure 7.3 Correction of raised international normalised ratio (INR) and/or bleeding secondary to overtreatment with warfarin. (Adapted from American College of Chest Physicians evidence-based clinical practice guidelines.)

(BCR), whilst the fragment from chromosome 9 that joins the BCR carries the ABL oncogene. The ABL oncogene forms a chimeric gene with the remaining part of the BCR, with the gene encoding a protein with tyrosine kinase activity. This BCR-ABL tyrosine kinase protein has a number of effects upon cellular differentiation that ultimately results in the leucocytosis that characterises CML. Any of a number of different molecular biology techniques may be used to detect this t(9; 22) mutation.

The mainstay of treatment in CML is with therapy that inhibits the tyrosine kinase activity of the BCR-ABL fusion protein, such as imatinib. However, such treatments appear to 'hold' the disease rather than cure it, and the natural history of CML is to progress to an accelerated/blast phase after approximately five years; the prognosis from this point is very poor. The only treatment that appears to be a feasible complete cure for the majority of patients is allogeneic stem cell transplantation.

The genetic abnormalities that form the other options for this question relate to other haematological diseases. Deletion of the long arm of chromosome 5 del(5q) is found in approximately 30% of those with myelodysplasia. Translocation between chromosome 15 and 17 t(15;17) is typical of acute promyelocytic leukaemia, a particular form of acute myeloid leukaemia (AML). Inversion of chromosome 16 inv(16) may also be found in certain forms of AML, whilst deletion of the long arm of 13q del(13q) has been found to be a poor prognostic marker in those with multiple myeloma.

Faderl S, et al. The biology of chronic myeloid leukaemia. N Engl J Med 1999; 341(3):164–172.

14. A Hypocalcaemia

Massive blood transfusion is defined as transfusion as more than 100% of a person's circulating blood volume in less than 24 hours. As well as the risks intrinsic to any transfusion of blood products (e.g. wrong component transfused), there are some complications specific to massive blood transfusion (**Table 7.9**).

Stainsby D, et al. Guidelines on the management of massive blood loss. Brit J Haematol 2006; 135(5):634–641.

Table 7.9		
Complication	**Details**	**Treatment**
Coagulopathy	Transfusion of large volumes of colloid/red blood cells may have a dilutional effect on plasma coagulation proteins/platelet count	Frequent monitoring of coagulation profile, and use of fresh frozen plasma, platelet transfusion, etc, as required
Hypocalcaemia	• Donated red blood cells are stored mixed with citrate as an anticoagulant. Citrate is a calcium chelator • Clinical manifestations of hypocalcaemia (e.g. tetany) and associated arrhythmias may be seen in severe cases • Citrate is metabolised by the liver, so especially a risk in patients with liver disease	Calcium chloride or calcium gluconate may be required
Hyperkalaemia	• Potassium slowly leaks out of the cytoplasm of red blood cells in storage • Patients with renal failure are particularly at risk	In patients at risk of hyperkalaemia, consider: • Red blood cells less than 5 days in storage • 'Washed' red blood cells (to remove extracellular potassium)
Metabolic alkalosis	May occur through the metabolism of citrate to bicarbonate	
Hypothermia	Blood products are stored chilled to prolong shelf-life	Prevented by transfusing products through a blood warmer

Table 7.9 Metabolic complications of massive blood transfusion.

15. E Prothrombin deficiency

The description of a young woman with two episodes of venous thrombosis from a family with a history of recurrent thrombosis strongly raises the possibility that she is suffering from an inherited thrombophilia. The major causes of inherited thrombophilia are:

- Antithrombin III deficiency.
- Factor V Leiden – the most common inherited thrombophilia, accounting for approximately 50% of all cases. This is a mutation to the Factor V gene (the 'Leiden mutation') that renders the protein resistant to the actions of activated protein. Since activated protein C normally acts to inhibit factor V, this mutation is associated with factor V over activity and hence a pro-coagulant state.
- Protein C deficiency.
- Protein S deficiency.
- Prothrombin gene mutation (G20210A) – the second most common cause inherited thrombophilia, accounting for approximately 10% of all cases. This mutation to the prothrombin gene is associated with overactivity of prothrombin, and hence a procoagulant state.

Whilst certain mutations to the prothrombin gene are associated with overactivity of the protein, other mutations are associated with deficiency of either the amount or the activity of the prothrombin synthesised ('hypoprothrombinaemia'). This latter group of mutations are associated with a propensity to excessive bleeding, making E the correct answer.

Antithrombin III, protein C and protein S deficiencies are diagnosed by laboratory immunological assays, whilst Factor V Leiden and prothrombin gene mutations are diagnosed by direct analysis of DNA. Most laboratories will also perform a number of additional tests as part of a 'thrombophilia screen', including for antiphospholipid antibodies, lupus anticoagulant, and, especially if arterial thrombosis has occurred, for hyperhomocysteinaemia.

Dahlbäck B. Advances in understanding pathogenic mechanisms of thrombophilic disorders. Blood 2008; 112:19–27.

16. A β-thalassaemia minor

Table 7.10 explains how iron studies can be used to help differentiate different causes of microcytic anaemia from each other.

The normal iron studies in this patient mean that an underlying haemoglobinopathy is the most likely explanation for the microcytic anaemia (option A). The thalassaemias are a collection of genetic disorders characterised by reduced or absent formation of the α or β-globin chains of haemoglobin, with the severity of the anaemia depending upon the exact mutations present. They are particularly found in people from the Mediterranean, Middle East, central Asia or the Far East. β-thalassaemia minor is an autosomal recessive condition, sufferers of which usually often experience only mild symptoms from their anaemia. The diagnosis of β-thalassaemia minor is usually first suspected from the finding of a microcytosis that seems out of proportion with the degree of anaemia present, as is the case here. Target cells may be seen on the blood film. The diagnosis is confirmed by haemoglobin electrophoresis, with HbA2 being > 3.5%. No treatment is usually required.

Rund D, Rachmilewitz E. Beta-thalassemia. N Engl J Med 2005; 353(11):1135–1146.

Table 7.10

	Iron-deficiency anaemia	Haemoglo-binopathies	Anaemia of chronic disease	Sideroblastic anaemia
Causes	• Poor dietary intake • Malabsorption – coeliac disease, atrophic gastritis, etc. • Excessive iron loss – menorrhagia, GI bleeding, hookworm infestation • Increased iron requirements – e.g. growth, pregnancy	Principally: • Sickle cell disease • Thalassaemia syndromes	Any cause of chronic disease may result in microcytic or normocytic anaemia	Conditions in which sideroblasts (nucleated erythrocyte precursors) are unable to metabolise iron normally. • Congenital – usually X-linked • Acquired – e.g. alcohol excess, drugs, copper deficiency, lead poisoning
Serum iron	Reduced	Normal	Reduced	Increased
Total iron binding capacity	Raised	Normal	Reduced	Normal
Ferritin	Reduced	Normal	Normal or increased	Increased
Other findings		Diagnosis usually confirmed by electro-phoresis	Ferritin may be increased as a reflection of underlying inflammation	Ring sideroblasts seen on examination of bone marrow

Table 7.10 Causes of microcytic anaemia

17. D Genetic screening for *JAK2* mutation

Polycythaemia rubra vera (PRV) is one of the myeloproliferative disorders, and is best characterised by an increased haemoglobin and red cell mass. The median age of onset is 60 years of age. Typical presenting features include pruritus (particularly found in relation to exposure to warm water) and the phenomenon of erythromelalgia. This is defined as a burning pain accompanied by pallor or cyanosis in the hands or feet, and appears to represent small vessel thrombosis in association with the disease. Other presentations can include thrombotic disorders or gastrointestinal complications (particularly peptic ulcer), although many cases are diagnosed during investigation for an incidental finding of a raised haemoglobin. Examination may reveal plethora as a consequence of the polycythaemia, with splenomegaly occurring in approximately 70% of cases.

Investigation of polycythaemia is a complex area. One of the particular difficulties is the large number of different causes of polycythaemia, haematological and otherwise (**Table 7.11**).

Table 7.11

Type of polycythaemia	Mechanism	Specific causes
Primary	Primary/clonal disorder	Polycythaemia rubra vera
Secondary	Chronic hypoxia (i.e. physiologically increased haemoglobin production)	• High altitude • Chronic lung/cardiac disease • Cigarette smoking
	Pathological erythropoietin overproduction	• Exogenous erythropoietin • Malignancy – renal cell carcinoma, hepatocellular carcinoma, uterine leiomyomas, etc.
Apparent	Reduced plasma volume	• Dehydration • Diuretics • 'Stress polycythaemia'

Table 7.11 Causes of polycythaemia.

However, this is an area that has undergone significant recent change. In particular, it is now recognised that the mutation *JAK2V617F* is present in approximately 95% of patients with polycythaemia rubra vera, and laboratory assays to detect this mutation are now widely available. As such, many current guidelines and diagnostic criteria now recommend that if the history and examination findings are very suggestive of PRV, and there is no obvious secondary cause for polycythaemia, then the next most appropriate investigation is assessing the patient for the presence of *JAK2* mutation.

If no mutation is detected, further investigation is necessary to decide if the patient is one of the few percent of patients with PRV that does not have the *JAK2* mutation, or if there is a secondary cause for polycythaemia. **Table 7.12** summarises the suitable investigations.

McMullin MF, et al. Amendment to the guideline for diagnosis and investigation of polycythaemia/erythrocytosis. Brit J Haematol 2007; 138(6): 821–822.
Vardiman JW, et al. The 2008 revision of the World Health Organisation (WHO) classification of myeloid neoplasms and acute leukaemia: rationale and important changes. Blood 2009; 114:937–951.

Table 7.12

Investigations for PRV	Investigations for secondary causes of polycythaemia
• Full blood count – raised platelet and leucocyte counts in approximately half of patients. Erythropoietin levels usually reduced • Red cell mass – if raised, helps to confirm the polycythaemia (rather than other causes of high blood counts) • Biochemistry – typical findings include raised neutrophil alkaline phosphatase, raised serum B_{12}/B_{12} binding capacity and raised urate • Bone marrow – characteristically hypercellular	• Arterial blood gas/lung function tests – to assess for chronic hypoxia • Abdominal ultrasound – to assess for occult malignancies

Table 7.12 Investigations for the cause of polycythaemia.

18. A Desmopressin

von Willebrand's disease is a disorder characterised by excessive bleeding, reflecting a qualitative and/or quantitative deficit in von Willebrand's factor (VWF). The majority of cases are inherited, although acquired forms are recognised too.

A number of different agents are used in the treatment of the disease. Desmopressin (an analogue of anti-diuretic hormone) acts to promote the release of VWF from the endothelial cells in which it is stored. There is a variety of different preparations available, including intranasal, subcutaneous and intravenous; all of these will increase VWF levels in plasma within several hours, although the degree to which they do so depends upon the amount used and the particular mutation/form of von Willebrand's disease that the patient has. The ability to administer the application intranasally or subcutaneously and for a quick response to be generated makes the ideal choice in this scenario, and hence option A is the correct answer. This would also be the correct choice for minor bleeding episodes.

The other major therapy is the use of the blood products containing von Willebrand's factor itself, including factor VIII concentrates and cryoprecipitate. These are extremely effective, but are expensive, can only be given intravenously, and require careful storage and preparation. They are particularly useful for patients with von Willebrand's disease who are undergoing a major bleed, as prophylaxis before significant surgery, or after failure of desmopressin. Other useful agents include antifibrinolytics (such as transexamic acid) and oestrogen therapy.

Prothrombin complex concentrates and vitamin K are useful for restoring the role of vitamin K dependent clotting factors (II, VII, IX and X), and are most often used in the context of bleeding related to warfarin overdose or decompensated liver disease; however, neither would be appropriate here. Protamine is useful in counteracting the anticoagulant effect of heparin, but has no role in increasing the concentration of von Willebrand's factor.

Nichols WL, et al. von Willebrand disease (VWD): evidence-based diagnosis and management guidelines, the National Heart, Lung, and Blood Institute (NHLBI) Expert Panel report (USA). Haemophilia 2008; 14(2):171–232.

19. D Continue with surgery, for regular follow-up in haematology clinic afterwards

One of the difficulties in managing chronic lymphocytic leukaemia (CLL) is that it has such a variable clinical spectrum – whilst many patients have disease with an indolent course, others suffer very rapid progression. CLL tends to affect elderly populations, and the treatments used for it may have a number of serious side effects; it is therefore important to be aware of factors associated with active and/ or advanced disease, so that treatment can be appropriately targeted at those who stand to benefit most. A range of different factors associated with more active disease may be established from the history, examination or investigations, and are summarised in **Table 7.13**.

Table 7.13	
Category	**Specific features of active and/or advanced disease**
History	Constitutional symptoms, including: • Unintentional weight loss (>10% of body weight lost within past 6 months) • Fatigue • Persistent fever (in the absence of other causes) • Night sweats (for > 1 month)
Examination	• Splenomegaly • Multiple sites of lymphadenopathy, or a single massive node (> 10 cm diameter)
Investigations	• Anaemia • Thrombocytopaenia • Progressive lymphocytosis (defined as 50% increase in less than 2 months, or 100% increase in less than 6 months) • High expression of CD38 on immunophenotyping • Unmutated immunoglobulin V_H (IgV_H) gene status • Diffuse involvement on bone marrow trephine

Table 7.13 Features of active and/or advanced chronic lymphocytic leukaemia.

Note that it is the rate at which the lymphocyte count increases over time – rather than the absolute degree of lymphocytosis at any single point – that is useful for establishing disease activity.

From the information given, this woman appears to have early disease. Most importantly of all, she has no symptoms – one of the key factors in deciding whether treatment is appropriate or not. A number of different trials have consistently found that there is no prolongation of survival of patients with the earliest stage of CLL treated with chemotherapy in comparison to those who are not given any treatment at all. Treating now would risk all the harm of medication side effects with no evidence that it would result in better disease control. As such, watchful waiting with regular follow-up in the haematology clinic is the most appropriate initial management for this patient. There is no obvious reason, why her surgery should not proceed.

All of the other options listed have a role in the treatment of CLL, but would not be appropriate at this point.

Gribben JC. How I treat CLL up front. Blood 2010; 115:187–197.
Hallek M et al. Guidelines for the diagnosis and treatment of chronic lymphocytic leukaemia: a report from the International Workshop on Chronic Lymphocytic Leukaemia updating the National Cancer Institute-Working Group 1996 guidelines. Blood 2008; 111:5446–5456.

20. C Haemolytic-uraemic syndrome

The blood count and blood film results are consistent with this man having a microangiopathic haemolytic anaemia (MAHA). This is a disease process whereby small blood vessels (such as those in the kidney) become lined with fibrin deposits and on which platelets aggregate, with erythrocytes becoming sheared as they pass through the narrowed vessels. There are a number of different causes.

Both anti-phospholipid syndrome and disseminated intravascular (DIC) are associated with thrombocytopaenia and may cause MAHA. However, the normal clotting screen denies these diagnoses – anti-phospholipid syndrome is usually accompanied by a prolonged activated partial thromboplastin time (APTT), whilst DIC is associated with both prothrombin time (PT) and APTT being significantly longer than usual. Scleroderma renal crisis is another cause of MAHA, but the lack of clinical features of systemic sclerosis and negative anti-nuclear antibodies (ANA) make this diagnosis unlikely (ANA is positive in up to 90% of cases of systemic sclerosis).

The other major group of conditions associated with MAHA are haemolytic-uraemic syndrome (HUS) and thrombotic thrombocytopaenic purpura (TTP). Clotting profiles are usually either normal (or at most show minor abnormalities) in both disorders. Differentiating these two conditions from each other can be difficult; current thought is that they represent different points on the same spectrum of disease. However, clinical clues can help to decide whether the condition at hand is more 'HUS-like' or 'TTP-like' (**Table 7.14**).

His illness came soon after dysenteric disease acquired in India, which may reflect *Escherichia coli* 0157 infection. There is severe kidney injury but no suggestion of neurological disease or fever. As such, the probable diagnosis is haemolytic-uraemic syndrome.

The typical blood film findings of microangiopathic haemolytic anaemia are illustrated in **Figure 7.4**.

Franchini M, Zaffanello M, Veneri D. Advances in the pathogenesis, diagnosis and treatment of thrombotic thrombocytopenic purpura and haemolytic uremic syndrome. Thromb Res 2006; 118(2): 177–184.

Table 7.14		
Category	**HUS**	**TTP**
Aetiopathogenesis	• Most strongly associated with infective diarrhoea, especially *Escherichia coli* 0157 dysentery, particularly in children. The most common cause of acute kidney injury in children • Many cases idiopathic	A number of different recognised triggers, including: • Vasculitis • Pregnancy/pre-eclampsia • Drugs, e.g. ciclosporin Many cases idiopathic
Clinical findings	• Microangiopathic haemolytic anaemia • Thrombocytopaenia • Acute kidney injury – normally much more severe in comparison to that of TTP	Classically, a pentad of: • Microangiopathic haemolytic anaemia • Thrombocytopaenia. • Fever • Neurological disease – a huge range, from the mild (e.g. irritability) to the serious (seizures, psychosis-like behaviour, etc.) • Acute kidney injury – normally mild in comparison to that in HUS ...Although it is rare in clinical practice to find more than three of these features together
Diagnosis	• Stool cultures for *Escherichia coli* 0157 are useful • Renal biopsy may be indicated in cases of diagnostic doubt	• Renal biopsy may be indicated in cases of diagnostic doubt
Treatment	Treatment of any underlying cause Fresh frozen plasma	Plasma exchange Renal replacement therapy

Table 7.14 Differentiating haemolytic-uraemic syndrome (HUS) from thrombotic thrombocytopaenic purpura (TTP).

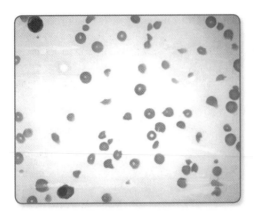

Figure 7.4 Microangiopathic haemolytic anaemia. Multiple red cell fragments may be noted on the film.

21. E Myelofibrosis

The history, examination and blood film findings are very suggestive of myelofibrosis. This is a myeloproliferative disorder characterised by clonal proliferation of the megakaryocytes that produce platelet-derived growth factor. As this proliferation continues, there is progressive fibrosis of the bone marrow and the development of extra medullary haematopoiesis. Whilst these extra medullary sites initially compensate for the function of bone marrow, they eventually begin to fail. As such, the disease has a poor prognosis, with survival usually less than two years from diagnosis.

The most common initial symptom in myelofibrosis is lethargy, although patients may also complain of fever, weight loss and night sweats. The major clinical finding is hepatomegaly and massive splenomegaly, with organomegaly becoming increasingly marked as extramedullary haematopoiesis progresses. The full blood count may show a raised white blood cell and platelet count early in the course of disease, although counts tend to drop as the disease progresses as a result of splenic sequestration, bleeding, and failure of extra medullary haematopoiesis. The finding that is most suggestive of myelofibrosis is the typical blood film result:

- Leukoerythroblastic blood films are those in which multiple immature blood cells (e.g. nucleated erythrocytes) are seen (**Figure 7.5**). These most commonly reflect bone marrow infiltration, either primary (e.g. fibrotic infiltration in myelofibrosis)

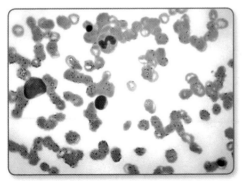

Figure 7.5 Leukoerythroblastic blood film. This film shows classical leucoerythroblastic features, including the presence of erythroblasts (primitive red blood cells, still containing nuclei) and myelocytes (early white blood cells).

or secondary (e.g. malignancy that has now metastasised to bone). This appearance may also be seen in critical illness (e.g. post-trauma, severe sepsis).
- Tear drop poikilocytes reflect extra-medullary haematopoiesis. These are most often seen in myelofibrosis, although may also been seen in thalassaemia. This patient's age and lack of prior medical history means that β-thalassaemia major is not the diagnosis here.

Other investigations also have a role in helping to confirm the diagnosis of myelofibrosis. Bone marrow aspiration is difficult because of marrow fibrosis, but marrow biopsy typically shows megakaryocyte proliferation and either reticulin or collagen fibrosis. *JAK2* mutations appear to be present in at least 40% of affected patients, and their presence in now part of many diagnostic criteria for the disease.

Vardiman JW, et al. The 2008 revision of the World Health Organisation (WHO) classification of myeloid neoplasms and acute leukaemia: rationale and important changes. Blood 2009; 114:937–951.

22. C Multiple myeloma

Howell–Jolly bodies are the name given to the presence of nuclear remnants in erythrocytes as seen on a blood film (**Figure 7.6**). Since such nuclear material is normally removed from erythrocytes by the spleen, their presence usually implies splenic dysfunction (hyposplenism). Other causes can reflect defects in erythropoiesis and include:

- Splenectomy
- Autosplenectomy – e.g. found eventually in almost all patients with sickle cell anaemia, as chronic sickling results in eventual splenic infarction
- Infiltrative disease – e.g. sarcoidosis, amyloidosis, lymphoma
- Gastrointestinal disease – e.g. 10% of patients with coeliac disease develop splenic atrophy. Also found in inflammatory bowel disease
- Myeloproliferative disease – the marked splenomegaly that accompanies these diseases results in eventual hyposplenism
- Defects in erythropoiesis – including myelodysplasia and megaloblastic anaemias
- Multiple myeloma is not a cause

Treatment of hyposplenism is with appropriate vaccination against encapsulated organisms, and prophylaxis for infection with daily antibiotics.

Bain BJ. Diagnosis from the blood smear. N Engl J Med 2005; 353(5):498.

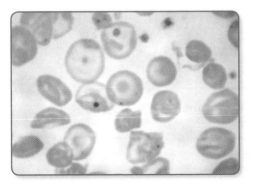

Figure 7.6 Howell–Jolly bodies.

23. E Waldenström's macroglobulinaemia

Waldenström's macroglobulinaemia is a low-grade lymphoma that is associated with IgM paraprotein production. It is most often found in the elderly, and slightly more common in men. Presenting features either relate to the underlying lymphoma (i.e. night sweats, weight loss, lymphadenopathy, hepatosplenomegaly, anaemia, etc) or to the presence of the paraprotein. In particular, the IgM paraprotein is associated with plasma hyperviscosity, and patients may present with features of a 'hyperviscosity syndrome':

- Limbs – deep vein thrombosis
- Central nervous system disease – including dizziness, headache, confusion and stroke-like syndromes
- Peripheral nervous system disease – typically a symmetrical distal sensorimotor peripheral neuropathy
- Retinal disease – visual disturbance may occur secondary to retinal vein thrombosis
- Excessive bleeding – despite the paraprotein causing an increased plasma viscosity, bleeding from the gums and easy bruising is frequently noted. This is believed to reflect the paraprotein interacting with glycoproteins on the surface of platelets and impairing their normal ability to aggregate

Although the serum immunoglobulin and electrophoresis results are very suggestive of Waldenström's macroglobulinaemia, examination of a bone marrow sample would be needed to confirm the diagnosis. Chronic lymphocytic leukaemia and chronic myeloid leukaemia are both unlikely, given the normal white blood cell count. Multiple myeloma is also unlikely, since this is almost always associated with paraproteins of IgG and IgA rather than IgM. Furthermore, renal and bone involvement are common in multiple myeloma but not in Waldenström's macroglobulinaemia, and this patient has a normal creatinine and corrected calcium. The diagnosis of monoclonal gammopathy of uncertain significance (MGUS) can only be made where there is only a small amount of paraprotein detectable and no features consistent with lymphoma – the presence of such high levels of paraprotein and features consistent with lymphoma (including anaemia and lymphadenopathy) means this cannot be the correct diagnosis here.

Treatment of the hyperviscosity syndrome is with plasmapheresis, whilst treatments for the underlying lymphoma include fludarabine and rituximab.

Dimopoulos MA, et al. Diagnosis and management of Waldenstrom's macroglobulinaemia. J Clin Oncol 2005; 23(7):1564–1577.

24. D Sequestration crisis

Patients with sickle cell disease may present with any of a variety of different emergency presentations. The most typical presentations are:

- Aplastic crisis: this is defined by sudden complete failure of bone marrow production of erythrocytes. It is associated with a low reticulocyte count, meaning that it cannot be the diagnosis here. It occurs in response to infection with parvovirus B19. It is usually self-limiting, with recovery occurring within two weeks.

- Vaso-occlusive crisis: microvascular occlusion within the bone marrow leads to severe acute bone pain. Any bone may be affected, and bones may undergo necrosis with recurrent crises. There is no mention of bone pain in this scenario, hence this is unlikely to be the diagnosis here.
- Sequestration crisis: thrombosis of the splenic vein leads to pooling of blood in the spleen, resulting in the development of tender splenomegaly. Tender hepatomegaly may also occur by the same mechanism. It is associated with a marked reticulocytosis, reflecting the bone marrow attempting to compensate for splenic sequestration. This form of crisis is particularly found in children and young adults with sickle cell disease, since recurrent sequestration crises may result in eventual splenic infarction at a young age. This patient's symptoms and investigation results are most consistent with sequestration crisis as the diagnosis here.

Whilst the bones, spleen and liver are the organs most commonly affected by sickle cell crises, microvascular occlusion can in fact occur in organ. For instance, papillary necrosis can occur as a result of occlusion of the vasa recta of the kidney; however, the lack of haematuria means that this cannot be the diagnosis here.

Rees DC, Williams TN, Gladwin MT. Sickle-cell disease. Lancet 2010; 376(9757):2018–2031.

25. B Gestational thrombocytopaenia

Thrombocytopaenia is by definition one of the key components of the pregnancy-associated HELLP (haemolysis, elevated liver enzymes, low platelets) syndrome, but this woman's normal liver function tests rules this out. Although there is an association between pre-eclampsia and thrombocytopaenia, the normal blood pressure and lack of proteinuria means that this cannot be the diagnosis. Similarly, whilst pregnancy may be a trigger for thrombotic thrombocytopaenic purpura (TTP) and disseminated intravascular coagulopathy (DIC), the lack of other features associated with these conditions (e.g. microangiopathic haemolytic anaemia on blood film in TTP, abnormal coagulation profile in DIC) makes these unlikely.

The answer is option B. Gestational thrombocytopaenia is a condition characterised by a mild ($> 70 \times 10^9$/L), asymptomatic, isolated thrombocytopaenia that is typically most marked in late pregnancy before completely resolving soon after delivery. It occurs in approximately 5% of pregnancies. Where gestational thrombocytopaenia is suspected, clinicians can only make the diagnosis after confirming that the neonate has no evidence of thrombocytopaenia, and after demonstrating that the mother's platelet count resolves completely between pregnancies; this confirmation is needed to exclude the possibility of immune thrombocytopaenia, the main differential diagnosis. No treatment is necessary.

Kadir RA, McLintock C. Thrombocytopenia and disorders of platelet function in pregnancy. Semin Thromb Hemost 2011; 37(6):640–652.

26. A Carcinoma of the breast

Long-term follow up of patients treated for Hodgkin's lymphoma with either chemotherapy, radiotherapy or both treatments in combination has confirmed that these patients are at risk of a number of late complications relating to their therapy. Such complications may develop up to decades after the original treatment.

These complications include cardiac disease (e.g. anthracycline cardiotoxicity), lung disease (e.g. radiation pneumonitis), endocrine disease (particularly thyroid dysfunction) and the increased risk of secondary malignancies. Patients previously treated for Hodgkin's disease are at increased risk of recurrent lymphoma, leukaemia and a wide variety of solid organ malignancies.

Recurrent lymphoma cannot be the correct answer, since it can explain lymphocytes in the pleural effusion but not adenocarcinoma cells. Meigs' syndrome is the combination of pleural effusion (usually right sided), ascites and ovarian fibroma; however, it also has no association with adenocarcinoma. Similarly, although several histological forms of thyroid carcinoma exist, none of these are adenocarcinoma. The risk for gastrointestinal malignancies is significantly increased in survivors of Hodgkin's disease, and oesophageal malignancy may manifest as adenocarcinoma, making this a viable option. However, epidemiological studies show that the malignancies that Hodgkin's disease survivors are most strongly at risk for are breast and lung malignancies, hence option A is the correct answer here.

van Leeuwen FE, et al. Long-term risk of second malignancy in survivors of Hodgkin's disease treated during adolescence or young adulthood. J Clin Oncol 2000; 18(3):487–497.

27. D Immediate intravenous piperacillin-tazobactam and amikacin

There are two key components to the definition of neutropenic sepsis:

- the detection of at least one temperature of 38.3°C, or two temperatures of 38°C at one hour apart, **and**
- a neutrophil count of $< 0.5 \times 10^9$/L, or a predicted neutrophil nadir of 0.5×10^9/L.

Neutropenic sepsis is a medical emergency with a significant associated mortality. It may be a difficult condition to diagnosis and manage, since patients may often not show the 'classical' features of a systemic inflammatory response, and only in the minority of cases is a causative organism isolated. Research has indicated that much of the mortality associated with sepsis – especially in neutropenic cohorts – is due to failure in making the diagnosis quickly enough and preventable delays in administering antibiotics. It was data of this nature that led the International Surviving Sepsis Campaign to issue guidance that the time between septic patients first presenting to medical services and receiving their first dose of antibiotics should ideally be less than 1 hour. Many national and international guidelines relating to the management of neutropenic sepsis have now adapted the policy of 'less than one hour door-to-needle' for the administration of antibiotics to be the gold standard of care.

This patient's fever and tachycardia are consistent with sepsis. He has a background of acute myeloid leukaemia and clinical features suggestive of significant bone marrow failure, including clinical anaemia and purpura that may suggest thrombocytopenia. The chemotherapy he recently underwent is likely to inhibit his bone marrow function even further, with cell counts typically lowest at 10–14 days post-chemotherapy. Given his relatively low neutrophil count prior to chemotherapy, it is therefore reasonable to assume – even without blood test results – that he is suffering from neutropenic sepsis. Broad-spectrum antibiotics should be given immediately if there is any suspicion of neutropenic sepsis; waiting for blood test results to become available will delay the administration of potentially life-saving therapy. Option D is therefore the correct answer.

Anti fungal agents are normally administered to patients with neutropenic sepsis if they remain febrile after 4 days of intravenous antibiotic therapy, whilst antiviral agents would be introduced usually only on the basis of culture results. Recombinant granulocyte–macrophage colony-stimulating factors (such as filgrastim) have a role in prophylaxis for patients at high-risk of neutropenic sepsis, but there is controversy as to whether they have any efficacy in the treatment of the condition.

Freifeld AG, et al. Clinical practice guidelines for the use of antimicrobial agents in neutropenic patients with cancer: 2010 update by the Infectious Diseases Society of America. Clin Infect Dis 2011; 52:e56–e93.

28. A α-fetoprotein and β-human chorionic gonadotropin

Tumour markers are proteins secreted by tumours into blood that may be detected by simple blood tests. A wide range of tumour markers are now available, but their presence or absence in a particular patient must be interpreted with caution. More specifically, many markers have a significant 'false positive' rate (i.e. other possible causes for the marker being detected) or 'false negative' rate (i.e. only a proportion of tumours secrete the protein). However, they are still useful in particular circumstances, one of which is in management of testicular tumours.

Testicular tumours may be divided up into germ cell and non-germ cell tumours, with germ cell tumours accounting for approximately 95% of the total. Of the germ cell tumours, approximately half are pure seminomas, whilst the other half are termed non-seminomatous germ cell tumours (NSGCTs). Teratomas account for a significant proportion of the NSGCTs. Of patients with seminoma, 10% have mildly raised β-human chorionic gonadotropin (β-hCG) levels, but α-fetoprotein (α-FP) is always normal. Amongst patients with NSGCTs, up to 90% have elevated β-hCG and/or α-FP levels. β-hCG and α-FP do not have high enough specificity or sensitivity to recommend them as part of the diagnostic investigations for testicular tumours; their main use is in monitoring for recovery after treatment. For example, serial decreases in β-hCG and α-FP following surgical resection of a teratoma imply successful surgical resection, whilst any subsequent increases could imply tumour recurrence.

β_2-microglobulin is useful as prognostic factor in certain haematological malignancies, whilst carbohydrate antigen (CA) 125 is useful as part of the diagnosis and follow-up for ovarian malignancies. Neither are raised in teratoma. As such, option A is the correct answer.

Sturgeon CM, et al. Serum tumour markers: how to order and interpret them. BMJ 2009; 339: b3527.

29. D Tumour lysis syndrome

The raised uric acid level may be consistent with gout, but there is no mention of any of the other characteristic clinical features of this disease (e.g. monoarthritis), making this unlikely. Polymyositis has an association with malignancy, and both polymyositis and rhabdomyolysis can present with muscular pain, acute kidney injury and the pattern of electrolytes found here. However, the normal creatine kinase suggests that this patient's muscular pain reflects electrolyte disturbance rather than muscle damage. The main side effect of vincristine is peripheral neuropathy, which could account for the patient's symptoms; however, it cannot account for the patient's abnormal biochemistry results.

The correct answer is option D. Tumour lysis syndrome is a collection of serious metabolic derangements that may occur in response to the massive destruction of tumour cells that accompanies the start of chemotherapy. Patients particularly at risk are those starting chemotherapy for aggressive lymphomas or acute lymphoblastic leukaemia, as these tumours tend to be highly proliferative and extremely sensitive to modern cytotoxic agents.

As tumour cells lyse, potassium and phosphate are released from the cell cytoplasm into blood, hence hyperkalaemia and hyperphosphataemia are characteristic. Phosphate binds with plasma calcium, and hypocalcaemia develops. Tumour cells also release large quantities of nucleic acid as they lyse, which is metabolised to uric acid and results in hyperuricaemia. Uric acid and calcium-phosphate precipitants may be deposited in the renal tubules and lead to acute kidney injury. Patients may develop uric acid renal calculi in certain cases.

The best management of tumour lysis syndrome is prevention of its occurrence, with intravenous hydration, allopurinol and rasburicase all of use. Rasburicase is a recombinant form of the urate oxidase enzyme found in many mammals but not in humans. Treating established tumour lysis syndrome is difficult, with management focused on correcting electrolyte abnormalities and providing renal replacement therapy as required.

Cairo MS, et al. Recommendations for the evaluation of risk and prophylaxis of tumour lysis syndrome (TLS) in adults and children with malignant diseases: an expert TLS panel consensus. Brit J Haematol 2010; 149(4):578–586.

30. B Dexamethasone

Chemotherapy-induced nausea and vomiting is one of the most common and distressing complications of this treatment. Cisplatin is a particularly emetogenic drug, with up to 90% of patients developing these symptoms in association with its use without appropriate prophylaxis or treatment. Trial data have demonstrated that 5-HT_3 receptor antagonists (such as ondansetron and granisetron) appear to be the single most effective class of antiemetics in this situation, with corticosteroids also appearing to provide significant benefit. 5-HT_3 antagonists and corticosteroids together appear to be a particularly effective combination, and hence B is the correct answer here. There is also evidence demonstrating the efficacy of neurokinin-1 receptor antagonists (e.g. aprepitant, fosepritant) in preventing chemotherapy induced nausea and vomiting, although these are not as yet widely available.

Hesketh PJ. Drug therapy: chemotherapy-induced nausea and vomiting. N Engl J Med 2008; 358:2482–2494.

Chapter 8

Neurology

1. An 18-year-old man presented to the emergency department with a 48-hour history of headaches, fevers and generally feeling unwell. He had no past medical history, and no recent history of travel or contact with anyone ill. On examination, he was alert and orientated and had some neck stiffness. His temperature was 37.5°C. There were no focal neurological abnormalities, but he was unable to tolerate funduscopy. There were no visible rashes.

    Investigations:

C-reactive protein	12 mg/L (<5)
CT head	normal

    He underwent a lumbar puncture for cerebrospinal fluid analysis:

opening pressure	15 cmH$_2$O
serum glucose	4.9 mmol/L

    Cerebrospinal fluid:

appearance	clear
protein	0.4 g/L
glucose	2.9 mmol/L
lymphocytes count	60 cells/mm^3 (<5)

    What is the most likely diagnosis?

    A   Bacterial meningitis
    B   Froin's syndrome
    C   Subacute sclerosing panencephalitis
    D   Tuberculous meningitis
    E   Viral meningitis

2. A 67-year-old woman presented with sudden onset slurred speech and weakness in the left arm that started 4 hours ago. Examination revealed a left-sided facial dropping and weakness in all muscle groups in the left arm. She remained dysphasic and there were no abnormalities when examining the eyes. There were no cerebellar signs.

    Investigations:

CT head	No evidence of haemorrhage

    Which of the following would best describe this condition?

A   Lacunar infarct
B   Left total anterior circulation infarct
C   Posterior circulation infarct
D   Right partial anterior circulation infarct
E   Right total anterior circulation infarct

3. A 60-year-old man, a builder, presented with tremor in the hands, which had been present for 3 months.

    Which one of the following would be most suggestive of benign essential tremor?

    A   Associated with rigidity
    B   Associated with titubation
    C   Improves on stretching out hands
    D   Improves with writing
    E   Worse with alcohol intake

4. A 32-year-old woman presented to the outpatient clinic with a 6-month history of headaches. She described the headaches as occurring intermittently, but with sudden onset, on the left side, and around the eye. During these episodes, her husband has noticed that the left eye in particular looked bloodshot and was very watery, with some drooping of the left eyelid. However, these disappeared when the headache resolved. The headaches were becoming more frequent and were making it difficult for her to continue with her job as a secretary. There was no significant past medical history. Physical examination was normal. Blood tests and CT scan head arranged by her general practitioner were normal.

    What is the most appropriate prophylactic medication for this patient?

    A   Amitriptyline
    B   Propranolol
    C   Short burst oxygen therapy
    D   Sumatriptan
    E   Verapamil

5. A 21-year-old man was referred to the neurology outpatient clinic with multiple skin lesions. These were sessile and pedunculated in character, measuring 2–4 cm in diameter, all over the body.

    Which one of the following is more in keeping with a diagnosis of neurofibromatosis type 2 disease, rather than type 1 disease?

    A   6 'café au lait' spots
    B   Axillary freckling
    C   Lisch nodules
    D   Optic glioma
    E   Vestibular schwannomas

6. A 45-year-old woman presented to the neurology clinic with worsening dysarthria over a period of 2 months. She had a nasal quality to her speech and described a choking sensation. On examination, the uvula was deviated to the right and the tongue was deviated to the left.

Which one of the following is the least likely cause?

A Botulinism
B Guillain–Barré syndrome
C Lyme disease
D Motor neurone disease
E Multiple sclerosis

7. A 73-year-old man presented with gait abnormalities for the past 4–5 months. A provisional diagnosis of normal pressure hydrocephalus had been made.

Which one of the following is least likely to be associated with this condition?

A Ataxic gait
B Frontal lobe dementia
C Papilloedema
D Parkinsonian gait mimic
E Urinary incontinence

8. An 84-year-old man presented to the medical assessment unit with a right-sided facial droop, which had started yesterday after developing pain behind his right ear. He had no previous medical history. On examination, he had weakness of the right side of the face including the forehead, was unable to close his right eye, and the right side of the mouth was drooping. There was no obvious rash. Apart from some change in taste sensation there were no other cranial nerve defects, and he had no limb weakness.

What is the most likely diagnosis?

A Bell's palsy
B Cholesteatoma
C Demyelination syndrome
D Ramsay–Hunt syndrome
E Stroke

9. A 36-year-old woman had recently been diagnosed with multiple sclerosis (MS).

Which one of the following drugs would be the most appropriate to reduce the progression of disability?

A Azathioprine
B Cyclophosphamide
C Intravenous immunoglobulin
D Linoleic acid
E Mitoxantrone

10. Which one of the following is most closely associated with carpal tunnel syndrome?

A Hyperthyroidism
B Conn's syndrome
C Rheumatoid arthritis
D Diabetes insipidus
E Systemic lupus erythematosus (SLE)

11. A 21-year-old man was reviewed in the epilepsy clinic. He had a 2-year history of myoclonic seizures and was currently taking sodium valproate. Although he was compliant with medication, he was experiencing an increase in the frequency of seizures. What is the next step in management?

    A   Carbamazepine and vigabatrin
    B   Carbamazepine alone
    C   Lamotrigine alone
    D   Sodium valproate and carbamazepine
    E   Sodium valproate and lamotrigine

12. A 21-year-old woman presented to the emergency department with muscle cramps and vomiting. She had recently been prescribed metoclopramide. On examination, her temperature was 38.2°C, pulse 110 beats per minute and blood pressure 169/100 mmHg. Examination of chest, heart, and abdomen showed no abnormality. She had increased tone throughout her arms and legs. Neuroleptic malignant syndrome was suspected.

    What is the most appropriate treatment?

    A   Dantrolene
    B   Domperidone
    C   Metoclopramide
    D   Glutamate
    E   Olanzapine

13. A 15-year-old boy was seen in the clinic due to difficulty in walking. He had had problems with his balance for a long-time, but it was becoming increasingly difficult for him to walk short distances. On examination, he had nystagmus and dysarthric speech. There were no pupillary defects and funduscopy demonstrated optic atrophy. He also had absent ankle jerks and extensor plantars. There was loss of proprioception and vibration sense over the feet. Romberg's test was positive. Blood tests, including haematinics were within normal range. Electromyography confirmed axonal neuropathy.

    What is the most likely diagnosis?

    A   Charcot–Marie–Tooth disease
    B   Friedreich's ataxia
    C   Motor neurone disease (MND)
    D   Multiple sclerosis
    E   Subacute combined degeneration of spinal cord

14. A 29-year-old man was noted to have downbeat nystagmus. He had a history of mitral valve prolapse. Apart from the nystagmus, he had no other neurological findings on examination.

    What is the most likely diagnosis?

    A   Acoustic neuroma
    B   Arnold–Chiari malformation

C Benign paroxysmal positional vertigo (BPPV)
D Cerebellar vermis lesion
E Multiple sclerosis

15. A 27-year-old man presented to the emergency department with an acutely painful left eye. He was otherwise fit and well with no past medical history. On examination, he was afebrile with pulse 60 beats per minute (regular), and blood pressure 126/65 mmHg. There was complete ptosis on the left with the position of the eye looking down and out. The pupil was fixed and dilated with diplopia in all directions, except to the left.

What is the most likely diagnosis?

A Horner's syndrome
B Multiple sclerosis
C Myasthenia gravis
D Optic nerve glioma
E Posterior communicating artery aneurysm

16. A 52-year-old man presented with visual disturbances that resulted in reduced visual field on the same side in both eyes. He was found to have a right-sided homonymous hemianopia.

Where is the site of the lesion?

A Left optic nerve
B Left optic tract
C Optic chiasm
D Right optic nerve
E Right optic tract

17. A 62-year-old woman was admitted to the intensive care unit for the management of respiratory failure and pneumonia. Prior to admission she described a prolonged history of weakness and fatigue. Myasthenia gravis was suspected.

Which one of the following is not useful in the diagnosis of myasthenia gravis?

A Antibodies to voltage gated calcium channels
B Antibodies to muscle-specific receptor tyrosine kinase (MuSK)
C Antibodies to acetylcholine receptor
D Single fibre electromyography testing
E Tensilon test

18. Which one of the following conditions is chorea most strongly associated?

A Hypothyroidism
B Hyperkalaemia
C Aortic sclerosis
D Anaemia
E Systemic lupus erythematosus (SLE)

19. A 36-year-old man with multiple sclerosis was reviewed in the neurology clinic. He complained of worsening urinary incontinence at night.

    What is the most appropriate management?

    A   Electrical stimulation of pelvic floor muscles
    B   Intranasal desmopressin
    C   Intravesical botulinum
    D   Prophylactic antibiotics
    E   Finasteride

20. A 20-year-old woman presented to her general practitioner with a 2-month history of intermittent headaches. They occurred throughout the day and felt like a band-like pressure across the forehead and occurred for 30 minutes at a time. She had difficulty tolerating bright lights, but no problems with vision. She had no vomiting or nausea. She took paracetamol with some relief, but the headaches were becoming more frequent. She had no previous medical history and was not on any other medication. Clinical examination was normal.

    What is the most likely diagnosis?

    A   Cluster headache
    B   Meningitis
    C   Migraine
    D   Raised intracranial pressure
    E   Tension headache

21. Which one of the following features is in keeping with sporadic Creutzfeldt–Jakob disease (CJD) rather than variant Creutzfeldt–Jakob disease (vCJD)?

    A   Age of onset 20–30 years
    B   Electroencephalogram (EEG) showing periodic sharp waves
    C   Myoclonus
    D   'Pulvinar' sign on MRI
    E   Duration of illness 18 months

22. A 36-year-old man presented with change in vision. On examination, there was a left inferior quadrantanopia defect.

    Where is the site of the lesion?

    A   Optic chiasm
    B   Left parietal lobe
    C   Left temporal lobe
    D   Right parietal lobe
    E   Right temporal lobe

23. A 42-year-old man presented with a sudden onset flaccid paraplegia and acute urinary retention. Examination revealed weakness in both lower limbs, loss of pain and temperature sensation below the level of T5. Joint position and

vibration senses were intact. However, the bladder was palpable and anal tone reduced.

What is the most likely diagnosis?

A Anterior spinal artery thrombosis
B Brown-Séquard syndrome
C Metastatic infiltration of spinal cord
D Prolapsed disc
E Syringomyelia

24. A 19-year-old man is seen in neurology clinic due to difficulty in walking.

Which one of the following features is most strongly associated with myotonic dystrophy?

A Autosomal recessive inheritance
B Cardiomyopathy
C Hyperthyroidism
D Male predominance
E Superoxide disutase 1 (*SOD1*) gene defect

25. A 40-year-old man was seen in the clinic due to difficultly in walking for approximately 4 months. He had noticed increasing weakness in his legs, but no specific pain or numbness. There were no bladder or bowel symptoms. On examination, his speech had a nasal quality and there was wasting of the facial muscles. In addition, there was spastic weakness of both legs with hyperreflexia, ankle clonus and extensor plantars. There were no sensory disturbances.

Which one of the following is most likely to be associated with this condition?

A Fourth nerve palsy
B Frontotemporal dementia
C Sixth nerve palsy
D Sphincter disturbances
E Third nerve palsy

26. A 38-year-old woman was seen in the neurology clinic with a 3-month history of dizzy spells. These episodes lasted for a couple of minutes at a time and came on with bending down to pick up things or with turning her head. When these spells occurred she felt like the room was spinning around. Occasionally, she experienced nausea. She had had no hearing problems, headaches or any recent illnesses. She was not taking any medications. Examination was unremarkable. ECG was normal sinus rhythm with rate 62 beats per minute.

What is the most likely diagnosis?

A Acoustic neuroma
B Benign paroxysmal positional vertigo (BPPV)
C Ménière's disease
D Multiple sclerosis
E Labyrinthitis

27. An 85-year-old man was found to have an ipsilateral VI nerve palsy, facial weakness with contralateral hemiplegia and a lateral conjugate gaze palsy; there were no cerebellar signs.

What is the most likely diagnosis?

A   Foville's syndrome
B   Millard–Gubler syndrome
C   Nothnagel's syndrome
D   Wallenberg's syndrome
E   Weber's syndrome

28. A 76-year-old man was referred with random, flinging movements of his arms. A diagnosis of hemiballismus was made.

Which one of the following locations within the brain is most likely to be affected?

A   Brainstem
B   Caudate nucleus
C   Cerebellum
D   Subthalamic nucleus
E   Substantia nigra

29. An 84-year-old man was seen in the memory clinic. He was accompanied by his son, who claimed that the patient was becoming increasingly forgetful over the past year. He scored 18/30 on a mini mental state examination. An MRI has been arranged, but not yet done.

Which one of the following is considered the least useful test to be carried out initially?

A   Calcium
B   Folate
C   Syphilis serology
D   Thyroid function
E   Vitamin B_{12}

30. A 35-year-old woman on labour ward suffered a seizure. She was 39 weeks pregnant. This was her first pregnancy. On examination, her Glasgow Coma Scale (GCS) was 15/15, temperature 35.6°C, pulse 120 beats per minute (regular), and blood pressure 176/108 mmHg. There was hyperreflexia in both lower limbs and mild peripheral oedema. Urine analysis: Protein ++.

What is the most appropriate next step in management?

A   Diazepam
B   Labetalol
C   Magnesium sulphate
D   Nifedipine
E   Phenytoin

Answers

1. E Viral meningitis

The differences between viral, bacterial (and tuberculous) meningitis are shown below in **Table 8.1.**

Table 8.1			
CSF	**Bacterial**	**Viral**	**Tuberculosis**
Appearance	Cloudy	Clear	Cloudy/clear/fibrin web
Predominant cells	Polymorphs	Lymphocytes	Lymphocytes
Cell count/mm³	90–1000	50–1000	10–1000
Protein (g/L)	>1.5	<1	1–5
Glucose	<50% of serum levels	>50% serum levels	<50% serum levels

Table 8.1 Cerebrospinal fluid (CSF) characteristics in viral, bacterial and tuberculous meningitis.

Froin's syndrome is an abnormality in the cerebrospinal fluid (CSF), which leads to a high protein content and production of yellow CSF. It is due to blockage (complete or partial) in the spinal cord leading to an increase in protein in the fluid below the level of the obstruction. The most likely cause of Froin's syndrome is a spinal cord tumour.

With no history of measles, very short duration, and an abnormal CSF, subacute sclerosing panencephalitis is an unlikely diagnosis. This rare form of encephalitis occurs as a result of chronic infection with the measles virus. It presents with mild behavioural changes, progressing to features such as myoclonus, pyramidal and extrapyramidal signs, ataxia, seizures and lateralising neurological signs. Diagnosis is through imaging with MRI, EEG and CSF examination. CSF is usually normal, or with a normal or mildly raised protein level and raised anti-measles antibody titres.

Garg RK. Subacute sclerosising panencephalitis. Postgrad Med J 2002; 78:63–70.

2. D Right partial anterior circulation stroke

This patient has had an ischaemic stroke, which can be further classified by the Oxfordshire Community Stroke Classification (also known as the Bamford Classification) (**Table 8.2**).

Total anterior circulation infarct (TACI)

This requires all three of the following:

1. A higher cortical dysfunction such as dyspraxia or dysphasia.

Table 8.2				
	Higher cortical dysfunction	**Visual field defect**	**Motor/sensory defect**	**Brainstem signs**
Clinical features	Aphasisa or neglect or dyspraxia		Face Arm Leg	Cranial nerve signs + Contralateral limb signs
TACI	✓	✓	✓ ≥ 2 out of 3 areas	
PACI	✓	✓	✓	
LACI		✓	✓	Ataxic hemiparesis
POCI		✓		✓

TACI, total anterior circulation infarct; PACI, partial anterior circulation infarct; LACI, lacunar infarct; POCI, posterior circulation infarct.

Table 8.2 Types of ischaemic stroke.

2. Contralateral homonymous hemianopia
3. Contralateral hemiparesis or weakness of at least two out of three of **ARM, FACE and LEG** (with or without contralateral hemisensory loss)

Partial anterior circulation infarct (PACI)

Two of the three TACI criteria must be present or 'limited' criteria present:

- Contralateral weakness of arm or leg or hand or face
- Higher cortical dysfunction alone (dysphasia or dyspraxia), which may be the only manifestation of PACI

Lacunar infarct (LACI)

- Pure motor affecting two out of three of face, arm and leg
- Pure sensory
- Sensorimotor (basal ganglia and internal capsule)
- Ataxic hemiparesis (ipsilateral cerebellar signs and contralateral hemiparesis)

Posterior circulation infarct (POCI)

- Cranial nerve palsies with contralateral motor/sensory loss
- Ocular palsies, isolated conjugate palsies
- Isolated homonymous hemianopia
- Isolated cerebellar stroke
- Bilateral motor or sensory loss

Bamford P et al. Classification and natural history of clinically identifiable subtypes of cerebral infarction. Lancet 1991; 337:1521–1526.

3. B Associated with titubation

Benign essential tremor can often be mistaken for Parkinsonism. It is a condition, which is inherited in an autosomal dominant manner. Although a benign tremor, it can often lead to functional impairment. The onset follows a bimodal distribution with peaks in the 20–29 and 60–69 year age groups.

It is characterised by a symmetrical rhythmic tremor that is present on exertion or with stress, and therefore not present at rest (differentiating it from Parkinsonian tremor). In a small minority, cogwheel rigidity may be present leading to difficulty in diagnosis.

The tremor worsens with physical or emotional stress and can be exacerbated by caffeine and some medications such as antidepressants. Often the tremor settles down with ingestion of alcohol and is an important feature as patients may be consuming excessive amounts to prevent symptoms.

Titubation (nodding movement of the head or body) is commonly present, contributing to the functional impairment.

Treatment is with beta-blockers such as propranolol or anticonvulsants such as primidone.

Benito-León J, Louis ED. Essential tremor: emerging views of a common disorder. Nature Clin Pract Neurol 2006; 2:666–678.

4. E Verapamil

Headaches are a common presentation to outpatient clinic. This scenario describes a history of cluster headaches. The distinct pattern of unilateral, sudden onset with neurological disturbance is highly suggestive over migrainous headaches.

The question specifically is asking about prophylaxis, as it is apparent this patient is not in the acute phase of the condition. The management of the acute phase is with short burst oxygen therapy and use of sumatriptan subcutaneous injections. However, preventative medications such as verapamil, lithium and steroids are more appropriate in this situation.

Propranolol may be used as prophylaxis for migraine management, whilst amitriptyline is a treatment option for trigeminal neuralgia.

Duncan CW, Watson DP, Stein A. Guideline Development Group. Diagnosis and management of headache in adults: summary of SIGN guideline. BMJ 2008; 337:a2329.

5. E Vestibular schwannomas

Neurofibromatosis (NF) is divided into two types (**Table 8.3**). NF-2 is much rarer than NF-1.

Gutmann DH, et al. The diagnostic evaluation and multidisciplinary management of neurofibromatosis 1 and neurofibromatosis 2. JAMA 1997; 278(1):51.
Bausch B, et al. Clinical and genetic characteristics of patients with neurofibromatosis type 1 and pheochromocytoma. N Engl J Med 2006; 354(25):2729–2731.

Table 8.3

	NF1	NF2
Inheritance	Autosomal dominant	Autosomal dominant
Gene	Chromosome 17	Chromosome 22

Clinical features and diagnosis	Positive diagnosis made with 2 of the following criteria
	• >2 neurofibromas
	• Lisch nodules*
	• Axillary freckling
	• >6 'café-au-lait' spots
	• Optic glioma
	• First-degree relative with NF-1
	• Sphenoid dysplasia
	• Phaeochromocytoma found in 1% of patients
		Positive diagnosis is made when either of the following is found
		1. Bilateral acoustic neuromas (vestibular schwannomas)
		2. First degree relative with unilateral vestibular schwannoma or the following
		  • Neurofibroma
		  • Juvenile posterior subcapsular lenticular opacity
		  • Glioma
		  • Menigioma

Management	Genetic counselling Yearly blood pressure monitoring and cutaneous surveying	Yearly hearing tests Surigical intervention for vestibular schwannoma
Complications	• Local effects of neurofibromas • Optic glioma (2%) • Malignant transformation • Epilepsy	• Local effects of schwannomas • Deafness • Malignant transformation (cutaneous)

*Lisch nodules are small, pigmented, hamartomas found on the iris.

Table 8.3 Differences between neurofibromatosis type 1 (NF1) and type 2 (NF2).

6. E Multiple sclerosis

This patient demonstrates a classical presentation of a bulbar palsy. Differentiating a bulbar palsy from a pseudobulbar palsy can be difficult.

Bulbar palsy occurs due to loss of motor function in the motor nuclei in the medulla, leading to lower motor neuron lesion signs. These include a flaccid tongue with fasciculations and speech is queit, with a nasal quality. It can involve cranial nerves IX, X, XI and XII. Causes of a bulbar palsy can be categorised according the mnemonic 'TIMID':

Toxic: *Clostridium botulinum*, tetanus
Inflammatory/Infective: Guillain–Barré, poliomyelitis, HIV, Lyme disease, myasthenia gravis
Malignancy: glioma
Infarction: medullary infarction
Degenerative: motor neuron disease, syringobulbia

Pseudobulbar palsy is an upper motor neuron lesion as a result of the involvement of corticobulbar tracts in the mid pons. It occurs more frequently than bulbar palsy. Patients report difficulty in chewing and swallowing, along with altered speech. On examination, jaw jerk is increased, with 'Donald Duck' speech.

A useful way of remembering the speech abnormalities in bulbar and pseudobulbar palsies is through the mnemonic '**BLOOMIN PUMPED**'.

BLMNN – Remembered as 'Bloomin'
Bulbar palsy
LOwer
Motor
Neuron lesion
Nasal speech

PUMp'D – Remembered as 'Pumped'
Pseudobulbar palsy
Upper
Motor neuron lesion
'**D**onald Duck' speech

Gillig PM, Sanders RD. Cranial Nerves IX, X, XI, and XII. Psychiatry (Edgmont) 2010; 7(5):37–41.

7. C Papilloedema

Normal pressure hydrocephalus is often misdiagnosed as either Parkinson's disease or Alzheimer's disease. It is characterised by the triad of:

- Dementia (frontal lobe)
- Urinary incontinence
- Gait abnormality

Dementia is predominantly of the frontal lobe type. The gait can be ataxic in nature but also may mimic a Parkinsonian gait and posture. Urinary incontinence presents as urgency and incontinence, and therefore alternative diagnoses are usually thought of first (such as urinary tract infection and benign prostatic hyperplasia).

Normal pressure hydrocephalus occurs as a result of a defect in the absorption of cerebrospinal fluid. It may be caused by meningitis, traumatic head injury, subarachnoid haemorrhage, malignancy or following neurosurgery.

Diagnosis is made with a combination of performing lumbar puncture (with a raised opening pressure), imaging with CT and/or MRI (T2/FLAIR sequence). Treatment is the insertion of a ventriculoperitoneal shunt.

Wilson RK, Williams MA. Normal pressure hydrocephalus. Clin Geriatr Med 2006; 22(4):935–51viii.

8. A Bell's palsy

The causes of facial nerve palsy are as follows:

'**DR POSTBAGS:**

Diabetes

Ramsay-Hunt syndrome

Parotid swellings
Otitis media and cholesteatoma
Stroke – brainstem
Trauma
Bell's palsy
Acoustic neuroma
Guillain–Barré syndrome (causing bilateral weakness) and other sequelae of infection (e.g. Lyme disease)
Sarcoid – neurosarcoid, leading to bilateral weakness

This patient does not have features of a stroke, particularly as there is no focal neurological abnormality in the peripheral nervous system or involvement of the forehead muscles; indicating a lower motor neuron lesion. Pain in the ear along with an inability to close an eye is compatible with Bell's palsy. The absence of a vesicular rash make Ramsay Hunt syndrome (varicella zoster infection) unlikely.

Bell's palsy is a result of a viral infection (likely herpes simplex type 1 and herpes zoster virus).

Gilden D. Bell's Palsy. N Engl J Med 2004; 351:1323–1331.

9. D Linoleic acid

Multiple sclerosis (MS) is a popular topic in the MRCP part 1 examination and thorough knowledge of the current guidelines is advised. This question specifically discusses treatments to prevent disease progression, rather than the management of acute flares of the disease.

The National Institute of Health and Clinical Excellence (NICE) guidelines recommend that patients with MS take 17–23 g of linoleic acid a day as this may reduce disease progression. The following treatments should only be used after consultation and evaluation of adverse events.

- Azathioprine
- Mitoxantrone (a chemotherapy agent)
- Intravenous immunoglobulin
- Plasma exchange

The following should not be used as there has been no evidence of benefits in the course of the condition:

- Cyclophosphamide
- Cladribine
- Long-term corticosteroids
- Linomide
- Hyperbaric oxygen
- Myelin basic protein

National Institute for Health and Clinical Excellence (NICE) Guidelines. Multiple sclerosis: Management of multiple sclerosis in primary and secondary care. NICE; 2003 http://guidance.nice.org.uk/CG8 (Last accessed May 2012).

10. C Rheumatoid arthritis

Carpal tunnel is the one of the most common mononeuropathies involving the median nerve, which leads to numbness and tingling in the lateral three and a half fingers. Causes of carpal tunnel syndrome include the following:

'**HARDTOP**':

Hypothyroidism
Acromegaly, amyloidosis
Rheumatoid arthritis
Diabetes mellitus
Trauma
Obesity
Pregnancy

It is also useful to recall the key anatomical features associated with this condition. The muscles innervated by the median nerve can be remembered by using the mnemonic '**LOAF**':

Lateral two lumbricals
Opponens pollicis
Abductor pollicis
Flexor pollicis brevis

Bland JD. Carpal tunnel syndrome. BMJ 2007; 335(7615):343–346.

11. C Lamotrigine alone

Recent UK guidelines have recommended that antiepileptic drugs (AEDs) should be initiated by a specialist, after thorough investigation to rule out additional causes of seizures.

Monotherapy, with a single AED should be used wherever possible (**Table 8.4**). If one monotherapy fails, then monotherapy with another agent should be trialled. Combination therapy should be considered once different monotherapies are unsuccessful. If an antiepileptic drug has been unsuccessful due to continued seizures or adverse effects, then a second agent should be started (either alternative first line or second line) being built up to an adequate or maximum tolerated dose, whilst the first agent is tapered down slowly. When prescribing sodium valproate alone or in combination with other AEDs to women and girls of present and future child-bearing potential, discussions must take place about the risk of possible neurodevelopmental impairments or malformations in the unborn child, particularly if prescribed at high doses. Also there are contraindications to prescribing carbamazepine to people of Thai or Han Chinese origins, therefore alternative AEDs should be prescribed.

National Institute for Health and Clinical Excellence (NICE). The epilepsies: the diagnosis and management of the epilepsies in adults and children in primary and secondary care. Clinical Guideline CG 137. London: NICE, 2012.

Table 8.4

Seizure type	First-line AEDs	Adjunctive AEDs	Other AEDs that may be considered on referral to tertiary care	Do not offer AEDs (may worsen seizures)
Generalised tonic–clonic	Carbamazepine Lamotrigine Oxcarbazepine[a] Sodium valproate	Clobazam[a] Lamotrigine Levetiracetam Sodium valproate Topiramate		(If there are absence or myoclonic seizures, or if JME suspected) Carbamazepine Gabapentin Oxcarbazepine Phenytoin Pregabalin Tiagabine Vigabatrin
Tonic or atonic	Sodium valproate	Lamotrigine[a]	Rufinamide[a] Topiramate[a]	Carbamazepine Gabapentin Oxcarbazepine Pregabalin Tiagabine Vigabatrin
Absence	Ethosuximide Lamotrigine[a] Sodium valproate	Ethosuximide Lamotrigine[a] Sodium valproate	Clobazam[a] Clonazepam Levetiracetam[a] Topiramate[a] Zonisamide[a]	Carbamazepine Gabapentin Oxcarbazepine Phenytoin Pregabalin Tiagabine Vigabatrin
Myoclonic	Levetiracetam[a] Sodium valproate Topiramate[a]	Levetiracetam Sodium valproate Topiramate[a]	Clobazam[a] Clonazepam Piracetam Zonisamide[a]	Carbamazepine Gabapentin Oxcarbazepine Phenytoin Pregabalin Tiagabine Vigabatrin
Focal	Carbamazepine Lamotrigine Levetiracetam Oxcarbazepine Sodium valproate	Carbamazepine Clobazam[a] Gabapentin[a] Lamotrigine Levetiracetam Oxcarbazepine Sodium valproate Topiramate	Eslicarbazepine acetate[a] Lacosamide Phenobarbital Phenytoin Pregabalin[a] Tiagabine Vigabatrin Zonisamide[a]	

Contd...

Contd...

Prolonged or repeated seizures and convulsive status epilepticus in the community	Buccal midazolam Rectal diazepam[b] Intravenous lorazepam		
Convulsive status epilepticus in hospital	Intravenous lorazepam Intravenous diazepam Buccal midazolam	Intravenous phenobarbital Phenytoin	
Refractory convulsive status epilepticus	Intravenous midazolam[b] Propofol[b] (not in children) Thiopental sodium[b]		

[a] At the time of the NICE guideline's publication (January 2012) this drug did not have UK marketing authorisation for this indication and/or population (see table 3 in the NICE guideline for specific details about this drug for this indication and population). Informed consent should be obtained and documented.

[b] At the time of the NICE guideline's publication (January 2012), this drug did not have UK marketing authorisation for this indication and/or population (see table 3 in the NICE guideline for specific details about this drug for this indication and population). Informed consent should be obtained and documented in line with normal standards in emergency care.

Table 8.4 Antiepileptic drug (AED) options by seizure type. From National Institute for Health and Clinical Excellence. CG 137 The epilepsies: the diagnosis and management of the epilepsies in adults and children in primary and secondary care. London: NICE 2012. Available from www.nice.org.uk/guidance/CG137. Reproduced with permission.

12. A Dantrolene

Neuroleptic malignant syndrome is a life-threatening neurological emergency as a characterised by fever, autonomic instability, muscle rigidity and change of mental status.

The pathogenesis is not completely clear, but it is likely that the condition is associated with dopamine receptor blockade, due to onset of symptoms with the use of medications that have dopamine receptor blockage activity. The use of haloperidol and chlorpromazine are also common causes. Levodopa can cause symptoms, if the dose is reduced abruptly. In addition, medications with antidopaminergic effects such as metoclopramide and domperidone can lead to this condition.

Olanzapine is a dopamine antagonist, whilst dopamine agonists work to inhibit release of glutamate.

The features of neuroleptic malignant syndrome therefore can be summarised by the mnemonic '**RECTAL**':

Rigidity
Elevated enzymes (creatinine kinase)
Confusion
Temperature, tremor
Autonomic instability
Leukocytosis

Management of the condition includes intravenous fluids to prevent onset of renal failure, along with other supportive measures. It is of course necessary to stop the offending medications. In some cases dantrolene and bromocriptine (dopamine agonist) may be used.

Bhanushali MJ, Tuite PJ. The evaluation and management of patients with neuroleptic malignant syndrome. Neurol Clin 2004; 22(2):389–411.

13. B Friedreich's ataxia

This patient has Friedreich's ataxia, an autosomal recessive spinocerebellar degenerative ataxia, accounting for half of all hereditary ataxias. It is the result of an increased number of GAA trinucleotide repeat sequences in the gene for frataxin, found on chromosome 9. Friedreich's ataxia does not follow the phenomenon of genetic anticipation

It is usually present from ages 5 to 15 years, but late onset Friedreich's ataxia has been reported to present in individuals aged 20–30 years. The features of the condition are consistent with spinocerebellar degeneration:

These can be remembered as '**LOANED**':

Loss of proprioception and vibration sense
Optic atrophy
Ataxia
Nystagmus
Extensor plantars, absent ankle jerks
Dysarthic speech

Other conditions associated with Friedrich's ataxia can be remembered as '**PACK(e)D**':

Pes cavus
Atrial fibrillation
Cardiomyopathy
Kyphoscoliosis
Diabetes mellitus

Table 8.5 outlines the key clinical features of this and similar neurological conditions.

Pandolfo M. Friedreich ataxia. Arch Neurol 2008; 65(10):1296–303.

Table 8.5

	UMN/LMN lesion	Peripheral neuropathy	Ankle jerks	Plantar response	Vibration and proprioception
Charcot–Marie–Tooth	Mixed	Minimal or absent	Absent	No response or down	Preserved
MND 1. Bulbar palsy 2. Amyotrophic lateral sclerosis 3. Progressive muscular atrophy	1. LMN 2. UMN and LMN 3. LMN	No sensory loss	1. N/A 2. Increased 3. Absent	1. N/A 2. Extensor 3. Down going	1. N/A 2. Preserved 3. Preserved
Friedreich's ataxia	Mixed	Spared	Absent	Extensor	Loss
Multiple sclerosis	UMN	May be present	Increased (or normal)	Extensor	Loss
SACD	Mixed	Present	Absent	Extensor	Loss

LMN, lower motor neuron lesion; MND, motor neurone disease; SACD, subacute combined degeneration of the spinal cord; UMN, upper motor neuron lesion.

Table 8.5 Clinical features of neurological conditions.

14. B Arnold–Chiari malformation

This patient has an Arnold–Chiari malformation. This is one of the only causes of downbeat nystagmus, along with other foramen magnum lesions. In view of his mitral valve prolapse, the unifying diagnosis is therefore Ehlers–Danlos syndrome.

An acoustic neuroma would usually present with additional neurological findings. Benign paroxysmal positional vertigo has horizontal, gaze evoked nystagmus. Cerebellar lesions present with upwards gaze nystagmus. Multiple sclerosis commonly has other neurological findings (although these may be subtle), but downbeat nystagmus is not a usual feature.

Wagner JN, et al. Downbeat nystagmus: aetiology and comorbidity in 117 patients. J Neurol Neurosurg Psychiatry 2008; 79(6):672–677.

15. E Posterior communicating artery aneurysm

The above describes a lone oculomotor, (third) nerve palsy and the causes are varied. The two main alternative options are posterior communicating artery aneurysm and multiple sclerosis. Myasthenia gravis would have a more insidious onset, with bilateral ptosis and fatigue as the predominant features (no pain). Disturbance of vision is the initial main complaint.

Therefore in view of the acute pain and third nerve palsy, an unruptured aneurysm of the posterior communicating artery best explains the findings. In this situation, the patient should be referred urgently to the neurosurgical team with a view to further imaging and surgery.

Understanding the anatomy of the oculomotor (third) nerve helps with identifying the signs and the causes. The nucleus of the third nerve is positioned in the midbrain and passes through the cerebral peduncles. It then passes anterior to the superior cerebellar and posterior cerebellar arteries. From here it runs along the posterior communicating artery, entering the cavernous sinus and through the superior orbital fissure into the orbit. Finally, it supplies the muscles of the eye (the inferior, superior and medial recti muscles, the inferior oblique, levator palpebrae and sphincter pupillae) apart from the superior oblique (IVth nerve) and lateral rectus (VIth) nerve.

Therefore, a third nerve palsy (**Figure 8.1**) will result in:

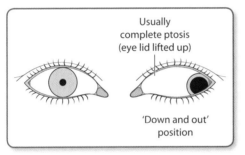

Figure 8.1 Third (oculomotor) nerve palsy.

- Complete ptosis
- 'Down and out' position of the eye (lateral rectus and superior oblique preserved)
- Fixed and dilated pupil

The causes of a third nerve palsy can be remembered using the following mnemonic, '**AVID SITCOM**':

Aneurysm (posterior communicating artery) – usually painful
Vascular lesions
Iatrogenic
Diabetes

Multiple **S**clerosis
Infection
Trauma
Cavernous sinus thrombosis
Post-**O**perative complication
Myasthenia gravis

Bruce BB, Biousse V, Newman NJ. Third nerve palsies. Semin Neurol 2007; 27(3):257–68.

16. B Left optic tract (Figure 8.2)

Right homonymous hemianopia means that the lesion is on the **LEFT**.

As a reminder, for quadrantanopsias: ='PITS'

Parietal lobe = Inferior quadrantanopia
Temporal lobe = Superior quadrantanopia

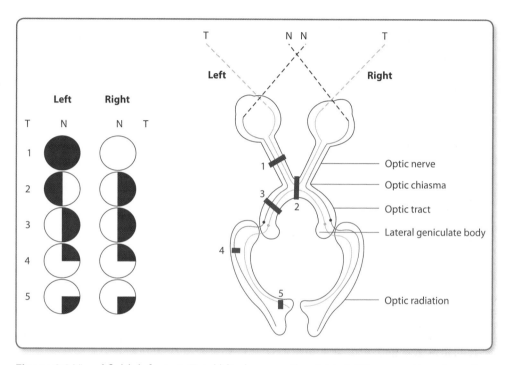

Figure 8.2 Visual field defects. 1. Total blindness on the right; 2. Bitemporal hemianopia; 3. Right homonymous hemianopia; 4. Right upper quadrantanopia; 5. Right lower quadrantanopia. Key: N, nasal field; T, temporal field.

17. A Antibodies to voltage gated calcium channels

Antibodies to voltage-gated calcium channels are used in the diagnosis of Lambert–Eaton syndrome. Diagnosis of myasthenia gravis relies on both serological and electrophysiological testing. Antibodies to the acetylcholine receptor is the test of choice. It has a sensitivity of 80–95%, but may be negative. Antibodies to muscle-specific receptor tyrosine kinase may be positive in those patients who are negative for acetylcholine receptor antibodies, particularly those with ocular-bulbar involvement.

Single fibre electromyography is much more selective than conventional electromyography and is the most sensitive measure of neuromuscular junction transmission.

Although traditionally the Tensilon test has been thought of the investigation of choice, it is not used widely in clinical practice. The Tensilon test is not as specific or sensitive as serological or electrophysiological testing.

Scherer K, Bedlack RS, Simel DL. Does this patient have myasthenia gravis? JAMA 2005; 293(15): 1906–1914.

18. E Systemic lupus erythematosus (SLE)

Thyrotoxicosis rather than hypothyroidism is a recognised cause of chorea.

Chorea is a continuous, non-rhythmic, purposeless jerking movement, flitting from limb to face with no specific pattern. Huntingdon's disease and rheumatic fever (Sydenham's chorea) are the two well-known causes, using the aid '**SHOPPER**':

SLE
Huntingdon's disease
Oral contraceptive pill and other medications (phenytoin)
Pregnancy (chorea gravidum)
Polycythaemia rubra vera
Endocrine – thyrotoxicosis
Rheumatic fever

Orzechowski NM, et al. Antiphospholipid antibody-associated chorea. J Rheumatol 2008; 35(11):2165–2170.

19. B Intranasal desmopressin

Bladder dysfunction is a major side effect of multiple sclerosis. Prophylactic antibiotics are not recommended for the management of chronic bladder dysfunction. In the initial management, acute infection should be ruled out in those with worsening urinary symptoms and a post-micturition bladder ultrasonography should be performed.

Intranasal desmopressin should be offered to any person with a history of nocturia, or those who have failed other treatments. Anticholinergics such as oxybutynin and tolterodine may be an option. If a large post micturition bladder volume is present, intermittent self-catheterisation could be an option (if the patient is able to perform this). Electric shock stimulation therapy can be used followed by a structured programme of pelvic floor muscle exercises. Intravesical botulinum infection is also a possibility. Ultimately long-term catheterisation may be required, but the patient's sexual function should be considered prior to this.

National Institute for Health and Clinical Excellence (NICE). Multiple sclerosis: Management of multiple sclerosis in primary and secondary care. Clinical Guideline CG8, London: NICE, 2003.

20. E Tension headache

The chronic nature of the headache, along with typical band like pressure description makes tension headaches the likely diagnosis.

Life-threatening headaches can be generally divided into the following three categories:

1. Meningitis
2. Subarachnoid haemorrhage
3. Raised intracranial pressure

The headache in meningitis occurs much more acutely, with associated fever and systemic symptoms. There is sometimes (but not always) the presence of photophobia and neck stiffness and, if severe can lead to drowsiness. Bacterial meningitis may have a petechial, non-blanching rash.

Subarachnoid haemorrhage (SAH) features an abrupt and sudden onset of the 'thunder clap headache', typically at the back of the head and sometimes associated with vomiting. The important information is to establish over what period the headache reached the maximum intensity. A headache reaching its peak at 15 minutes and lasting over 1–2 hours, makes the diagnosis unlikely (but certainly not impossible). **Figure 8.3** is a CT scan of a subarachnoid haemorrhage.

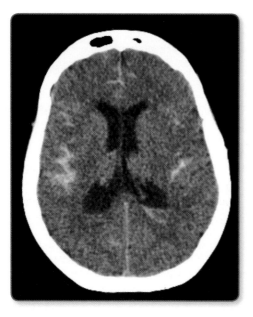

Figure 8.3 CT head showing subarachnoid haemorrhage.

Diagnosing raised intracranial pressure (secondary to an intracranial lesion) is clinically difficult. The key features however are headaches, which get worse on coughing or bending, and are particularly severe in the mornings. The presence of seizures or personality changes certainly necessitates urgent investigation.

Tension headache presents as a band like pressure around the head, with a non-pulsating and tightening quality. It is intermittent in its onset, normally does not last longer than a few hours and may be accompanied with photophobia during the acute exacerbations.

Duncan CW, Watson DP, Stein A; Guideline Development Group. Diagnosis and management of headache in adults: summary of SIGN guideline. BMJ 2008; 337:a2329.

21. B EEG showing periodic sharp waves

Creutzfeldt–Jakob disease (CJD) is rare but fatal neurodegenerative disease caused by a protein called prion. Rapidly progressive dementia is one of the first features of the condition and quickly progresses to further neurological and cognitive abnormalities.

The different forms of the condition include sporadic, variant (acquired form) and a rarer form, familial. It is important to differentiate the features of sporadic and variant CJD, particularly as variant CJD has become much more of an issue in recent years (**Table 8.6**).

Table 8.6		
	Sporadic CJD	**Variant CJD**
Mean presenting age	60 years	28 years
Mean duration of disease	5 months	14 months
Clinical features*	Myoclonus	Myoclonus
	Behavioural/personality changes	Pyramidal signs
	Sleep disorders	Cerebellar signs
	Visual disturbances/hallucinations	Vertical gaze palsy
'Pulvinar' sign** on MRI (T2 DWI, FLAIR sequences)	Usually absent	Present in a significant proportion (up to 90% of cases)
EEG findings	Periodic wave complexes	Slow wave complexes
* Please note in some cases these features can be interchangeable between the different forms. ** 'Pulvinar' sign is a radiological finding, which is highly specific and sensitive for variant CJD and is a characteristic abnormality of symmetrical hyperintensity of the posterior thalamic region.		

Table 8.6 Differences between sporadic and variant Creutzfeldt–Jakob disease (CJD).

Although it is said that definitive diagnosis of CJD can only occur once an autopsy is performed, improvement in imaging and diagnostic tests mean that along with clinical features, an accurate diagnosis of CJD can be made during a patient's lifetime. In addition to the clinical history and examination, as well as ruling out other causes of dementia the following diagnostic tools are used in identifying CJD.

- Electroencephalogram (EEG)
- Cerebrospinal fluid examination for 14-3-3 protein
- MRI (T2-weighted images)
- PET scan
- The diagnosis of familial CJD is through testing for the *PRNP* (prion protein) gene

There are no current proven treatments for Creutzfeldt–Jakob disease.

Belay ED, Schonberger. Variant Creutzfeldt–Jakob disease and bovine spongiform encephalopathy. Clin Lab Med 2002; 22(4):849–862.
Collie DA, Summers DM, Sellar RJ, et al. Diagnosing variant Creutzfeldt–Jakob disease with the pulvinar sign: MR imaging findings in 86 neuropathologically confirmed cases. AJNR Am J Neuroradiol 2003; 24(8):1560–1569.

22. D Right parietal lobe

Parietal lobe = inferior quadrantanopia
Temporal lobe = superior quadrantonopia (see **Figure 8.4**)

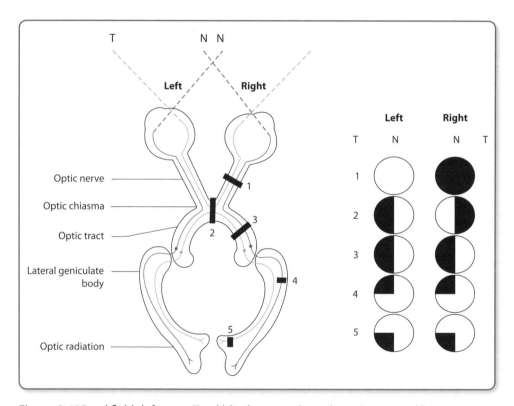

Figure 8.4 Visual field defects; 1. Total blindness on the right; 2. Bitemporal hemianopia; 3. Left homonymous hemianopia; 4. Left upper quadrantanopia; 5. Left lower quadrantanopia. T, temporal field; N, nasal field.

23. A Anterior spinal artery thrombosis

Anterior spinal artery thrombosis leads to damage to the corticospinal and spinothalamic tracts causing loss of pain and temperature. As the dorsal column lies posteriorly, vibration and proprioception remains intact. A patient with anterior spinal artery thrombosis will present with acute flaccid paraplegia, urinary retention and loss of pain and temperature below the level of the lesion.

Brown-Séquard syndrome or hemicord syndrome, results in involvement of the descending corticospinal tract leading to ipsilateral upper motor neuron weakness below the lesion and ascending dorsal column involvement causing ipsilateral joint position and vibration loss. In addition, there is contralateral loss of pain and temperature because of crossed ascending spinothalamic fibres involved.

Metastatic infiltration and prolapsed disc will cause extrinsic cord compression with predominant motor signs. In addition, prolapsed disc at thoracic levels is uncommon.

Spinothalamic tracts are always involved in syringomyelia and results in the earliest signs. The dorsal column is spared. The syrinx usually originates at the cervical cord causing bilateral wasting and weakness in the small muscles of the hand due to compression of T1 roots.

Suzuki K, Meguro K, Wada M, et al. Anterior spinal artery syndrome associated with severe stenosis of the vertebral artery. AJNR Am J Neuroradiol 1998; 19(7):1353–1355.

24. B Cardiomyopathy

There are various forms of myotonic dystrophy, however type 1 is by far the most common type. It is an autosomal dominant condition, with a prevalence of approximately 1 in 8000 with a trinucleotide sequence expansion. Myotonic dystrophy also follows the phenomenon of genetic anticipation as the trinucleotide expansion increases in successive generations.

Myotonic dystrophy type 1 is caused by a defect in the *DMPK* (dystrophia myotonica-protein kinase) gene on chromosome 19 and distal weakness is more prominent.

Myotonic dystrophy type 2 is caused by a defect on the *ZNF9* (zinc finger protein) gene located on chromosome 3, and proximal weakness is more prominent.

The features and associated conditions with myotonic dystrophy involve many systems. Typical onset is at around 25 years of age (equal male to female ratio) with myotonia, weakness, muscle wasting in the face. Additional features which can be remembered by going from '**head to toe**' as illustrated in **Figure 8.5**.

SOD1 (superoxide dismutase) gene defect is associated with motor neurone disease (amyotrophic lateral sclerosis)

Turner C, Hilton-Jones D. The myotonic dystrophies: diagnosis and management. J Neurol Neurosurg Psychiatry 2010; 81(4):358–367.

25. B Frontotemporal dementia

Motor neuron disease (MND) is a progressive neurodegenerative disease, with degeneration of the neurons of the spinal cord ventral horn. This patient has motor neurone disease, with a mixture of upper and lower motor neuron signs; therefore the most likely diagnosis is amyotrophic lateral sclerosis, which is the most common form of motor neuron disease. The different forms are:

- Amyotrophic lateral sclerosis
- Bulbar palsy – this is a lower motor neuron lesion leading to a nasal speech, difficultly in swallowing and a flaccid and fasciculating tongue

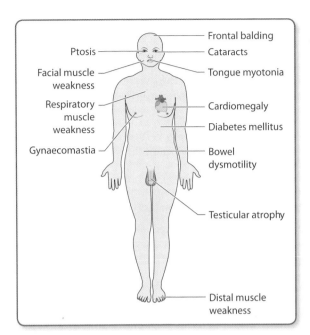

Figure 8.5 Clinical features of myotonic dystrophy.

- Progressive muscular atrophy – anterior horn lesion. It has a better prognosis than amyotrophic lateral sclerosis and typically affects the distal before proximal muscles.

In motor neuron disease there is an absence of sensory and sphincter disturbances. There is no involvement of external eye movements (III, IV and VI cranial nerves).

Frontotemporal dementia is seen in up to 35% of cases.

Lillo P, Hodges JR. Frontotemporal dementia and motor neurone disease: Overlapping clinic-pathological disorders. J Clin Neurosci 2009; 16(9):1131–1135.

26. B Benign paroxysmal positional vertigo (BPPV)

Dizzy spells are a common complaint and associated with a wide differential diagnosis. Benign paroxysmal positional vertigo (BPPV) is one of the most common inner ear conditions.

Vertigo is a distinct symptom and a particular type of dizziness – a feeling of movement of the patient or surroundings when the patient is stationary. Vertigo is always exacerbated by movement. Therefore, vertigo and dizziness may sometimes be used as interchangeable terms and it essential to obtain a detailed description of the symptoms.

BPPV can be triggered by infection, trauma or vasculitis and is probably caused by debris in the inner ear. The key feature is recurrent vertigo with change of position such as bending forward and turning in bed. Additionally these episodes occur for a short period (a few minutes) and are self-limiting, occasionally accompanied by nausea. Diagnosis is by the Hallpike manoeuvre, which in summary is performed by sitting the patient upright and moving the patient's head by forty five degrees towards the ear being tested, whilst keeping the patients eyes focused on the examiner's eyes. A positive result is with the presence of rotational nystagmus on testing. Formal consent must be obtained prior to the procedure.

Acute labyrinthitis is caused by inflammation of the inner ear and may be associated with hearing loss and tinnitus. It occurs with rapid onset severe vertigo, with the presence of nystagmus on examination.

Acoustic neuroma presents with hearing loss, with vertigo a feature later on in the disease course. There is also cranial nerve involvement (ipsilateral V, VI, IX and X), along with ipsilateral cerebellar signs.

Ménière's disease is characterised by fluctuating sensorineural hearing loss, tinnitus and vertigo. Episodes of vertigo are prolonged (can last to 30 minutes, if not longer).

Furman JM, Cass SP. Benign paroxysmal positional vertigo. N Engl J Med 1999; 341:1590–1596.

27. A Foville's syndrome

These are a collection of eponymous syndromes related to brainstem infarction.

Foville's syndrome is involvement in the pons leading to ipsilateral VI nerve palsy, facial weakness with contralateral hemiplegia and a lateral conjugate gaze palsy.

Millard–Gubler syndrome is the as Foville's syndrome but **without** the lateral conjugate gaze palsy.

Nothnagel's syndrome is involvement in the midbrain, leading to ipsilateral III nerve palsy and cerebellar ataxia.

Weber's syndrome is also in the midbrain leading to ipsilateral III nerve palsy and contralateral hemiplegia.

Wallenberg's syndrome (or lateral medullary syndrome) is characterised by:

Ipsilateral: Horner's syndrome (descending sympathetic tract)
                Cerebellar signs (cerebellum)
                Reduced trigeminal temperature and pain sensation (V)
                IX and X nerve palsy leading to palatial paralysis

Contralteral: spinothalamic tract involvement resulting in reduced pain and temperature sensation

Hubloue I, Laureys S, Michotte A. A rare case of diplopia: medial inferior pontine syndrome or Foville's syndrome. Eur J Emerg Med 1996; 3(3):194–198.

28. D Subthalamic nucleus

Hemiballismus is a random, severe, flinging movement of the limbs occurring contralateral to the side of the lesion. The most common site of the lesion is the subthalamic nucleus. Although rarer, lesions at other sites may cause hemiballismus.

It occurs most commonly in patients with hypertension, diabetes and those who have had a stroke.

Handley A, et al. Movement disorders after stroke. Age Ageing 2009; 38(3):260–266.

29. C Syphilis serology

The basic screen for dementia at the initial presentation includes:

- Routine haematology
- Biochemistry (glucose, calcium, liver function tests, electrolytes and renal function)
- Serum vitamin B_{12} and folate levels
- Thyroid function

The following should not be performed routinely, unless there are risk factors, or clinical signs

- Syphilis serology
- HIV test
- Cerebrospinal fluid analysis

National Institute for Health and Clinical Excellence (NICE). Dementia: supporting people with dementia and their carers in health and social care. Clinical Guideline CG42. London: NICE, 2006.

30. C Magnesium sulphate

This patient has eclampsia presenting with a seizure. Eclampsia is defined the occurrence of one or more seizures on the background of pre-eclampsia. The recommendations for control of seizures in eclampsia is firstly to assess the patient's airway and seek appropriate help. The patient should be placed in the left lateral position. Intravenous magnesium is the therapy of choice to control seizures, initially with a loading dose over 10 minutes, followed by a continuous infusion over 24 hours. Diazepam and phenytoin should not be used as first line treatment. Signs of magnesium toxicity (respiratory depression and loss of deep tendon reflexes) along with serum levels should be monitored. If there is evidence of magnesium toxicity, calcium gluconate infusion should be started.

Pre-eclampsia is pregnancy-induced hypertension with proteinuria (>0.3 g over 24 hours). In this setting, severe hypertension is classed as systolic blood pressure >170 mmHg and diastolic blood pressure >110 mmHg on two separate occasions. Therefore, the features of pre-eclampsia are:

- Hypertension
- Proteinuria
- Severe headache
- Visual disturbance
- Papilloedema
- Epigastric pain
- Clonus
- HELLP syndrome (haemolysis, elevated liver enzymes and low platelets)

In pre-eclampsia, without the presence of seizures, anti-hypertensives should be started with a systolic blood pressure > 160 mmHg and diastolic blood pressure > 110 mmHg, although treatment could be started if the clinical condition warrants it. The following are recommended:

- Intravenous or oral labetalol
- Intravenous or oral nifedipine
- Intravenous hydralazine
- Intravenous or oral methyldopa

In moderate hypertension, alternative agents which the clinician is comfortable with, can be used. However diuretics, angiotensin-converting enzyme inhibitors (ACEi), angiotensin receptor blocking (ARB) medications should be avoided in pregnancy.

Altman D, Carroli G, Duley L, et al. Do women with pre-eclampsia, and their babies, benefit from magnesium sulphate? The Magpie Trial: a randomised placebo-controlled trial. Lancet 2002; 359: 1877–1890.
Royal College of Obstetricians and Gynaecologists (RCOG). The management of severe pre-eclampsia/ eclampsia. Guideline No. 10A. London: RCOG, 2010.

Chapter 9

Ophthalmology

1. A 56-year-old man attended the rapid access eye clinic complaining of his vision being tinted with a blue hue. His past medical history included chronic obstructive pulmonary disease, type 2 diabetes mellitus, hypertension, paroxysmal atrial fibrillation, and erectile dysfunction. Slit lamp examination revealed normal anterior chamber, lens, vitreous humour and retina.

    Which drug is the most likely cause of the blue vision?

    A   Amlodipine
    B   Bendroflumethiazide
    C   Digoxin
    D   Metformin
    E   Sildenafil

2. A 56-year-old man was seen in the hypertension clinic. Funduscopy showed multiple flame-shaped haemorrhages and a few cotton wool spots with normal optic discs bilaterally.

    Investigations:

urine analysis	protein 1+
	glucose 1+
	blood negative

    What is the most likely diagnosis?

    A   Grade I hypertensive retinopathy
    B   Grade II hypertensive retinopathy
    C   Grade III hypertensive retinopathy
    D   Malignant hypertension
    E   Pre-proliferative diabetic retinopathy

3. A 30-year-old woman was referred to the ophthalmology clinic after diabetic changes were found at her routine retinal screening. She explained that she had noticed worsening of her vision in the right eye in recent months. She was found to have proliferative retinopathy in her right eye without involvement of the macula and pre-proliferative retinopathy in the left eye.

    What is the most appropriate treatment?

    A   Intravitreal triamcinolone acetate
    B   Laser photocoagulation to left eye

   C   Panretinal photocoagulation to right eye
   D   Ruboxistaurin
   E   Vitrectomy

4. A 57-year-old man attended his annual diabetic review in clinic. Funduscopy revealed dot/blot haemorrhages, cotton wool spots and venous beading in both eyes.

   Which one of the following is the least likely cause?

   A   Macrovascular retinal changes related to poor diabetic control
   B   Basement membrane thickening
   C   Capillary endothelial cell damage
   D   Hyperglycaemia-induced loss of vascular pericytes
   E   Increased platelet aggregation

5. A 70-year-old Caucasian woman was seen in the eye clinic complaining of distorted central vision that had come on rapidly over the last 2 weeks. She described straight lines appearing wavy when reading.

   What is the most significant predisposing risk factor for the likely underlying eye condition?

   A   Age > 60 years
   B   Family history
   C   Female sex
   D   Myopia
   E   Smoking

6. A 45-year-woman presented to her general practitioner because her partner had noticed that her right pupil was larger than her left pupil. On examination, she had abnormal pupillary reflexes as below.

   Investigations:

	Direct reflex	Consensual reflex	Accommodation
Left pupil	Sluggish	Sluggish	Slow
Right pupil	Normal	Normal	Normal

   What is the most likely diagnosis?

   A   Congenital anisocoria
   B   Left Argyll Robertson pupil
   C   Left Holmes–Adie pupil
   D   Left Horner's syndrome
   E   Left optic neuritis

7. A 34-year-old man presented to the rapid access eye clinic with a painful right eye. He described right eye photophobia, increased lacrimation and blurred vision. On examination, he had a red eye with a small fixed oval right pupil, blurred vision on the right side without any staining of the cornea with fluorescein.

What is the most likely diagnosis?

A   Acute angle closure glaucoma
B   Acute anterior uveitis
C   Conjunctivitis
D   Corneal abrasion
E   Scleritis

8. A 58-year-old man presented to the emergency department complaining of headache and sudden onset of painless blurred vision. He suffered with hypertension, for which he took amlodipine. On examination, in the left eye he had reduced visual acuity to 6/12, and loss of vision in the lower nasal field. Examination of the right eye was normal.

Investigations:

erythrocyte sedimentation rate   8 mm/1st hour (<20)

What is the most likely diagnosis?

A   Acute optic neuritis
B   Branch retinal artery occlusion
C   Branch retinal vein occlusion
D   Central retinal artery occlusion
E   Central retinal vein occlusion

Answers

1. E Sildenafil

This man is complaining of blue vision, also known as cyanopsia. There are two main causes of this phenomenon:

1. Post cataract removal – The normal eye lens is naturally tinted yellow to reduce the intensity of blue light reaching the retina. After cataract removal, the replacement artificial lens is clear, so it allows more blue light to fall on the retina, thus causing cyanopsia. Studies have shown that cyanopsia tends to last only for a few weeks to months post cataract removal, implying that some method of neural adaptation or colour constancy occurs.
2. Sildenafil – This is primarily a phosphodiesterase (PDE)-5 inhibitor but in high doses, can inhibit PDE-6. Phosphodiesterase-6 is involved in regulating the function of rod cells, which are most sensitive to light of wavelengths near 498 nm (i.e. blue-green light), so inhibition of PDE-6 enhances rod cell sensitivity to blue light. There is also a risk of altitudinal visual field loss with sildenafil use.

Xanthopsia refers to yellow vision due to yellowing of the optic media of the eye. The principal cause is digoxin toxicity causing cataracts that produce a yellow filtering effect.

The other medications are not known to affect colour perception.

Jordan DR, Valberg JD. Dyschromatopsia following cataract surgery. Can J Ophthalmol 1986; 21(4):140-143.

2. C Grade III hypertensive retinopathy

Hypertensive retinopathy is classified as shown in **Table 9.1**.

Disc swelling is not synonymous with papilloedema, which is a term that should only be applied to bilateral disc swelling secondary to raised intracranial pressure. It is commonly incorrectly used to describe disc swelling of any cause.

Table 9.1	
Grade	**Funduscopic changes**
I	Mild generalised narrowing of arterioles
II	Arteriovenous (AV) nipping
	Moderate narrowing of arterioles
III	Flame-shaped haemorrhages and cotton wool spots (signifying infarction of nerve fibre layer of retina)
	Marked arteriolar narrowing ('copper wiring')
IV	Disc swelling from 'accelerated-phase' or 'malignant' hypertension
	Severe arteriolar narrowing ('silver wiring')

Table 9.1 Grades of hypertensive retinopathy.

Grade IV hypertensive retinopathy needs urgent treatment with antihypertensives because it can cause severe target organ damage and increased mortality.

Hypertension can also predispose to retinal vein occlusion and retinal artery macroaneurysms.

Keith NM, Wagener HP, Barker NW. Some different types of essential hypertension: their course and prognosis. Am J Med Sci 1974; 268(6):336.
Wong TY, et al. Retinal microvascular abnormalities, and their relation to hypertension, cardiovascular diseases and mortality. Surv Ophthalmol 2001; 46: 59–80.

3. C Panretinal photocoagulation to right eye

Treatment of diabetic retinopathy depends on what stage of diabetic eye disease the patient has reached as shown in **Table 9.2**.

Mohamed Q, Gillies MC, Wong TY. Management of diabetic retinopathy: a systematic review. JAMA 2007; 298(8):902.

Table 9.2

Stage of diabetic retinopathy	Funduscopic appearance	Treatment
Background	Microaneurysms Dot/blot haemorrhages Hard exudates (leakage of lipids and lipoproteins)	No local treatment is usually required other than adequate control of diabetes
Maculopathy (More common in type 2 diabetes)	Microaneurysms, dot/blot haemorrhages and hard exudates in the macular area in close proximity to the fovea	1. Macular oedema close to the fovea risks damage to central vision and requires laser photocoagulation 2. Intravitreal triamcinolone is a long-acting steroid that can reduce diabetic macular oedema not responding to repeated laser treatment. The preparation lasts for 3 months, so repeated injections may be needed. Complications include steroid-induced glaucoma, cataracts and endophthalmitis 3. Ruboxistaurin is a protein kinase C-β inhibitor that has been proposed to work on diabetic macular oedema but is not currently licensed yet. It is only an investigational drug at present so option D is incorrect
Pre-proliferative	As background retinopathy changes plus cotton wool spots (axonal ischaemia), venous dilatation, venous beading	Currently deferment of laser treatment is advocated, based on previous randomised controlled trials

Contd...

Contd...

Proliferative (more common in Type I diabetes)	Retinal neovascularisation at the disc and the vascular arcades Vitreous haemorrhage Tractional retinal detachment Iris neovascularisation (may be complicated by glaucoma)	1. Proliferative retinopathy can be treated with laser photocoagulation, which aims to stop the production of vascular endothelial growth factor (VEGF) from the ischaemic retina at visible lesions and cause regression of new vessels 2. Panretinal photocoagulation (PRP) involves the creation of 1500–2000 burns in the peripheral retina, which effectively destroys the peripheral retinal tissue. Whilst laser photocoagulation targets specific lesions, PRP is applied over extensive areas of the retina. This will reduce the oxygen demand and VEGF production from the retina. Patients undergoing PRP may lose some of their peripheral vision; patients undergoing bilateral PRP may not be able to legally drive and should inform the appropriate authorities. Patients can also experience a reduction of contrast and night vision. However, PRP has been shown to lower the risk of severe vision loss by 50% 3. Vitrectomy is indicated when there is severe vitreous haemorrhage or retinal detachment from proliferative diabetic retinopathy

Table 9.2 Features and management of diabetic retinopathy.

4. A Macrovascular retinal changes related to poor diabetic control

Diabetic retinopathy is due to microvascular, rather than macrovascular, retinal changes. The pathological changes that cause increased vascular permeability are:

- Intramural death of pericytes due to hyperglycaemia (via protein kinase C-β signalling) causes a reduction in the structural architecture of the vessel wall, which leads to disruption of the blood–retina barrier and predisposes to the formation of microaneurysms
- Capillary endothelial cell damage leads to the formation of hard exudates on the retina
- Basement membrane thickening from carbohydrate and glycogen deposition
- Increased platelet aggregation

Neovascularisation is thought to be caused by the production of growth factors, e.g. vascular endothelial growth factor (VEGF), in response to retinal ischaemia.

Strict control of diabetes and any concurrent hypertension, as well as smoking cessation, are key to reducing the sequelae of diabetic retinopathy at all stages.

Ciulla TA, Amador AG, Zinman B. Diabetic retinopathy and diabetic macular edema: pathophysiology, screening, and novel therapies. Diabetes Care 2003; 26(9):2653–2664.

5. A Age > 60 years

This woman has age-related macular degeneration (AMD). This is a degenerative disease of the macula (the centre of the retina). There are two forms of the disease:

1. Dry AMD – Early on this is characterised by drusen, which appear as yellow spots on fundus examination. These are formed by build-up of debris within Bruch's membrane (lying under the retina) due to reduced phagocytosis with ageing. Later on atrophy of the retinal pigment epithelium occurs, which leads to gradual vision loss through loss of photoreceptors (rods and cones) at the macula. 90% of patients with AMD have the dry form, for which there is no treatment. However 10% develop wet AMD.
2. Wet AMD – This occurs due to choroidal neovascularisation. This leads to growth of abnormal blood vessels under/within the retina. These vessels are fragile and can leak fluid or blood. Leakage at or near the foveal centre can present suddenly as central distortion or blurring, or as a central scotoma (blind spot). If not treated promptly this can lead to irreversible photoreceptor damage and scarring. Treatment is now available for wet AMD, through intravitreal injection of anti-vascular endothelial growth factor injections (e.g. ranibizumab), which should be given promptly to avoid visual deterioration.

All the above risk factors are involved in AMD but age is the biggest risk factor and smoking is the most modifiable.

Klein R, et al. Fifteen-year cumulative incidence of age-related macular degeneration: the Beaver Dam Eye Study. Ophthalmol 2007; 114(2):253–262.
Chakravarthy U, et al. Clinical risk factors for age-related macular degeneration: a systematic review and meta-analysis. BMC Ophthalmology 2010; 10:31.

6. C Left Holmes–Adie pupil

This woman has a left Holmes–Adie pupil. It is a benign condition, being unilateral in 80% of cases and affecting women more than men (2:1). It is caused by denervation of the postganglionic supply to the sphincter pupillae and ciliary muscle, and may follow a viral illness. The affected pupil does eventually react to accommodation but over a much longer duration of time than normal. This pupillary defect can be associated with absent ankle and knee reflexes, giving the Holmes–Adie syndrome. Congenital anisocoria (unequal pupils) would produce normal light/accommodation reflexes on either eye. Argyll Robertson pupil is a complication of neurosyphilis and usually causes bilateral asymmetric small irregular pupils which react to both light and accommodation. Horner's syndrome causes a large pupil which reacts normally to light and accommodation, associated with a mild ptosis. Optic neuritis can cause reduced light reflexes (afferent papillary defect) but with no anisocoria.

Lee A. Tonic pupil. In: Basow DS (ed), UpToDate. Waltham, MA: UpToDate, 2011. http://www.uptodate.com (Last accessed 1 May 2012).

7. B Acute anterior uveitis

All of the options are causes of painful red eye. Option B is the most likely given the associated symptoms of photophobia, lacrimation and blurred vision with a small pupil. The small pupil occurs due to posterior synechiae, which describes adhesions between the pupil and the anterior surface of the lens. This occurs due to increased fibrinous exudation in the anterior chamber as a result of inflammation. Treatment of uveitis involves topical steroids and cycloplegic agents (to break the posterior synechiae). Acute angle closure glaucoma also presents with pain and reduced vision but typically other features are semi-dilated pupil, hazy cornea and the patient sees haloes. Conjunctivitis tends to be bilateral and there is usually discharge (purulent if bacterial and clear if viral). Corneal abrasions would stain with fluorescein on testing with blue light, and the pupil would be unaffected. Scleritis presents with an intensely red tender eye with severe throbbing pain, which can wake up the patient at night; the pupil again would be unaffected.

Howard M, Leibowitz MD. The Red Eye. N Engl J Med 2000; 343:345–351.

8. B Branch retinal artery occlusion

There is a left lower nasal field defect suggesting occlusion of the superior temporal branch of the left retinal artery – a branch retinal artery occlusion.

Table 9.3					
Trauma	Toxic	Infectious	Inflammatory	Compressive	Congenital
	Alcohol	Any cause of meningitis	Autoimmune – Sjögren's SLE	Abscess	Leber's hereditary optic neuropathy
	Tobacco			Glioma	
	Vitamin B_1 and B_{12} deficiency	Lyme disease	Paraneoplastic	Meningioma	
		Syphilis	Sarcoidosis	Thyroid ophthalmopathy	
		Toxoplasma			

SLE, systemic lupus erythematosus.

Table 9.3 Causes of optic neuritis.

Occlusion of the central retinal artery causes retinal infarction and thus sudden, profound, painless visual loss in the corresponding area supplied. On funduscopy one would expect to find a pale oedematous retina with a cherry-red spot at the fovea (although this latter feature, caused by the choroidal reflex showing through the fovea where the retina is thinner, only tends to last for 48 hours). Treatment is to induce vascular dilatation by rebreathing to cause hypercarbia or reducing intraocular pressure.

The clinical signs of central retinal vein occlusion include loss of vision, relative afferent pupillary defect, multiple retinal haemorrhages (giving a 'blood and thunder' appearance on funduscopy), retinal venous dilatation, cotton wool spots, vascular sheathing and neovascularisation.

Acute optic neuritis is a demyelinating, inflammatory condition that causes painful, usually monocular, visual loss and has a strong association with multiple sclerosis. Gadolinium-enhanced MRI will show optic nerve inflammation in 95% of patients. Methylprednisolone hastens recovery, which is usually complete. There are other causes of optic neuritis that can be remembered by the mnemonic 'TIC' as shown in **Table 9.3**.

Hedges T. Central and branch retinal artery occlusion. In: Basow DS (ed), UpToDate. Waltham, MA: UpToDate, 2012. http://www.uptodate.com (Last accessed 1 May 2012).
Osborne B, Balcer L. Optic neuropathies. In: Basow DS (ed), UpToDate. Waltham, MA: UpToDate, 2012. http://www.uptodate.com (Last accessed 1 May 2012).

Chapter 10

Psychiatry

1. A 78-year-old man was referred to clinic because of worsening confusion. He was accompanied by his daughter, who said that his behaviour had changed over the past year, fluctuating between episodes where he was completely well to those where he was not able to do even basic activities. During the past few weeks, he had also described seeing his mother at home, even though she had died over 20 years ago. He had had two falls at home over the past 2 months, but previously had no history of falls. He had no problems with his vision, which had been recently checked by an optician. He had no past medical history of note and took no regular medications.

   What is the most likely diagnosis?

   A   Alzheimer's disease
   B   Charles Bonnet syndrome
   C   Frontotemporal dementia
   D   Lewy body dementia
   E   Vascular (multi-infarct) dementia

2. A 48-year-old woman was referred to the neurology clinic because of recurrent left arm paraesthesia. She had undergone extensive investigations previously including blood tests, nerve conduction studies, Doppler studies, and magnetic resonance imaging of her head, spine and left shoulder with no cause found. The symptoms had been present for 18 months, but had been particularly persistent since her divorce 1 year ago. She had no other past medical history, took no regular medication, and neither smoked nor drank alcohol. Examination of the arms was normal.

   What is the most likely diagnosis?

   A   Conversion disorder
   B   Generalised anxiety disorder
   C   Hypochondriacal disorder
   D   Post-traumatic stress disorder
   E   Somatisation disorder

3. A 62-year-old man was admitted to hospital after a fracture of his right radius following a road traffic accident. He denied any past medical history and his only regular medication was thiamine supplements. He underwent uncomplicated surgery and returned to the ward with the aim of several days of physiotherapy prior to discharge. Two days post-operatively, the patient developed nausea and sweating, and was noted by the nurses to be agitated and disorientated.

Examination revealed the patient to be afebrile, but with a regular pulse of 112 beats per minute, blood pressure 170/100 mmHg, and a marked rest tremor. The patient also described seeing 'shapes at the end of my bed that come and go'.

Investigations:

haemoglobin	132 g/L (130–180)
mean cell volume	106 fL (80–96)
white cell count	10.4×10^9/L (4.0–11.0)
serum sodium	137 mmol/L (137–144)
serum potassium	3.6 mmol/L (3.5–4.9)
serum urea	2.7 mmol/L (2.5–7.0)
serum creatinine	108 µmol/L (60–110)
serum C-reactive protein	21 mg/L (<10)
urine analysis	negative
chest X-ray	normal
ECG	sinus rhythm, rate 112 beats per minute
CT head	involutional changes, no haemorrhage

What is the most appropriate treatment?

A   Adenosine
B   Chlordiazepoxide
C   Metoprolol
D   Quetiapine
E   Zopiclone

4. A 42-year-old man was assessed because of a 1-year history of low mood, irritability and anxiety. He was accompanied by his wife who described recent episodes of confusion and frequent 'twitching' movements in his arms and legs. He had no previous medical history and took no regular medications. His brother and mother were both well, but his father had been under follow-up by a neurologist for an unknown condition before committing suicide aged 56. Examination revealed a man with low affect and poor eye contact. There were some involuntary, non-stereotyped, jerk-like movements in his arms and legs but tone, power and reflexes were normal.

What is the most likely diagnosis?

A   Catatonic schizophrenia
B   Gilles de la Tourette syndrome
C   Huntington's disease
D   Parkinson's disease
E   Severe depression

5. A 34-year-old woman was referred because of debilitating tiredness, generalised myalgia and painful lymph nodes. These symptoms started after an upper respiratory tract infection 8 months ago and had never resolved. She had been

on long-term sick leave from work ever since. She had undergone extensive investigation by a number of different physicians but no cause for her symptoms had been found. She was given a diagnosis of chronic fatigue syndrome.

What is the most appropriate management?

A   Antiretroviral therapy
B   Corticosteroids
C   Doxycycline
D   Eye movement desensitisation and reprocessing
E   Graded exercise therapy

6.   A 38-year-old woman presented to her general practitioner with a 3-day history of constant anxiety, insomnia, and persistent pacing up and down. Four days ago, she was on holiday abroad when an earthquake occurred, killing a number of people in the town in which she was staying. She and her husband had sustained no injuries. According to her husband, there had been no change in her mood. She had no other past medical history and took no regular medications.

What is the most likely diagnosis?

A   Acute stress disorder
B   Adjustment disorder
C   Generalised anxiety disorder
D   Panic disorder
E   Post-traumatic stress disorder

7.   A 40-year-old man was brought to the emergency department by the police with confusion. He had been found by a member of the public at a bus stop, and could neither remember his name or address nor how he got to the bus stop. He denied any past medical history, and claimed not to drink alcohol, smoke, or take recreational drugs. He was apyrexial, looked well, and physical examination was normal. Mental state examination revealed that he was orientated to time and person but not place.

What is the most likely diagnosis?

A   Alzheimer's disease
B   Bipolar affective disorder
C   Depersonalisation
D   Dissociative fugue
E   Schizophrenia

8.   A 32-year-old man was brought to hospital with superficial lacerations to all of his limbs. They were caused by him jumping from a wall because of auditory hallucinations telling him that he was worthless and deserved to die. He was under psychiatric follow-up, and suffered with depression which had not responded to fluoxetine or citalopram. After being cleared medically, he was admitted under the psychiatrists for observation. He still harboured suicidal thoughts and refused to eat or drink.

What is the most appropriate treatment?

    A   Amitriptyline
    B   Cognitive behavioural therapy (CBT)
    C   Dosulepin
    D   Electroconvulsive therapy (ECT)
    E   Trazodone

9. A 66-year-old man underwent investigation for a 6-month history of progressive memory decline, confusion, low mood and anxiety. He used to be an intravenous heroin abuser, but did not drink alcohol and no longer used illicit drugs. He was a homosexual, but did not have a regular partner at present. Neurological examination was normal, with pupils equal and reactive to light and accommodation.

Investigations:

haemoglobin	132 g/L (130–180)
mean cell volume	92 fL (80–96)
white cell count	3.2×10^9/L (4.0–11.0)
neutrophil count	2.6×10^9/L (1.5–7.0)
lymphocyte count	0.1×10^9/L (1.5–4.0)
monocyte count	0.3×10^9/L (<0.8)
eosinophil count	0.10×10^9/L (0.04–0.40)
basophil count	$<0.1 \times 10^9$/L (<0.1)
CT brain	diffuse cerebral atrophy, widened sulci, enlarged ventricles

What is the most appropriate next investigation?

    A B_{12} level
    B   HIV serology
    C   Brain MRI
    D   Syphilis serology
    E   Thyroid function tests

10. Which one of the following is the 'positive' symptom most suggestive of schizophrenia?

    A   Alogia
    B   Avolition
    C   Delusional perception
    D   Neologisms
    E   Visual hallucinations

11. Which one of the following symptoms is most likely to support a diagnosis of mania rather than hypomania?

    A   Elevated mood
    B   Flights of ideas
    C   Grandiose delusions

D   Increased appetite
E   Insomnia

12. Which one of the following features is not characteristic of post-traumatic stress disorder?

A   Avoidance of stimuli relating to war
B   Emotional numbing
C   Hypervigilance
D   Inability to work
E   Persistence of symptoms for 3 weeks

13. An 18-year-old woman was brought to the emergency department by her parents with abdominal pain and vomiting. She reported being on a diet because she was training for a triathlon. She claimed that her eating patterns were very irregular but when she did eat, she ate lots. On examination, she was very thin with body mass index 19, and had very dry skin, erosion of dental enamel, parotid gland swelling and calluses on the dorsum of her right hand. Her abdomen was soft and tender in the epigastrium. Examination revealed a temperature of 36.5°C, regular pulse of 120 beats per minute, blood pressure 85/48 mmHg and oxygen saturation of 99% on air.

What is the most likely diagnosis?

A   Acute gastroenteritis
B   Anorexia nervosa
C   Binge-eating disorder (BED)
D   Bulimia nervosa
E   Pregnancy

14. What biochemical abnormality is consistent with anorexia nervosa?

A   High testosterone
B   High T3
C   Low cortisol
D   Low follicle stimulating hormone (FSH)
E   Low growth hormone

15. A 28-year-old woman was seen in the surgery of her general practitioner along with her husband. She had given birth 3 weeks ago, but had been suffering bad mood swings and had difficulty interacting with the baby. The husband was concerned that the patient was suffering from auditory hallucinations by claiming to hear voices.

What is the most likely diagnosis?

A   Baby blues
B   Bipolar disorder
C   Postnatal depression

D Psychotic depression
E Puerperal psychosis

16. A 34-year-old man was brought to the emergency department with agitation, fever and palpitations. He was previously diagnosed with depression and had recently been started on moclobemide. Examination revealed a temperature of 38.5°C, regular pulse of 130 beats per minute and blood pressure 89/50 mmHg. He had increased tone and hyperreflexia in both his upper and lower limbs.

What is the most appropriate next step in management?

A Give activated charcoal
B Start cyproheptadine
C Start dantrolene
D Start methysergide
E Stop moclobemide

Answers

1. D Lewy body dementia

The combination of dementia, fluctuation of cognitive function and visual hallucinations is very typical of Lewy body dementia. Falls are another characteristic feature, usually reflecting the extrapyramidal motor deficit and/or autonomic dysregulation that both occur in the disease.

Alzheimer's disease and vascular dementia are the two most common causes of dementia, but many patients have a mixture of both pathologies. Vascular dementia may be the more dominant pathology if the patient has a past medical history of ischaemic heart disease, stroke, or risk factors for these conditions, such as hypertension, dyslipidaemia or diabetes mellitus. Although a 'step-wise' decline in cognition was previously described as a specific feature of vascular dementia (presumed to reflect discrete episodes of cerebral infarction), this is no longer felt to be the case. The characteristic clinical feature of frontotemporal dementia (aside from the decline in cognition) is a change in a person's personality and behaviour, e.g. loss of inhibition. The history given here is inconsistent with this diagnosis.

Charles Bonnet syndrome is the phenomenon of visual hallucinations occurring in people with people with chronic visual impairment. This is most commonly elderly people with macular degeneration, but can be due to any ophthalmic deficit. Sufferers do not technically have true hallucinations, as they have insight that the images they are seeing are not real. The recent normal ophthalmic examination in this patient's case makes this unlikely to be the diagnosis here.

McKeith I, et al. Dementia with Lewy bodies. Lancet Neurol 2004; 3(1):19–28.

2. A Conversion disorder

Medically unexplained physical symptoms (MUPS) are common in clinical practice and also occur frequently in examination questions. MUPS may be the manifestation of any one of a number of psychiatric disorders, including:

- Conversion disorder: this is characterised by the persistence of a single symptom that mimics physical disease in the absence of any organic pathology. It is believed to occur through patients with intolerable persistent psychic stress unconsciously 'converting' their stress into more bearable physical symptoms. This psychic stress is often an adverse life event which the patient has found difficult to progress from. The temporal relationship between this patient's divorce and her symptoms, along with the long list of negative investigations for numbness, makes it likely that this is the diagnosis here.
- Somatisation disorder: this condition is characterised by at least two years of multiple physical symptoms, spanning many organ systems, with no organic cause ever identified. this is more common in women.
- Hypochondriacal disorder: this is the persistent belief by the patient that they have at least one specific serious illness (often cancer) despite multiple normal

investigations, and despite attempts at reassuring them that there is nothing to support their beliefs.
- Factitious disorder: deliberately feigning symptoms in the context of a severe personality disorder without obvious motivation is known as Munchausen's syndrome. Malingering is the deliberate feigning of symptoms with the intent of secondary gain, e.g. state financial support, leave from work, etc.

Treatment of medically unexplained physical symptoms is difficult, but psychotherapy is normally the mainstay of treatment. However, it may be difficult to get the patient to accept the idea that their symptoms have a psychological basis. None of the features in options B or D are present in the scenario given.

LaFrance WC. Somatoform disorders. Semin Neurol 2009; 29(3):234–246.

3. B Chlordiazepoxide

The investigation results make several of the more common causes of acute postoperative confusion – such as sepsis, electrolyte disturbance and dehydration/renal failure–unlikely. There are a number of clues that this man has a background of alcohol excess and that his presentation may be related to withdrawal, including the fact that he is prescribed thiamine supplements, the presence of macrocytosis, and the description of involutional changes to the brain in a relatively young man. The description of him sustaining his injury in a road traffic incident raises the possibility that he is drink-driving.

Delirium tremens is a syndrome that affects 5% of those who withdraw from alcohol. Symptoms begin within 2–3 days of the patient's last drink, and tend to last for 5 days. Early prominent manifestations include autonomic features (anxiety, tachycardia, sweating, hypertension, nausea, tremor, fever, etc.), with later features including disorientation and confusion, hallucinations/illusions, delusions and insomnia. The most appropriate treatment to minimise symptoms is long-acting benzodiazepines, such as chlordiazepoxide.

Adenosine would be effective if this man had supraventricular tachycardia and metoprolol if this man had an atrial arrhythmia, but there is no suggestion that either would help significantly here. Quetiapine and zopiclone would provide a temporary symptomatic relief only.

Kosten TR, O'Connor PG. Management of drug and alcohol withdrawal. N Engl J Med 2003; 348(18):1786–1795.

4. C Huntington's disease

The presence of involuntary movements means this cannot be purely depression. Rather than demonstrating excessive motor activity (as does the patient here), patients with catatonic schizophrenia demonstrate a lack of motor function (e.g. waxy flexibility – being able to place the patient in an unusual posture with them able to maintain it without obvious difficulty). Gilles de la Tourette syndrome is a condition characterised by recurrent motor and verbal tics that by almost all definitions first manifests before the age of 21 years, so is not the diagnosis here. Involuntary movements (especially rest tremor) are found in Parkinson's disease, but there is no suggestion of the other key extrapyramidal features of this disease in the scenario. Furthermore, cognitive decline is a late feature of Parkinson's disease, and it is unlikely that this man would have advanced Parkinson's disease at such a young age.

Huntington's disease (HD) is an autosomal dominant disorder characterised clinically by choreiform movements, affective symptoms and eventual cognitive decline. It was until recently thought to be very rare, but there is an increasing recognition that cases may have been missed previously because of the diagnosis not being considered (e.g. misdiagnosis as depression); the suicide of this patient's father and unclear neurological problems may represent a missed Huntington's disease diagnosis. It is a trinucleotide repeat disorder, and is associated with expansion (i.e. more trinucleotide repeats in each generation) and anticipation (i.e. younger age of onset in each successive generation). The only current treatment for the disease is symptomatic.

Walker FO. Huntington's disease. Lancet 2007; 369(9557):218–228.

5. E Graded exercise therapy

A wide range of different treatment modalities have been investigated in the management of chronic fatigue syndrome (CFS), but only cognitive behavioural therapy (CBT) and graded exercise therapy (GET) appear to produce any sustained improvement in fatigue. A recent large parallel-group randomised trial has given further evidence that both of these therapies produce significant symptom improvement when compared with supportive medical care alone.

Because of a prior suggestion that material from retroviruses (especially xenotropic murine leukaemia virus-related virus (XMRV) and *Borrelia burgdorferi* (the causative agent of Lyme disease) were more prevalent in the population with CFS than the healthy population, antiretrovirals and antibiotics respectively were suggested as possible useful treatments. However, there has been no evidence to suggest any significant efficacy. Corticosteroids have also been trialled because of a hypothesised link between CFS and neurally-mediated hypotension, but without success. Eye movement desensitisation and reprocessing is a treatment indicated in certain cases of post-traumatic stress disorder.

White PD, et al. Comparison of adaptive pacing therapy, cognitive behaviour therapy, graded exercise therapy, and specialist medical care for chronic fatigue syndrome (PACE): a randomised trial. Lancet 2011; 377 (9768):823–836.

6. A Acute stress disorder

Acute stress disorder is the sudden onset of anxiety and dissociative symptoms (e.g. wandering aimlessly, appearing disorientated as if 'cut off' from one's own body) occurring within minutes to hours of a sudden intensely stressful event. Triggers include natural disasters, accidents (e.g. train crash), or extreme life events (e.g. being a victim of terrorist activity). Symptoms usually begin to resolve without intervention within days. Brief cognitive behavioural therapy (CBT) interventions may shorten the course of symptoms.

Adjustment disorder is the term for the occurrence of a combination of anxiety and depressive symptoms after an adverse life event, e.g. divorce. Symptoms first occur within weeks of the adverse event and last up to 6 months. Treatment is with CBT. The lack of depressive symptoms means this is not the diagnosis in this scenario.

Post-traumatic stress disorder (PTSD) has similar features to acute stress disorder (i.e. anxiety symptoms occurring after an intensely stressful event – with symptom onset up to years after the event), but also has certain unique features. Therapy includes CBT, debriefing therapy, eye movement desensitisation and reprocessing (EMDR), and the use of antidepressant medications. Since symptoms must be present for 1 month for the diagnosis of PTSD to be made, this cannot be the diagnosis here.

Panic disorder is characterised by recurrent panic attacks occurring without a precipitant. The diagnosis requires three panic attacks to occur within 3 weeks; this patient's anxiety symptoms are happening in response to a clear trigger and are not episodic, so this cannot be the diagnosis.

Generalised anxiety disorder describes persistent excessive anxiety for at least 6 months; the presence of symptoms for only a few days means that this diagnosis cannot be made here. Both conditions are treated with a combination of psychological treatments and pharmacotherapy.

Cardeña E, Carlson E. Acute stress disorder revisited. Ann Rev Clin Psychol 2011; 7:245–267.

7. D Dissociative fugue

Dissociative states are psychiatric conditions characterised by a temporary but profound change in sense of identity, awareness, and perception. These conditions often occur at an emotionally challenging time for the patient (e.g. breakdown in relationship), with the current understanding being that they are a psychological means of minimising further emotional strain. This scenario is a classic description for dissociative fugue, i.e. the physical abandonment of familiar surroundings and one's own identity in response to an emotional stressor, with the failure to differentiate between one's identity now from that previously.

Depersonalisation is another dissociative state, the condition characterised by the sensation of being 'cut off' from the world / 'looking in from elsewhere', as if the patient had been taken out of their physical body. There are no mentions of manic, depressive or psychotic features, making options B and E unlikely. Option A is unlikely as the patient has complete retrograde amnesia, not just loss the memory loss for recent events that defines early cognitive decline in Alzheimer's disease.

Spiegel D et al. Dissociative disorders in DSM-5. Depress Anxiety 2011;28(12):E17–E45.

8. D Electroconvulsive therapy (ECT)

This man has depression with psychotic features that now threaten his life, and requires a treatment with rapid onset.

Cognitive behavioural therapy (CBT) has efficacy in the treatment of depression (particularly of mild to moderate severity), but requires at least several weeks of therapy before its efficacy becomes significant, meaning it is not the correct choice here.

The patient has not shown any improvement with two serotonin-selective reuptake inhibitors (SSRIs). The temptation may be to try a different class of antidepressant; the other antidepressants listed are tricyclic antidepressants (options A and C) or tricyclic-related (option E), all with a sedative effect that may be of some use in this situation. However, the fact that the anti-depressant effect of these medications may take several weeks to become apparent, along with the risk of toxicity in overdose, means that this is not an appropriate choice. Antipsychotic medications, however, may be appropriate to consider in this scenario.

The major indication for ECT is severe depression with life-threatening features (such as suicidal intent or failure to eat or drink), with other indications including severe anxiety or psychotic disorders. Although there is a perception even within the medical community of questionability about its efficacy, there is now strong data for an improvement in symptoms for the majority of patients with psychotic depression in which ECT is used. In contrast to the other options listed, the improvement in symptoms with ECT begins within days, making this the most appropriate option from those given.

Lisanby SH. Electroconvulsive therapy for depression. N Engl J Med 2007; 357:1939–1945.

9. B HIV serology

The presence of combined progressive cognitive decline and affective symptoms – in the context of this man being a former intravenous drug user with profound isolated lymphopenia – strongly raises the possibility of this man being HIV positive and now suffering from HIV-associated dementia. HIV-associated dementia in its earlier stages is characterised by a progressive worsening of cognition and affective symptoms. The latter stages are accompanied by a more generalised neurological decline, including ataxia, paraparesis, speech disturbance, and incontinence. The disease most frequently develops in patients with advanced HIV disease, as characterised by a decline in CD4 lymphocyte count and/or increase in HIV viral load. The changes described on the CT are the characteristic CT findings, although these changes do not have a high specificity for HIV-associated dementia in particular. There is no definitive diagnostic test, with the diagnosis usually only made once other possible causes of confusion in HIV positive patients have been excluded (e.g. by lumbar puncture to assay for opportunistic infections). There is no specific treatment, but the huge reduction in incidence of this disease since the advent of highly-active antiretroviral therapy (HAART) means that this is the therapy of choice. Another differential diagnosis that may be considered is neurosyphilis. Neurosyphilis tends to present with marked neurological deficits as well as cognitive impairment – the normal neurological examination in this scenario makes this unlikely to be the diagnosis, but does not fully exclude it. The diagnosis is made through the detection of a cerebrospinal fluid (CSF) white cell count of > 20 cell/μL, and a CSF assay that is positive for VDRL. **Table 10.1** summarises some of the effects upon the nervous system of syphilis infection.

Ances BM, Ellis RJ. Dementia and neurocognitive disorders due to HIV-1 infection. Semin Neurol 2007; 27(1):86–92.
Marra CM. Update on neurosyphilis. Curr Infect Dis Rep 2009; 11(2):127–134.

Table 10.1

System	Features
Eye	• Includes uveitis, iritis, retinitis, and optic atrophy
Cranial nerves	• Classically, palsies of cranial nerves II, VI, VII and VIII as a result of endarteritis • Argyll Robinson pupils are bilateral, small, irregular pupils, usually of different sizes, that classically react normally to accommodation, but slowly or not at all to light

Spinal cord	• Tabes dorsalis reflects syphilitic involvement of the dorsal columns and posterior roots of the spinal cord. This manifests clinically as:
	   – Lower motor neurone signs
	   – Loss of proprioception and vibration sense. Over time, this leads to neuropathic (Charcot's) joints, i.e. deformed joints with marked crepitus
	   – Positive Romberg's sign, with ataxic, wide-based gait

Brain	• Taboparesis is characterised by all the features of tabes dorsalis, but also spastic paraparesis occurring as a result of cortical atrophy. As such, patients demonstrate mixed upper and lower motor neurone symptoms • Progressive endarteritis can result in meningoencephalitis within 3–4 years of the primary infection, and a dementia-like disease ('dementia paralytica') after at least 20 years of infection

Table 10.1 Clinical features of neurosyphilis.

10. C Delusional perception

Delusional perception is one of Schneider's first rank symptoms, the presence of which, although not pathognomonic, is strongly suggestive of schizophrenia. A useful mnemonic for Schneider's first rank symptoms is:

'**Hell** and **Dell Pass**ed **T**ogether'

- **Hall**ucinations
  - Third person auditory hallucinations
  - Thought echo ('echo de la pensée')
  - 'Running commentary' on patient's behaviour
- **Del**usional perception
  - Two stage process involving firstly perception of a normal object then a secondary delusional interpretation of the object as personally significant
- **Pass**ivity phenomenon
  - Actions, feelings, impulses or bodily sensations under the control of an external influence
- **T**hought disorder
  - Thought broadcasting
  - Thought insertion
  - Thought withdrawal

Alogia and avolition are both 'negative' symptoms that can be associated with schizophrenia, as are anhedonia and blunting of affect but these can be seen in other disorders like depression too. Neologisms, lack of insight, catatonia and the 'negative symptoms' are other features that can be apparent in schizophrenia. The negative symptoms can be remembered by the **4 A's**:

- **A**ffective blunting
- **A**nhedonia (inability to experience pleasure from activities previously found enjoyable)
- **A**logia (poverty of speech)
- **A**volition (poor motivation)

Taylor MA. Schneiderian first-rank symptoms and clinical prognostic features in schizophrenia. Arch Gen Psychiatry 1972; 26(1):64–67.

11. C Grandiose delusions

Hypomania and mania are both mood disorders where the patient has pathologically elevated mood. The distinguishing features of each are summarised in **Table 10.2**.

Symptoms common to both disorders are summarised in **Table 10.3**.

Stovall J. Bipolar disorder in adults: Pharmacotherapy for acute mania, mixed episodes, and hypomania. In: Basow DS (ed), UpToDate. Waltham, MA: UpToDate, 2012. http://www.uptodate.com (Last accessed 1 May 2012).

Table 10.2

Features	Hypomania	Mania
Delusions of special ability or status	Absent	Present
Grandiose delusions	Absent	Present
Auditory hallucinations	Absent	Present
Timescale for diagnosis	≥ 4 days	≥ 1 week
Effect on functioning	Mildly impaired	Impaired

Table 10.2 Features of hypomania and mania.

Table 10.3

Mood	Speech and thoughts	Behaviour
Elevated or irritable	Flight of ideas	Increased appetite without weight gain
	Inflated self esteem	Increased libido
	Over-optimistic ideas	Insomnia
	Poor attention / concentration	Loss of social inhibition – sexual promiscuity, risk-taking, overspending
	Pressured speech	Overactivity

Table 10.3 Common features of hypomania and mania.

12. E Persistence of symptoms for 3 weeks

The Diagnostic and Statistical Manual of Mental Disorders IV (DSM-IV) criteria for diagnosing post-traumatic stress disorder can be remembered by the mnemonic **TRAUMA**:

- **T**raumatic event
- **R**e-experience (flashbacks, nightmares)
- **A**voidance and emotional numbing (avoidance of behaviours, places, or people that might lead to distressing memories and decreased ability to feel certain feelings)
- **U**nable to function (e.g. inability to work or have social relations)
- **M**onth or more of symptoms (if all the symptoms but less than a month, this is diagnosed as acute stress disorder)
- **A**rousal increased (hypervigilance, difficulty falling or staying asleep)

American Psychiatric Association. Diagnostic and statistical manual of mental disorders: DSM-IV. American Psychiatric Association; 1994.
Khouzam HR. A simple mnemonic for the diagnostic criteria for post-traumatic stress disorder. West J Med 2001; 174(6):42.

13. D Bulimia nervosa

Bulimia nervosa (BN) is an eating disorder characterised by binge-eating and subsequent compensatory actions to prevent weight gain, e.g. intentional vomiting, misuse of laxatives/enemas/diuretics, excessive exercise or strict diets. Binge-eating disorder is binge-eating without the inappropriate compensatory actions.

Common examination signs in BN include hypotension, tachycardia, xerosis, parotid gland swelling, erosion of dental enamel and Russell's sign (calluses on the dorsum of the hand due to the pressure of the teeth on the skin from stimulation of the gag reflex to induce vomiting).

In BN females are affected more than males and the cause is multifactorial. Patients should be referred to a specialist unit for care. Cognitive behavioural therapy (CBT) is considered first-line therapy and support groups are used too. There is some evidence that antidepressants may work – fluoxetine being the one of choice. The long term efficacy of antidepressants in bulimia is unknown.

Mitchell JE, Crow S. Medical complications of anorexia nervosa and bulimia nervosa. Curr Opin Psychiatry 2006; 19(4):438.
Mitchell J, Zunker C. Bulimia nervosa and binge eating disorder in adults: medical complications and their management. In: Basow DS (ed), UpToDate. Waltham, MA: UpToDate, 2012. http://www.uptodate.com (Last accessed 1 May 2012).

14. D Low follicle stimulating hormone (FSH)

Anorexia nervosa is an eating disorder that involves:

- Intense fear of gaining weight (and body image distortion)
- Refusal to maintain a weight >85% of the expected weight for a given weight and age

Females are more affected (F > M by 10:1) and they tend to have a body mass index <17.5 through avoiding 'fattening' foods and vomiting, purging and exercise.

There are certain physiological adaptations to the starvation as shown in **Table 10.4**.

Mehler P. Anorexia nervosa in adults and adolescents: medical complications and their management. In: Basow DS (ed), UpToDate. Waltham, MA: UpToDate, 2011. http://www.uptodate.com (Last accessed 1 May 2012).

Table 10.4

High levels	Low levels
Amylase (from frequent vomiting)	Albumin
Carotene	FSH and LH
Cholesterol	Oestrogens
Cortisol	Potassium
Glucose (impaired glucose tolerance)	Testosterone
Growth hormone	T3
FSH, follicle stimulating hormone; LH, luteinising hormone.	

Table 10.4 Physiological adaptations in anorexia nervosa.

15. E Puerpural psychosis

This woman has puerperal psychosis and needs urgent admission to hospital for psychiatric investigation and management. **Table 10.5** shows the differences between the various post-partum mental health problems.

Brockington I. Postpartum psychiatric disorders. Lancet 2004; 363:303.
Lusskin S, Misri S. Postpartum blues and depression. In: Basow DS (ed), UpToDate. Waltham, MA: UpToDate, 2012. http://www.uptodate.com (Last accessed 1 May 2012).

16. E Stop moclobemide

This patient has serotonin syndrome. Diagnosis is made on clinical grounds. There are many causes of this either alone or in combination, such as selective serotinin reuptake inhibitors (SSRIs) such as fluoxetine, monoamine oxidase inhibitors (MAOIs, e.g. moclobemide, and opioids like pethidine, which all cause excess serotonergic activity at central nervous system and peripheral serotonin receptors. In all cases, the first line treatment should be to stop the offending drug (moclobemide in this case) and certainly not to add any more serotonergic drugs. Supportive treatment should be given to preserve haemodynamic stability, control the agitation (benzodiazepines), autonomic instability and hyperthermia. Activated charcoal is useful if given within

Table 10.5

	Baby blues	Postnatal depression	Puerpural psychosis
Percentage of mothers affected	60–80	5–20	0.2
Time of onset after birth	3–7 days	Usually begins within first month and peaks at 3 months	Usually within first 2–3 weeks
Features	Anxious Irritable Tearful	Anhedonia Appetite disturbance Decreased concentration Guilt Low energy Low mood Psychomotor changes Sleep disturbance Suicidal thoughts Weight disturbance	Altered perception, e.g. auditory hallucinations Severe mood swings (like in bipolar disorder)
Management	Reassurance and health visitor review	Reassurance and health visitor review Cognitive behavioral therapy Selective serotonin reuptake inhibitors (SSRIs), e.g. paroxetine	Admission to hospital

Table 10.5 Postpartum psychiatric disorders.

1 hour of the overdose. Serotonin antagonists like cyproheptadine and methysergide may be useful. Dantrolene can be used to treat malignant hyperthermia secondary to neuroleptic malignant syndrome but has not been shown to be effective in serotonin syndrome.

Boyer EW, Shannon M. 'The serotonin syndrome'. N Engl J Med 2005; 352 (11): 1112–1220.

Chapter 11

Renal medicine

1. A 30-year-old African man presented to the medical assessment unit with bilateral leg swelling. He was diagnosed with HIV 2 years ago, but had been lost to follow-up.

   Investigations:

haemoglobin	104 g/L (130–180)
mean cell volume	88 fL (80–96)
white cell count	5.4×10^9/L (4.0–11.0)
serum sodium	134 mmol/L (137–144)
serum potassium	4.5 mmol/L (3.5–4.9)
serum urea	10 mmol/L (2.5–7.0)
serum creatinine	154 µmol/L (60–110)
serum albumin	25 g/L (37–49)
serum cholesterol	2.2 mmol/L (<5.2)
CD4 count	78 x 10^6/L (430–1690)
urine protein	10 g/day (<0.2)
ultrasound urinary tract	left kidney 14 cm, right kidney 14.5 cm, both with increased echogenicity

   What is the most likely diagnosis?

   A   Amyloidosis
   B   Focal segmental glomerulosclerosis
   C   Membranous nephropathy
   D   Minimal change nephropathy
   E   Nephritic syndrome

2. A 61-year-old woman was diagnosed with autosomal dominant polycystic kidney disease (ADPKD). The rest of her family was advised to be screened for the condition.

   Which one of the following findings would fit minimum ultrasound criteria for diagnosis of ADPKD type 1 in this woman?

   A   2 renal cysts unilaterally
   B   2 renal cysts bilaterally
   C   3 cysts bilaterally
   D   4 cysts bilaterally
   E   5 cysts bilaterally

3. A 35-year-old woman was referred to the nephrology clinic with a suspicion of diagnosis of autosomal dominant polycystic kidney disease (ADPKD).

Which one of the following statements regarding genetic transmission is least likely?

A   The gene product of *PKD1* is polycystin-1
B   The gene product of *PKD2* is polycystin-2
C   The *PKD1* gene is located on chromosome 17
D   The *PKD2* gene is located on chromosome 4
E   The *PKD3* gene's chromosomal location is unknown

4. A 35-year-old man presented to the emergency department with right loin pain that radiated to his groin. He was diagnosed with renal stones.

What is the most appropriate drug to minimise the risk of further calcium renal stones?

A   Bicarbonate
B   Cholestyramine
C   Citrate
D   Pyridoxine
E   Thiazide diuretics

5. A 28-year-old woman presented to the medical admissions unit with weakness and abdominal pain.

Investigations:

serum sodium	139 mmol/L (137–144)
serum potassium	2.3 mmol/L (3.5–4.9)
serum chloride	115 mmol/L (95–107)
serum creatinine	186 µmol/L (60–110)
serum bicarbonate	10 mmol/L (20–28)
serum pH	7.30 (7.35–7.45)
urinary pH	7.0 (5–7)
abdominal X-ray	bilateral renal calculi

What is the least likely cause of this type of renal tubular acidosis (RTA)?

A   Hypercalcaemia
B   Lithium toxicity
C   Sjögren's syndrome
D   Systemic lupus erythematosus (SLE)
E   Wilson's disease

6. A 21-year-old man, who was a jockey, attended the emergency department with abdominal pain and diarrhoea for 5 days. His mother was known to suffer from congestive cardiac failure. On examination, he was clinically dehydrated but apyrexial. Pulse was regular at 90 beats per minute and blood pressure 110/63 mmHg. Abdomen was soft and diffusely tender but there was no organomegaly.

Investigations:

serum sodium	138 mmol/L (137–144)
serum potassium	2.3 mmol/L (3.5–4.9)
serum creatinine	83 μmol/L (60–110)
serum magnesium	0.4 mmol/L (0.75–1.05)

Blood gas on air:

pH	7.55 (7.35–7.45)
pCO_2	3.6 kPa (4.7–6.0)
pO_2	12 kPa (11.3–12.6)
bicarbonate	32 mmol/L (21–29)

urine sodium	160 mEq/L (136–145)
urine potassium	35 mEq/L (25–120)
24 hour urinary calcium	50 mg (100–300)

What is the most likely diagnosis?

A   Bartter's syndrome
B   Gitelman's syndrome
C   Laxative abuse
D   Liddle's syndrome
E   Thiazide diuretic abuse

7. A 24-year-old woman was admitted with acute kidney injury following a paracetamol overdose. She was clinically well and haemodynamically stable. Her urine output was 25 mL/h.

Investigations:

serum sodium	128 mmol/L (137–144)
serum potassium	7.1 mmol/L (3.5–4.9)
serum urea	15.1 mmol/L (2.5–7.0)
serum creatinine	650 μmol/L (60–110)
serum C-reactive protein	100 mg/L (<10)
serum alanine aminotransferase	1100 U/L (5–35)
international normalised ratio	1.6 (<1.4)

Which one of the following is the strongest indication for dialysis?

A   Creatinine 650 μmol/L
B   Hyperkalaemia
C   Oliguria
D   Paracetamol overdose
E   Urea 15.1 mmol/L

8. A 50-year-old man who had a renal transplant 3 months ago presented to the emergency department with fever and loin pain. He was on ciclosporin. On examination, his temperature was 38°C, pulse 97 beats per minute, and blood pressure 136/84 mmHg.

Investigations:

haemoglobin	105 g/L (130–180)
mean cell volume	80.4 fL (80–96)
white cell count	9.8×10^9/L (4.0–11.0)
neutrophil count	7.5×10^9/L (2.5–7.0)
serum sodium	137 mmol/L (137–144)
serum potassium	3.8 mmol/L (3.5–4.9)
serum creatinine	360 µmol/L (baseline 180 µmol/L) (60–110)
ultrasound kidneys, ureters and bladder	normal
renal transplant biopsy	immune cell infiltrate and tubular damage

What is the most likely diagnosis?

A   Acute rejection
B   Chronic allograft nephropathy
C   Ciclosporin nephrotoxicity
D   Polyomavirus infection
E   Vascular thrombosis

9. A 35-year-old man with autosomal dominant polycystic kidney disease and on haemodialysis, was seen in the renal transplant clinic. His father had had renal cell carcinoma. He was on ramipril 10 mg once daily, atenolol 50 mg once daily and amlodipine 10 mg once daily. On examination, his temperature was 36.8°C, pulse 86 beats per minute, and blood pressure 163/92 mmHg.

Investigations:

urine dipstick	blood 1+ protein 2+ leucocytes 3+ nitrites positive
ultrasound kidneys, ureters and bladder	left kidney 19.5 cm right kidney 19.7 cm no evidence of hydronephrosis multiple cysts in both kidneys

What is the single strongest indication for recipient nephrectomy prior to transplant in this patient?

A   Age
B   Blood pressure 163/92 mmHg
C   Family history of renal malignancy
D   Massive polycystic kidneys
E   Positive urine dipstick

10. Which is the strongest contraindication to renal transplantation?

A   ABO blood group incompatibility
B   Age > 75 years

C Circulating anti-glomerular basement membrane (anti-GBM) antibodies
D Hepatitis B sAg positive
E Ischaemic heart disease

11. A 65-year-old man was referred to the renal clinic for investigation of hypertension. His blood pressure was 170/104 mmHg despite treatment with amlodipine, bendroflumethiazide and doxazosin. He had a medical history of ischaemic heart disease and had undergone femoral-popliteal bypass surgery 2 years ago. He smoked 20 cigarettes and drank two pints of lager per day.

Investigations:

serum sodium	134 mmol/L (137–144)
serum potassium	4.8 mmol/L (3.5–4.9)
serum urea	10 mmol/L (2.5–7.0)
serum creatinine	190 µmol/L (60–110)
ultrasound kidneys, ureters and bladder	left kidney of 11.8 cm diameter, right kidney of 9.3 cm diameter, no evidence of urinary tract obstruction

What is the most appropriate diagnostic investigation?

A CT abdomen and pelvis
B Magnetic resonance angiography (MRA) of the renal arteries
C Renal biopsy
D Renal radionuclide imaging with ^{99m}Tc-dimercaptosuccinic acid (DMSA)
E Urine cytology

12. A 44-year-old woman with diffuse cutaneous systemic sclerosis presented to the emergency department with an acute severe headache and blurred vision. She took no regular medications. Funduscopy revealed bilateral optic disc swelling. Her blood pressure was 204/120 mmHg.

Investigations:

haemoglobin	98 g/L (115–165)
white cell count	10.8×10^9/L (4–11)
platelet count	48×10^9/L (150–450)
reticulocyte count	244×10^9/L (25–85)
serum sodium	137 mmol/L (137–144)
serum potassium	4.8 mmol/L (3.5–4.9)
serum urea	18 mmol/L (2.5–7.0)
serum creatinine	448 µmol/L (104 µmol/L one year earlier) (60–110)
CT brain	no evidence of space occupying lesion

What is the most appropriate treatment for this patient?

A Bendroflumethiazide
B Doxazosin
C Indapamide

    D   Metoprolol
    E   Ramipril

13. A 58-year-old man underwent investigation for several months of progressive bilateral leg oedema. He had a past medical history of bronchiectasis, which required several hospital admissions each year because of infective exacerbations.

Investigations:

serum urea	7.0 mmol/L (2.5–7.0)
serum creatinine	170 µmol/L (60–110)
serum albumin	20 g/L (37–49)
urine dipstick	protein +3
ultrasound kidney, ureters and bladder	bilaterally enlarged, echogenic kidneys

What is the most likely diagnosis?

    A   Aminoglycoside nephrotoxicity
    B   Cor pulmonale
    C   Focal segmental glomerulosclerosis
    D   IgA nephropathy
    E   Renal amyloidosis

14. A 72-year-old man presented with fever and lethargy. He had a past medical history of myocardial infarction, and had undergone coronary angioplasty 3 weeks earlier. On examination, his temperature was 38°C, and he had livedo reticularis on the lower extremities along with dusky-appearing toes.

Investigations:

white cell count	17×10^9/L (4–11)
neutrophil count	14×10^9/L (1.5–7.0)
eosinophil count	1.01×10^9/L (0.04–0.40)
erythrocyte sedimentation rate	78 mm/1st hour (<20)
serum sodium	141 mmol/L (137–144)
serum potassium	5.3 mmol/L (3.5–4.9)
serum urea	8.5 mmol/L (2.5–7.0)
serum creatinine	230 mmol/L (130 mmol/L three weeks earlier) (60–110)
serum complement C3	45 mg/dL (65–190)
serum complement C4	10 mg/dL (15–50)
antineutrophil cytoplasmic antibodies	negative
antinuclear antibodies	negative
urine dipstick	protein +1, blood trace
urine microscopy	urinary eosinophils, scanty casts

What is the most likely diagnosis?

A   Cholesterol atheroembolisation
B   Churg–Strauss syndrome
C   Contrast-induced nephropathy
D   Henoch–Schönlein purpura
E   Systemic lupus erythematosus (SLE)

15. A 38-year-old man presented to the emergency department with severe sudden onset right flank pain and frank haematuria. A diagnosis of membranous nephropathy had been made 1 month earlier, and he was taking prednisolone and ramipril. There was no family history of haematuria or renal disease.

Investigations:

serum urea	7.5 mmol/L (2.5–7.0)
serum creatinine	190 µmol/L (142 µmol/L two months earlier) (60–110)
serum albumin	23 g/L (37–49)
urine dipstick	protein +3, blood +3

What is the most likely diagnosis?

A   Carcinoma of the prostate
B   IgA nephropathy
C   Renal artery stenosis
D   Renal vein thrombosis
E   Thin basement membrane nephropathy (benign familial haematuria)

16. A 23-year-old man presented with a 2-week history of progressive bilateral leg oedema. He had a similar episode 3 years ago and underwent a renal biopsy that demonstrated minimal-change nephropathy. He made a rapid and complete recovery following previous treatment but was on no regular medications at present.

Investigations:

serum albumin	22 g/L (37–49)
urine dipstick	protein +3

What is the most appropriate next step in management?

A   Azathioprine
B   Ciclosporin
C   Prednisolone
D   Renal biopsy
E   Renal ultrasound

17. A 65-year-old man with carcinoma of the lung was undergoing investigation to assess suitability for surgery. He took no regular medications, but was prescribed a course of penicillin 2 weeks earlier for a streptococcal throat infection. On examination, he had bilateral below knee oedema. Blood pressure was 126/84 mmHg.

Investigations:

serum sodium	141 mmol/L (137–144)
serum potassium	4.7 mmol/L (3.5–4.9)
serum creatinine	170 mmol/L (120 mmol/L two years earlier) (60–110)
serum albumin	21 g/L (37–49)
urine dipstick	protein +3
ultrasound kidneys, ureter and bladder	no evidence of obstructive uropathy

What is the most likely diagnosis?

A   Acute interstitial nephritis
B   Diffuse proliferative glomerulonephritis
C   IgA nephropathy
D   Membranous nephropathy
E   Retroperitoneal fibrosis

18. A 19-year-old man was injured in a road traffic accident and underwent emergency surgery for stabilisation of an open femoral fracture. He had no past medical history and took no regular medications. He was catheterised and transferred to the high dependency unit post-operatively. Later that day, his urine output was only 10 mL/h and he was given an intravenous fluid challenge. The rest of his physical observations were normal.

Investigations:

serum sodium	141 mmol/L (137–144)
serum potassium	5.9 mmol/L (3.5–4.9)
serum creatinine	184 mmol/L (104 mmol/L on admission) (60–110)
plasma osmolality	295 mOsmol/kg (278–300)
urinary sodium	54 mmol/L (<20)
urinary osmolality	324 mOsmol/kg (350–1000)
urine dipstick	trace of protein

What is the most likely cause of this patient's acute kidney injury?

A   Acute tubular necrosis
B   Blocked urinary catheter
C   Minimal change nephropathy
D   Membranoproliferative glomerulonephritis
E   Pre-renal failure/hypovolaemia

19. A 30-year-old man presented to the emergency department with 3 days of shortness of breath and haemoptysis. He had no past medical history. On examination, he had bilateral leg oedema and a blood pressure of 190/120 mmHg.

Investigations:

serum sodium	139 mmol/L (137–144)
serum potassium	5.9 mmol/L (3.5–4.9)
serum creatinine	510 mmol/L (60–110)
urine dipstick	protein +2, blood +3
chest X-ray	pulmonary infiltrates, consistent with recent haemorrhage
renal biopsy	crescentic changes with linear IgG deposition

What is the most likely diagnosis?

A   Churg–Strauss syndrome
B   Goodpasture's syndrome
C   Granulomatosis with polyangiitis (Wegener's)
D   IgA nephropathy
E   Systemic lupus erythematosus (SLE)

20. A 21-year-old man underwent a renal biopsy for investigation of the cause of his oedema, haematuria, and proteinuria. He had a past medical history of partial lipodystrophy.

What is the most likely finding on renal biopsy?

A   Focal segmental glomerulosclerosis
B   IgA nephropathy
C   Membranous nephropathy
D   Mesangiocapillary glomerulonephritis
E   Minimal change disease

21. A 54-year-old man presented to the emergency department with a 2-week history of worsening lethargy, nausea and dyspnoea. He had no past medical history of note.

Investigations:

serum sodium	136 mmol/L (137–144)
serum potassium	7.8 mmol/L (3.5–4.9)
serum creatinine	560 mmol/L (105 mmol/L three months earlier) (60–110)
ECG	small P waves, widened QRS complexes, peaked T waves

What is most appropriate next step in management?

A   Calcium gluconate
B   Calcium polystyrene sulphonate
C   Insulin–dextrose infusion
D   Nebulised salbutamol
E   Sodium bicarbonate

22. A 38-year-old man presented to the emergency department with severe, acute right sided colicky abdominal pain radiating between his loin and the

suprapubic area. He was diagnosed with ureteric colic by intravenous urogram. His only past medical history was Crohn's disease, which was currently being treated with a reducing dose of prednisolone because of a recent flare of this condition.

Investigations:

urine culture	no growth

What is the most likely composition of the ureteric calculi?

A   Calcium oxalate
B   Cholesterol
C   Cystine
D   Struvite (magnesium–ammonium–phosphate)
E   Uric acid

23. A 50-year-old man presented with a 1-week history of lethargy and nausea. One year ago, he had a renal transplant for membranous nephropathy. His current immunosuppression regimen was mycophenolate mofetil, ciclosporin and prednisolone. He was fully compliant with his immunosuppression and drug levels were therapeutic when last seen in clinic 1 month earlier. He had been well apart from an episode of oral candidiasis 2 weeks earlier which was treated with a course of fluconazole. Examination revealed a non-tender renal transplant graft and normal physical observations.

Investigations:

serum creatinine	250 mmol/L (130 mmol/L one month earlier) (60–110)
serum albumin	38 g/L (37–49)
urine dipstick	protein trace
ultrasound kidneys, ureters and bladder	no evidence of haematoma/collection, normal Doppler flow

What is the most likely cause of the deterioration of his renal function?

A   Acute interstitial nephritis in association with fluconazole
B   Ciclosporin toxicity
C   Disseminated candidiasis
D   Graft rejection
E   Recurrence of membranous nephropathy

24. A 60-year-old homeless man with a history of alcohol excess was admitted after being found collapsed in the street. On examination, he had a tender area over the lateral left forearm. There was a postural drop in blood pressure. He had a urinary catheter inserted and passed a residual volume of 200 mL of urine before passing 10 mL of dark urine in the next hour. Despite being given a fluid challenge with intravenous fluids he remained oliguric.

Investigations:

Blood tests:

serum sodium	141 mmol/L (137–144)
serum potassium	6.0 mmol/L (3.5–4.9)
serum urea	18.2 mmol/L (2.5–7.0)
serum creatinine	383 mmol/L (76 mmol/L six months earlier) (60–110)
serum corrected calcium	1.9 mmol/L (2.2–2.6)
serum phosphate	2.9 mmol/L (0.8–1.4)
serum creatine kinase	50,224 U/L (24–195)

Arterial blood gas on air:

pH	7.30 (7.35–7.45)
pCO_2	4.4 kPa (4.7–6.0)
pO_2	11.5 kPa (11.3–12.6)
bicarbonate	14 mmol/L (21–29)
lactate	3.5 mmol/L (0.5–1.6)

What is the most appropriate initial therapy?

A   Dopamine infusion
B   Haemofiltration
C   Intravenous mannitol
D   Intravenous saline
E   Urinary alkalinisation with sodium bicarbonate

25. A 28-year-old woman underwent a routine pre-employment medical assessment and was found to have a blood pressure of 170/98 mmHg. She had no history of hypertension, but she had a past medical history of recurrent urinary tract infections and nocturnal enuresis as a child. She was on no regular medication. Her mother had kidney problems and suffered with hypertension.

Investigations:

serum sodium	140 mmol/L (137–144)
serum potassium	5.5 mmol/L (3.5–4.9)
serum urea	22.1 mmol/L (2.5–7.0)
serum creatinine	482 mmol/L (60–110)
serum albumin	38 g/L (37–49)
urine dipstick	protein +2, leucocytes +1
ultrasound kidneys, ureters and bladder	bilateral small kidneys with possible renal scarring, no evidence of obstruction

What is the most likely diagnosis?

A   Alport's disease
B   Hypertensive renal disease
C   IgA nephropathy
D   Minimal change nephropathy
E   Reflux nephropathy (chronic pyelonephritis)

26. A 24-year-old man with sickle cell disease was admitted to hospital because of several days of severe generalised bone pain that had failed to respond to simple analgesia. Whilst in the ward, he had had an episode of left-sided loin pain and frank haematuria. He had no other past medical history. Abdominal examination was normal, blood pressure was 124/88 mmHg, and there was no peripheral oedema.

Investigations:

serum sodium	141 mmol/L (137–144)
serum potassium	5.3 mmol/L (3.5–4.9)
serum urea	8.2 mmol/L (2.5–7.0)
serum creatinine	152 mmol/L (60–110)
serum albumin	39 g/L (37–49)
urine dipstick	protein +1, blood +3, no nitrites or leucocytes
intravenous urogram	clubbing of left upper polar calyces, with 'cup and pencil' appearance

What is the most likely diagnosis?

- **A** Carcinoma of the bladder
- **B** IgA nephropathy
- **C** Membranoproliferative glomerulonephritis
- **D** Papillary necrosis
- **E** Urinary tract infection

27. A 24-year-old man was admitted to hospital because of acute right-sided flank pain and haematuria. He had a past medical history of epilepsy and learning disability. Examination of the abdomen revealed some right loin tenderness but no peritonism. Dermatological examination revealed a number of abnormalities, including the presence of salmon-coloured nodules in the region of the nasolabial folds and hypopigmented macules over the trunk and buttocks.

Investigations:

CT urogram	Multiple bilateral renal cysts Haemorrhagic change in the right kidney 3 cm mass at the base of the right kidney, with an appearance suggestive of angiomyolipoma

What is the next most useful diagnostic investigation?

- **A** Flexible cystoscopy and ureteroscopy
- **B** Hamartin and tuberin gene testing
- **C** Intravenous urogram
- **D** Renal radionuclide imaging with ^{99m}Tc-dimercaptosuccinic acid (DMSA)
- **E** Urine cytology

28. A 78-year-old man presented with a 2-month history of worsening lower back pain and lethargy. The pain had failed to resolve despite the use of increasingly potent analgesia. He had no past medical history. Examination revealed conjunctival pallor and tenderness over the region of the lumbar spine.

Investigations:

haemoglobin	83 g/L (130–180)
mean cell volume	92 fL (80–96)
platelet count	180 × 10⁹/L (150–450)
erythrocyte sedimentation rate	94 mm/1st hour (<20)
blood film	rouleaux appearance
serum sodium	142 mmol/L (137–144)
serum potassium	5.2 mmol/L (3.5–4.9)
serum urea	24.1 mmol/L (2.5–7.0)
serum creatinine	304 mmol/L (76 mmol/L one year earlier) (60–110)
serum corrected calcium	3.1 mmol/L (2.2–2.6)
international normalised ratio	1.2 s (<1.4)
activated partial thromboplastin time	33 s (30–40)

What is the most likely diagnosis?

A Haemolytic–uraemic syndrome
B Multiple myeloma
C Rheumatoid arthritis
D Sarcoidosis
E Thrombotic thrombocytopenic purpura

29. A 54-year-old man presented to his general practitioner with a 3-month history of dull lower back pain. His only past medical history was recurrent migraine, for which he had taken regular medication for many years. Physical examination was normal.

Investigations:

serum sodium	142 mmol/L (137–144)
serum potassium	5.1 mmol/L (3.5–4.9)
serum urea	13.8 mmol/L (2.5–7.0)
serum creatinine	235 mmol/L (60–110)
serum corrected calcium	2.4 mmol/L (2.2–2.6)
serum phosphate	1.2 mmol/L (0.8–1.4)
urine dipstick	negative
ultrasound kidney, ureters and bladder	bilateral proximal hydroureter, and medial deviation of the ureters

What is the most likely diagnosis?

A Focal segmental glomerulosclerosis
B Multiple myeloma
C Renal artery stenosis
D Renal calculi
E Retroperitoneal fibrosis

30. A 28-year-old man presented to his general practitioner complaining of recurrent episodes of dark-coloured urine. Two days ago he had had a sore throat but that was resolving. On examination, he had a blood pressure of 180/94 mmHg. The rest of the physical examination was normal.

Investigations:

urine dipstick   blood +2, protein +2

What is the most likely finding on renal biopsy?

A   IgA nephropathy
B   Membranous nephropathy
C   Minimal change nephropathy
D   Normal biopsy
E   Post-streptococcal glomerulonephritis

Answers

1. B Focal segmental glomerulosclerosis

HIV associated nephropathy (HIVAN) is a kidney disease that occurs predominantly in individuals of Afro-Caribbean ethnicity and can occur at any stage of HIV infection, but is more common in those with advanced infection and low CD4 counts. The most common type of HIVAN is focal segmental glomerulosclerosis. As in this case, it is characterised by hypoalbuminaemia, oedema and heavy proteinuria (often >10 g/day). In classical nephrotic syndrome, the cholesterol level is usually normal/high, however in this case the cholesterol level is low reflecting malnutrition. The typical picture on renal ultrasound is normal size to enlarged kidneys, even in those cases with persistent disease.

Renal biopsy may show:

- Podocyte swelling
- Segmental collapse of glomerular tuft
- Focal segmental scarring
- Interstitial inflammation
- Interstitial microcyst formation
- Negative immunofluorescence

Wilson D, et al. Handbook of HIV Medicine, 2nd edition. Oxford: OUP, 2008, p. 320.
Ray PE, et al. A 20-year history of childhood HIV-associated nephropathy. Paediatr Nephrol 2004; 19:1075–1092.

2. D 4 cysts bilaterally

Ultrasound is commonly used to screen for patients at risk of autosomal dominant polycystic kidney disease (ADPKD) type 1.

Table 11.1 shows the criteria required for diagnosis of ADPKD type 1 in individuals at risk (i.e. those with affected family members).

Ultrasound may be equivocal in patients under the age of 20 years, so it is not usually done until patients reach that age.

Ravine D, et al. Evaluation of ultrasonographic diagnostic criteria for autosomal dominant polycystic kidney disease 1. Lancet 1994; 343(8901):824–827.

Table 11.1

Age (in years)	Unilateral or bilateral	Number of cysts
<30	Unilateral or bilateral	≥ 2
30–59	Bilateral	≥ 2
≥ 60	Bilateral	≥ 4

Table 11.1 Diagnostic criteria for autosomal dominant polycystic kidney disease.

3. C The *PKD1* gene is located on chromosome 17

Autosomal dominant polycystic kidney disease (ADPKD) is one of the most common hereditary disorders with an incidence of between 1 and 2 per 1000 live births. There are at least three different genes causing ADPKD:

- *PKD1* gene, situated on chromosome 16, encoding polycystin-1, is involved in regulation of cell cycle and intracellular calcium transport in epithelial cells.
- *PKD2* gene, situated on chromosome 4, encoding polycystin-2, is similar to the alpha1 subunit of voltage-gated calcium and sodium channels.
- *PKD3* has been postulated but its chromosomal location has not been identified to date. In Europe, *PKD1* is the cause in roughly 85% of cases and *PKD2* the cause in 15%.

Boucher C, Sandford R. Autosomal dominant polycystic kidney disease (ADPKD, MIM 173900, PKD1 and PKD2 genes, protein products known as polycystin-1 and polycystin-2). Eur J Hum Genet 2004; 12: 347–354.

4. E Thiazide diuretics

Although thiazide diuretics can cause hypercalcaemia, they can help in preventing the formation of calcium renal calculi. They do so by increasing distal tubular calcium reabsorption (hence leading to potential hypercalcaemia) and therefore lowering calcium concentration in the urine. **Table 11.2** shows that different stone consistencies have different methods of treatment.

Curhan G. Prevention of recurrent calcium stones in adults. In: Basow DS (ed), UpToDate. Waltham, MA: UpToDate, 2010. http://www.uptodate.com (Last accessed 1 May 2012).
Reilly R, Peixoto A, Desir G. The evidence-based use of thiazide diuretics in hypertension and nephrolithiasis. Clin J Am Soc Neurol 2010; 5(10):1893–1903.

Table 11.2

Type of stone	Treatment
Calcium	High fluid intake
	Thiazide diuretics, e.g. chlorthalidone
	Low-salt diet and low-protein diet
Oxalate	Reduce urinary oxalate secretion with: cholestyramine, citrate and pyridoxine
Uric acid	Allopurinol
	Urinary alkalinisation using oral bicarbonate
Cystine	High fluid intake
	Urinary alkalinisation
	Cystine chelation (to increase its solubility) with D-penicillamine or tiopronin

Table 11.2 Different types of renal calculi and their treatment.

5. E Wilson's disease

This is a case of Type 1 (distal) renal tubular acidosis (RTA) as evidenced by the severe acidosis, hypokalaemia, inability to acidify the urine and nephrocalcinosis.

Type 1 and Type 2 RTAs both cause hyperchloraemic normal anion gap acidosis.

Table 11.3 illustrates the differences between Type 1 and Type 2 RTA.

Emmett M. Etiology and diagnosis of distal (type 1) and proximal (type 2) renal tubular acidosis. In: Basow DS (ed), UpToDate. Waltham, MA: UpToDate, 2011. http://www.uptodate.com (Last accessed 1 May 2012).

Table 11.3		
	Type 1	**Type 2**
Primary defect	Impaired urinary acidification	Impaired HCO_3 reabsorption
Site of defect	Distal tubule	Proximal tubule
Plasma K	Low	Low/normal
Plasma HCO_3	<10 mmol/L	14–20 mmol/L
Urine acidification	Not possible	Possible
Causes	Primary – genetic/idiopathic	Idiopathic
	Secondary to autoimmune diseases – SLE, Sjögren's syndrome, chronic active hepatitis, rheumatoid arthritis	With Fanconi syndrome – cystinosis, Wilson's disease, fructose intolerance, Sjögren's syndrome
	Tubulointerstitial disease – transplant rejection, obstructive uropathy	Tubulointerstitial disease – interstitial nephritis, myeloma, amyloidosis
	Medullary sponge kidney	Drugs – tetracyclines, streptozotocin, heavy metals, e.g. lead and mercury, acetazolamide, sulphonamides
	Hypercalcaemia	
	Drugs – lithium, toluene, amphotericin, ifosfamide	
Complications	Renal calculi	Rickets in children
	Nephrocalcinosis	Osteomalacia in adults
Features	Growth failure	Phosphaturia
	Urine infection	Aminoaciduria
	Hypocitraturia	Glycosuria
	Hypercalciuria	
SLE, systemic lupus erythematosus.		

Table 11.3 Differences between Type 1 and Type 2 renal tubular acidosis.

6. B Gitelman's syndrome

Both Bartter's and Gitelman's syndromes are characterised by metabolic alkalosis and hypokalaemia with normal blood pressure. **Table 11.4** shows the differences in these two syndromes.

Liddle's syndrome is a rare autosomal dominant condition caused by a mutation in the highly selective epithelial sodium channel (ENaC) in the distal nephron. It is characterised by hypokalaemia with hypertension. The overactive ENaC causes increased sodium uptake with accompanying increased water uptake, thus blood volume is increased causing secondary hypertension.

Both thiazide diuretic abuse and laxative abuse are associated with hypokalaemia and normotension as in this case. However, urinary sodium and potassium are normal (as water will follow the electrolytes) in thiazide diuretic abuse, and laxative abuse tends to cause low urinary sodium and potassium, with low serum bicarbonate, owing to gastrointestinal losses. Some jockeys may use thiazide diuretics to lose weight for races, but the biochemical picture does not fit this case.

Emmett M. Bartter and Gitelman syndromes. In: Basow DS (ed), UpToDate. Waltham, MA: UpToDate, 2011. http://www.uptodate.com (Last accessed 1 May 2012).

Table 11.4

	Bartter's syndromes	Gitelman's syndromes
Site of defect	$Na^+ K^+ 2Cl^-$ cotransporter in the ascending loop of Henle	Thiazide-sensitive Na^+Cl^- transporter in the distal convoluted tubule
Age of onset	Infancy	Adolescence/early adulthood
Dysmorphic features	May be present	None
eGFR	Low/Normal	Normal
Serum magnesium	High/Normal	Low
Urine sodium	Low	High
Urine calcium	High	Normal/Low

Table 11.4 Differences between Bartter's syndrome and Gitelman's syndrome.

7. B Hyperkalaemia

In this case, the patient has hyperkalaemia refractory to treatment, which is an indication for dialysis. A useful mnemonic for indications of dialysis is **AEIOU**:

A- Acidosis (refractory to treatment)

E- Electrolyte disturbances, e.g. hyperkalaemia (refractory to treatment)

I- Ingestion of toxins – **B**arbiturates, **L**ithium, **A**lcohol, **S**alicylate, **T**heophylline (mnemonic **BLAST**)

O- Oedema (refractory to treatment with diuretics)

U- Uraemic complications, e.g. pericarditis or encephalopathy

Palevsky PM. Renal replacement therapy I: indications and timing. Crit Care Clin 2005; 21(2):347–356.

8. A Acute rejection

Acute rejection occurs in about 30% of all renal transplants and should be sought for in the early weeks post-transplantation. It is usually characterised by fever, graft pain and a rising serum creatinine. The definitive investigation is a graft biopsy that shows a T-cell infiltrate and structural damage to the transplanted tissue. An episode of acute rejection if recognised early and treated promptly with pulsed intravenous methylprednisolone rarely leads to permanent graft failure. As long as renal function returns to baseline, acute rejection does not cause irreparable damage or impact long-term graft survival. Steroid-resistant cases occur in 5% and require treatment with antithymocyte globulin or muromonab-CD3 antibody.

Chronic allograft nephropathy and polyomavirus infections (e.g. BK or JC virus) are causes of chronic graft dysfunction and tend to occur 4 months post-transplantation onwards. Vascular thrombosis would be demonstrated on ultrasound scan of the transplanted vessels.

Madden RL, et al. Completely reversed acute rejection is not a significant risk factor for the development of chronic rejection in renal allograft recipients. Transpl Int 2000; 13:344.

9. D Massive polycystic kidneys

Indications for recipient nephrectomy prior to transplantation are:

- Massive polycystic kidneys (normal size of a kidney is 9–13 cm)
- Pyonephrosis or any suppuration in the urinary tract
- Renal or urothelial malignancy: patients must be free of recurrence for >2 years prior to transplantation
- Uncontrollable hypertension

Wagner MD, Prather JC, Barry JM. Selective, concurrent bilateral nephrectomies at renal transplantation for autosomal dominant polycystic kidney disease. J Urol 2007; 177:2250.

10. C Circulating anti-glomerular basement membrane (anti-GBM) antibodies

Goodpasture's syndrome is characterised by anti-GBM antibodies and may progress to end stage renal disease, requiring dialysis or renal transplantation. The latter tends to be delayed until circulating anti-GBM antibody levels have been undetectable for at least 1 year and there has been quiescent disease for at least 6 months post-treatment (without cytotoxic agents).

Transplants to ABO blood group incompatible patients are possible with the use of plasma exchange and B-lymphocyte suppressive therapy in the recipient a week or so prior to transplantation.

Age is not an absolute contraindication but owing to co-morbidities, few patients >75 years are subsequently listed. All dialysis patients should be immunised from hepatitis B infection.

Ischaemic heart disease is not in itself a contraindication to renal transplantation per se, but patients should undergo cardiovascular screening prior to referral with echocardiography (Left ventricular ejection fraction > 30%) and myocardial perfusion scan or stress echocardiography (to look for reversible ischaemia).

European best practice guidelines for renal transplantation (Part 2). Nephrol Dial Transplant 2002; 17(Suppl 4):16.

11. B Magnetic resonance angiography (MRA) of the renal arteries

The scenario given is highly suggestive of underlying renal artery stenosis (RAS). Up to 70% of patients with ischaemic heart disease and 60% with peripheral vascular disease may be affected, reflecting their shared pathological basis of progressive atheroma deposition. The clinical presentation is typically with treatment-resistant hypertension (accounting for approximately 80% of cases of secondary hypertension) and chronic renal failure; another typical presentation (especially in postgraduate examinations!) is of 'flash' pulmonary oedema occurring within a few days of starting an angiotensin-converting enzyme (ACE) inhibitor, reflecting ACE inhibitor-related acute renal failure. Ultrasound of the urinary tract showing a discrepancy in renal diameter of at least 2 cm in the absence of obstructive pathology is highly suggestive of unilateral renovascular disease.

The most commonly used screening test for investigating RAS is magnetic resonance angiography (MRA) of the renal arteries. Option A is the incorrect answer as although CT angiography will provide the diagnosis, the risk of contrast nephropathy secondary to contrast media and high radiation dose makes this less preferable to MRA. Although radionuclide imaging techniques are useful for demonstrating the relative level of function of each kidney, it does not diagnose the underlying cause of renal failure, making option D incorrect. Neither option C nor E would in any way contribute to making the diagnosis. It is worth noting that although renal angiography is viewed as the 'gold standard' for making the diagnosis of RAS (especially since it allows renal artery angioplasty +/- stenting at the same time), the high level of radiation exposure and need for nephrotoxic contrast medium means that the technique is usually only employed if there is thought to be a strong indication for treatment of renal artery stenosis.

Dworkin LD, Cooper CJ. Renal-Artery Stenosis. N Engl J Med 2009; 361:1972–1978.

12. E Ramipril

The most likely diagnosis in this case is scleroderma renal crisis, a complication of systemic sclerosis that is characterised by the combination of acute renal failure, accelerated-phase hypertension (as evidenced by the eye changes) and microangiopathic haemolytic anaemia.

Trials evaluating the treatment of scleroderma renal crisis have consistently found angiotensin-converting enzyme (ACE) inhibitors to offer greater antihypertensive efficacy, better preservation of renal function and lower mortality rates than all other classes of antihypertensive therapy; hence E is the correct answer. Although it might intuitively be expected that angiotensin receptor blockers are of similar efficacy to ACE inhibitors, there is little trial data comparing the two, and so ACE inhibitors remain the first-line recommendation at present. There is also an emerging role for the use of prostaglandin analogues.

Penn H, Denton CP. Diagnosis, management and prevention of scleroderma renal disease. Curr Opin Rheumatol 2008; 20 (6):692–696.

13. E Renal amyloidosis

This patient has nephrotic syndrome – hypoalbuminaemia, proteinuria and oedema. Although the history of bronchiectasis requiring frequent courses of antibiotics is suggestive of option A, aminoglycosides (such as gentamicin) in fact cause nephrotoxicity primarily through tubular disease and loss of renal concentrating ability rather than through glomerular damage. Similarly, although diseases characterised by chronic hypoxia such as bronchiectasis are associated with the development of cor pulmonale and consequently bilateral oedema, option B cannot explain the presence of the other features of the nephrotic syndrome.

Options C, D and E may all be associated with the nephrotic syndrome. The key to answering the question correctly is recognising that enlarged, echogenic kidneys on urinary tract ultrasonography is highly suggestive of renal amyloidosis. All chronic inflammatory diseases – including chronic infective/inflammatory diseases (such as bronchiectasis), as well as rheumatological diseases – may be complicated by the development of secondary (AA) amyloidosis. This is a disorder characterised by the extracellular deposition of fibrils composed of fragments of the acute phase reactant serum amyloid A protein, with proteinuria or nephrotic syndrome being the most common presentations. The diagnosis may be confirmed via renal biopsy, with amorphous extracellular material that shows red-green birefringence when stained with Congo red and viewed under cross-polarised light being the classic findings. Prevention of progression of AA amyloidosis is through treatment of the underlying infective or inflammatory process.

Dember LM. Amyloidosis-associated kidney disease. J Am Soc Nephrol 2006; 17(12):3458–3471.

14. A Cholesterol atheroembolisation

Cholesterol atheroembolisation occurs in patients with a high burden of atheromatous disease after manipulation of large vessels, typically after vascular surgery or angiography/angioplasty. These procedures result in the rupture of unstable atheromatous plaque and the release of cholesterol crystal showers that embolise to smaller arterial beds, including the renal vasculature and the distal peripheries. The effects of the embolisation may peak at up to several months after the initial procedure (compared to contrast-induced nephropathy, which classically peaks within several days of the use of contrast).

Patients typically present with a combination of acute kidney injury and systemic features (including rash and fever) that may mimic a vasculitic illness. The constellation of eosinophilia, fever, a raised erythrocyte sedimentation rate and low serum complement levels could suggest conditions with an autoimmune/ vasculitic basis (such as B, D and E). However, these are all also characteristic features of cholesterol atheroembolisation, reflecting immune system activation from exposure to the core of atheromatous plaques. The negative antinucleic antibodies and antineutrophil cytoplasmic antibodies make it unlikely that these findings represent an autoimmune process, whilst the lack of significant proteinuria and haematuria make a nephritic process unlikely. Urinary eosinophilia is most often a reflection of cholesterol atheroembolisation or acute interstitial nephritis.

Scolari F, Ravani P. Atheroembolic renal disease. Lancet 2010; 375(9726):1650–1660.

15. D Renal vein thrombosis

Renal vein thrombosis is secondary to the hypercoagulable state associated with this patient's nephrotic syndrome. The mechanism for this is complex, but includes the urinary loss of the natural anticoagulant antithrombin III. This hypercoagulable state may manifest in any of a number of ways, the most common of which are as deep vein thrombosis, pulmonary embolism and renal vein thrombosis. The presentation of renal vein thrombosis may range from the asymptomatic through to a severe syndrome characterised by severe flank pain, frank haematuria and a sudden decline in renal function as described here. The diagnosis is made either through Doppler ultrasound, the venous phase of renal angiography, or through CT or MRI; treatment is through management of the underlying nephrotic process, and with anticoagulation.

Renal artery stenosis is the incorrect answer as this could not explain the sudden pain. IgA nephropathy can certainly explain frank haematuria and proteinuria, but it is very unlikely that the patient has developed another cause of nephrotic syndrome. Urinary tract malignancies can present with frank haematuria, but this is often painless, and tends to be found in older patients than is the case here. Thin membrane basement nephropathy is a benign disease, most often inherited in an autosomal dominant manner, which is most often diagnosed during investigations after the incidental finding of persistent microscopic haematuria; however, it may present as a syndrome of acute flank pain and frank haematuria. The absence of a family history of haematuria and the presence of significant acute renal failure and proteinuria are all inconsistent with this diagnosis.

Crew RJ, Radhakrishnan J, Appel G. Complications of the nephrotic syndrome and their treatment. Clin Nephrol 2004; 62(4):245–259.

16. C Prednisolone

The presence of rapidly-progressive oedema in the context of hypoalbuminaemia and proteinuria is highly suggestive that the patient is undergoing a relapse of minimal-change nephropathy. Up to 75% of patients with minimal-change nephropathy relapse at least once, with approximately 20% relapsing frequently.

Although no information is given as to what treatment he was given before, up to 90% of patients under complete remission with glucocorticoid therapy, making this the treatment likely to have been used 3 years ago. Those patients who have responded to glucocorticoid therapy previously are very likely to respond to it again during subsequent relapses, and hence this is the correct answer.

A variety of other immunosuppressants (including ciclosporin, azathioprine and mycophenolate mofetil) have efficacy in inducing remission in minimal-change nephropathy, but are usually only trialled after failure of glucocorticoid therapy. Given the very high suspicion that the diagnosis is a relapse of minimal-change disease, neither a renal biopsy nor renal ultrasound would immediately help the patient's management.

Waldman M, et al. Adult minimal-change disease: clinical characteristics, treatment and outcomes. Clin J Am Soc Nephrol 2007; 2(3):445–453.

17. D Membranous nephropathy

Malignancy is associated with a variety of renal/urinary tract disorders, including urinary tract obstruction, tubulo-interstitial pathology (e.g. as a consequence of hypercalcaemia, or as a result of chemotherapeutic drug use), and glomerular disease. Whilst there is some relationship between malignancy and most forms of glomerulonephritis, the strongest association between malignancy and glomerular disease is with membranous nephropathy.

The presence of oedema and significant proteinuria immediately suggests underlying glomerular disease; penicillin can cause acute interstitial nephritis but has no strong association with glomerular disease. Both the history of malignancy and the recent streptococcal throat infection may make the candidate consider glomerulonephritis (such as options B and C), but the absence of haematuria and normal blood pressure makes a nephritic process very unlikely. The very low serum albumin gives further support to this patient having nephrotic syndrome, with membranous nephropathy being the option given most strongly associated with this finding. A normal urinary tract ultrasound makes retroperitoneal fibrosis very unlikely.

A useful mnemonic for causes of membranous nephropathy is **MAID**:

- **M**alignancy
- **A**utoimmune diseases – especially systemic lupus erythematosus
- **I**diopathic, or **i**nfections – particularly hepatitis B and C
- **D**rugs – especially agents used in rheumatology, including gold, penicillamine and non-steroidal anti-inflammatory drugs (NSAIDs)

Humphreys BD, Soiffer RJ, Magee CC. Renal failure associated with cancer and its treatment: an update. J Am Soc Nephrol 2005; 16(1):151–161.

18. A Acute tubular necrosis

The presence of only a protein trace on the urine dipstick and the absence of haematuria make options C and D respectively unlikely. A blocked catheter is a common cause of apparent oliguria in clinical practice, but it would not be associated with changes in the renal handling of sodium (as the investigation results here imply) unless the blockage had been present for a significant period of time.

Both prerenal failure and acute tubular necrosis (ATN) are possible in the context of the scenario given, but the investigations help to differentiate them (**Table 11.5**). In prerenal failure, tubules are intact and act to reabsorb as much of the filtered sodium as possible in order to preserve fluid volume, meaning that urine is produced in small volumes but is highly concentrated. In ATN, damage to tubular cells results in the failure of sodium reabsorption and the ability to concentrate urine, hence the findings of elevated urinary sodium and a reduced urinary osmolality. The biochemical findings that help differentiate prerenal failure from ATN are summarised in **Table 11.5**.

Lameire N, Van Biesen W, Vanholder R. Acute renal failure. Lancet 2005; 365 (9457):417–430.

Table 11.5

	Prerenal	ATN
Urinary sodium (mmol/L)	<20	>40
Urinary osmolality (mOsmol/kg)	>500	<350
Fractional sodium excretion (%)	<1	>2
Urine: plasma osmolality	1.5:1	1.1:1
Urine: plasma creatinine	>40:1	<20:1

Table 11.5 Differentiating prerenal failure from acute tubular necrosis (ATN).

19. B Goodpasture's syndrome

Goodpasture's syndrome is a rare disease, with a prevalence of approximately one case per million of population. The characteristic presentation is of a 'pulmonary–renal' syndrome, with the pulmonary involvement most often in the form of pulmonary haemorrhage and the renal manifestation as rapidly progressive glomerulonephritis. All of the options offered may give a pulmonary–renal syndrome; however, the pulmonary component of Churg–Strauss syndrome tends to be an asthma-like disease, whilst pulmonary involvement in systemic lupus erythematosus is typically pleuritis, leading to pleural effusions.

The diagnosis of Goodpasture's syndrome may be confirmed via two routes:

- Firstly, the findings on renal biopsy of crescentic glomerulonephritis with linear IgG deposition are almost pathognomonic of Goodpasture's syndrome. Renal biopsies from patients with IgA nephropathy tend to show predominant IgA deposition. Lupus nephritis usually demonstrates deposition of the full range of immunoglobulin classes. In contrast, granulomatosis with polyangiitis

(Wegener's) and Churg–Strauss often show a 'pauci-immune' biopsy pattern, i.e. only very scanty immune complex staining.
- Secondly, testing for plasma anti-glomerular basement membrane (anti-GBM) antibodies is both a sensitive and specific way of confirming the diagnosis.

Initial aggressive treatment with plasma exchange (to remove the anti-GBM antibody) or immunosuppression may stabilise renal function, but a high proportion of patients still end up requiring dialysis or transplantation.

Pusey CD. Anti-glomerular basement membrane disease. Kidney Int 2003; 64(4):1535–1550.

20. D Mesangiocapillary glomerulonephritis

There is a well-recognised association between type II mesangiocapillary glomerulonephritis (also known as membranoproliferative glomerulonephritis), acquired partial lipodystrophy, and low levels of serum complement factor C3. The low serum C3 levels may either be caused by complement factor H deficiency, or through the presence of antibodies to the C3 convertase C3bBb. In either case, the result is excessive activation of the alternative complement pathway. None of the options offered other than D has a significant association with lipodystrophy.

Type I and type II mesangiocapillary glomerulonephritis are associated with autoimmune diseases (especially systemic lupus erythematosus), infections (including malaria, and subacute bacterial endocarditis) and cryoglobulinaemia (itself often associated with hepatitis C).

Mesangiocapillary glomerulonephritis tends to be rapidly progressive, with half of patients having end stage renal failure by 10 years following diagnosis, and 90% by twenty years.

Appel GB, et al. Membranoproliferative glomerulonephritis type II (dense deposit disease): an update. J Am Soc Nephrol 2005; 16(5):1392–1403.

21. A Calcium gluconate

This biochemical profile in the absence of any past medical history and a recently normal plasma creatinine is consistent with severe acute kidney injury. The very elevated plasma potassium concentration and hyperkalaemic ECG changes are indications for immediate treatment of the hyperkalaemia. Calcium salts like calcium gluconate and calcium chloride act within a few minutes of administration to antagonise the effects of hyperkalaemia on excitable membranes (including the myocardium), and hence are the most appropriate immediate therapy in someone with hyperkalaemic ECG changes. Insulin therapy (normally co-administered with dextrose, to prevent hypoglycaemia) and nebulised β_2-adrenoceptor agonists are both very effective at reducing hyperkalaemia via their action of driving potassium into cells; however, both take approximately 30–60 minutes to act, so should always take 'second place' to the immediate administration of calcium salts. There is still considerable debate as to the efficacy of sodium bicarbonate in treating hyperkalaemia, and it certainly appears to be less effective than other medical therapies. Cation exchange resins (such as calcium polystyrene sulphonate) only reduce serum potassium after prolonged administration and are associated with a number of gastrointestinal side effects, meaning that they are not the best option here.

Kim HJ, Han SW. Therapeutic approach to hyperkalaemia. Nephron 2002; 92 (1):33–40.

22. A Calcium oxalate

Stones formed principally of calcium oxalate account for approximately 80% of all renal calculi, and an even higher percentage of those found in the population with Crohn's disease. In the presence of reduced fat absorption (either through Crohn's disease or any number of different causes), free fatty acids remain within the intestinal lumen and bind free calcium. Since oxalate normally binds calcium within the lumen to form insoluble calcium oxalate crystals, diseases that reduce luminal free calcium leave oxalate free for absorption across the intestinal lumen and subsequently into plasma. As oxalate is excreted by the kidneys, elevated plasma oxalate levels are associated with hyperoxaluria and an increased propensity for oxalate stone formation. The dehydration that may accompany a Crohn's flare is another factor increasing the likelihood of stone formation. Patients are advised to increase their fluid intake and to avoid oxalate-rich foods (such as spinach and rhubarb) to minimise their risk of stone recurrence.

Struvite stones (5% of all calculi) are found in association with upper urinary tract infection with urease-forming organisms, such as *Proteus* or *Klebsiella*; the negative urine culture result makes this unlikely. Cystine stones are relatively rare (only 2% of all stones) and normally occur in association with rare inherited renal tubular defects. Calculi composed of uric acid (10% of all stones) are associated with those conditions associated with crystal arthropathies, none of which are mentioned here. Cholesterol may be a component of gallstones but not urinary calculi; the remaining few percent of ureteric stones not composed of the substances already described are made of a variety of substrates.

Parks JH, et al. Urine stone risk factors in nephrolithiasis patients with and without bowel disease. Kidney Int 2003; 63(1):255–265.

23. B Ciclosporin toxicity

Although membranous nephropathy may recur in the transplanted kidney, the absence of any of the features of nephrotic syndrome and the fact that the immunosuppression appears to have been adequate up until now make option E very unlikely. The compliance with immunosuppressive treatment, non-tender graft and normal ultrasound scan make option D unlikely.

Although immunosuppression increases the vulnerability to opportunistic infections such as *Candida*, it is very unlikely that the patient would have a normal examination if disseminated candidiasis was the diagnosis; furthermore, the patient seems to have received appropriate therapy by his general practitioner. Thus, option C is unlikely too.

Acute interstitial nephritis has a huge range of possible causes but is often attributable to the introduction of new medications. Whilst some antifungals such as amphotericin are well-recognised as causing acute interstitial nephritis, there is no significant association between fluconazole and the disease. As such, option A is unlikely.

Fluconazole is, however, understood to be a cytochrome P450 enzyme inhibitor. Calcineurin inhibitors such as ciclosporin are medications with narrow therapeutic window and a range of possible toxic effects including nephrotoxicity, hence the rationale for close therapeutic drug monitoring in transplant patients. The temporal relationship between starting fluconazole and deterioration in renal function makes elevated plasma ciclosporin levels and associated nephrotoxicity the likely diagnosis in this case.

Naesens M, Kuypers DR, Sarwal M. Calcineurin inhibitor nephrotoxicity. Clin J Am Soc Nephrol 2009; 4(2):481–508.

24. D Intravenous saline

The finding of a combination of acute kidney injury, elevated creatine kinase and hyperphosphataemia in a patient who has experienced a 'long lie' is a typical presentation of rhabdomyolysis. Crush and ischaemic muscular injuries are amongst the most common causes of rhabdomyolysis, with the full list of causes memorable via the mnemonic **InSIDE:**

- **In**jury
- **S**nake bites
- **I**nherited myopathies, e.g. McCardle's syndrome
- **D**rugs, e.g. statins
- **E**ndocrine and metabolic causes, e.g. hypothyroidism; metabolic myopathies

The most appropriate option from those given for limiting any further deterioration in renal function is aggressive administration of fluids. Fluids help to better perfuse the kidney (thereby limiting any further ischaemic injury and tubular necrosis) and are also useful in washing out any obstructing tubular casts. The description of postural hypotension and metabolic/lactic acidosis is also consistent with this patient being significantly intravascularly depleted and requiring further fluid administration. It would be inappropriate to administer inotropic support whilst there was obvious intravascular depletion, hence option A is incorrect. Similarly, renal replacement therapy may potentially be required at some point, but would only be considered if medical therapies – including aggressive fluid replacement – had produced no benefit, rather than it being the appropriate initial therapy.

The presence of metabolic acidosis may makes option E plausible but although myoglobin is more soluble in alkaline urine (pH > 6.5), there is no good data to demonstrate that alkaline diuresis (e.g. by the administration of intravenous sodium bicarbonate) has any greater efficacy than saline diuresis. Furthermore, alkaline diuresis may potentially exacerbate hypocalcaemia and fluid overload; as such, it is not the most appropriate initial therapy. Mannitol – as osmotic diuretic – is used in some centres as a means of increasing tubular fluid flow, but there is conflicting trial evidence as to its efficacy.

Bosch X, Poch E, Grau JM. Rhabdomyolysis and acute kidney injury. N Eng J Med 2009; 361(1):62–72.

25. E Reflux nephropathy (chronic pyelonephritis)

Reflux nephropathy is a chronic tubulo-interstitial disease that is strongly related to vesicoureteric reflux (VUR) early in a person's life. Vesicoureteric reflux has a significant genetic component (at least a quarter of the children of sufferers have it themselves), and is closely associated with childhood urinary tract infections and nocturnal enuresis.

The ultimate effect of prolonged VUR is renal interstitial scarring. The diagnosis of VUR is often made in childhood (i.e. as part of investigation for recurrent urinary tract infection), when action can be taken to minimise the extent of reflux nephropathy. Unfortunately, chronic VUR may only first be recognised when adults present with the sequelae of renal interstitial scarring, including hypertension, proteinuria and chronic renal failure. A useful investigation to aid diagnosis in children is detecting the presence of reflux on micturating cystogram. In adults, nuclear medicine imaging (e.g. dimercaptosuccinic acid [DMSA] renal scanning) has been found to be a sensitive means of demonstrating renal scars. Treatment involves antibiotic prophylaxis and possible surgical intervention (e.g. ureteric reimplantation) when VUR is diagnosed in children, but is essentially standard chronic renal failure management when diagnosed in adults.

The presence of severe hypertension and a relevant family history suggest option A, but this option could not explain all the findings of this scenario; the hypertension here is likely a consequence of the renal failure. Option A is certainly genetically inherited (with X-linked dominance accounting for approximately 80% of cases), but is also associated with haematuria, along with other systemic features not mentioned here (including sensorineural deafness, eye disease, etc.). Both options C and D may present as nephrotic syndrome, but there is no evidence of oedema or significant hypoalbuminaemia.

Dillon MJ, Goonasekera CD. Reflux nephropathy. J Am Soc Nephrol 1998; 9(12):2377–2383.

26. D Papillary necrosis

Sickle cell disease is associated with a number of renal complications. The mechanism in most cases is sickling in the renal medulla within the vasa recta, reflecting the vulnerability of the renal medulla to hypoxia. Papillary necrosis occurs when there is total occlusion of the vasculature supplying the papillary areas of the kidney and a resultant sloughing off of these regions. The most common presentation is gross haematuria (either with no pain or minimal loin pain), although the condition may present as urinary tract infection or urinary tract obstruction. Other renal manifestations of sickle cell disease include a diminished tubular concentrating ability and distal renal tubular acidosis. The conventional means of confirming the diagnosis is by looking for the characteristic 'cup and pencil' appearance on intravenous urogram (IVU), reflecting calyceal clubbing in response to ischaemia.

Option B is associated with frank haematuria and option C with proteinuria and haematuria, but both seem unlikely given the lack of typical features of both either nephrotic or nephritic syndromes, and neither can explain the IVU findings. This patient is too young for carcinoma of the bladder to be a likely cause of his symptoms, but it should be remembered that young patients who have been exposed to *Schistosoma* are at increased risk of squamous cell bladder carcinoma, even at a young age. There is neither the mention of lower urinary tract symptoms nor the presence of nitrites and leucocytes in the urine dipstick, making urinary tract infection an unlikely diagnosis.

Pham PT, et al. Renal abnormalities in sickle cell disease. Kidney Int 2000; 57(1):1–8.

27. B Hamartin and tuberin gene testing

The features given are collectively very suggestive of underlying tuberous sclerosis. This is an autosomal dominantly inherited condition associated with mutations either in the hamartin gene (chromosome 9) or tuberin (chromosome 16), although 65% of cases are caused by spontaneous mutations. The presence of angiomyolipomata – in the kidney or otherwise – is highly suspicious of the condition. A wide range of organ systems may be affected, including (**Table 11.6**)

Curatolo P, Bombardieri R, Jozwiak S. Tuberous sclerosis. Lancet 2008; 372(9639):657–668.

Table 11.6	
Organ	**Features**
Skin	Includes adenoma sebaceum (salmon – coloured nodules in the nasolabial folds), periungual fibroma (nodular lesions adjacent to nails), shagreen patches (depositions of collagen with a cobblestone-like appearance found in the lumbosacral region) and ash-leaf macules (hypopigmented lesions found particularly in the region of the trunk and buttocks).
Eyes/central nervous system	Learning disability (up to 50% of patients), seizures (up to 75% of patients), cerebral tubers, cerebral tumours (e.g. astrocytoma), retinal hamartoma.
Renal	Renal cysts, renal hamartoma, renal angiomyolipomata
Respiratory	Lung cysts, with propensity to pneumothorax
Cardiac	Cardiac rhabdomyomata (may give propensity to arrhythmia)
Gastrointestinal	Hepatic/intestinal hamartomata, angiomyolipomata

Table 11.6 Clinical features of tuberous sclerosis.

28. B Multiple myeloma

Multiple myeloma is a haematological malignancy caused by the uncontrolled proliferation of a single clone of plasma cells, and hence huge overproduction of a monoclonal immunoglobulin. The constellation of clinical findings (bone pain, symptomatic anaemia) and biochemical findings (unexplained anaemia, hypercalcaemia, renal failure) are highly suggestive of the disease, especially in a patient of this age. Useful investigations include looking for a monoclonal immunoglobulin band (on either serum or urine electrophoresis), and examining a bone marrow aspirate or trephine for plasma cell morphology and immunophenotyping. Other supportive investigations include the presence of a significantly elevated plasma protein level, and a blood film showing a rouleaux pattern (i.e. red blood cells rounded and adhesive to each other as a result of elevated immunoglobulin levels).

Options A and E are both associated with anaemia and renal failure, but would be expected to be accompanied by thrombocytopenia and the presence of a microangiopathic haemolytic anaemia. Option D is incorrect as sarcoidosis tends to present in younger patients, and also cannot account for the blood film findings. Option C normally first presents with peripheral arthritis rather than back pain, and would not cause hypercalcaemia.

Laubach J, Richardson P, Anderson K. Multiple myeloma. Ann Rev Med 2011; 62:249–264.

29. E Retroperitoneal fibrosis

Retroperitoneal fibrosis (RPF) is a disease characterised by progressive extrinsic compression of the lower and middle thirds of the ureters through excessive fibrotic extracellular matrix deposition within the retroperitoneum. The probable pathogenesis involves fibrosis deposition as an exaggerated inflammatory response to lipid leakage from atheromatous plaques of the abdominal aorta. The other factor most commonly associated with onset of the disease is the use of certain medications, including ergot-derived drugs (such as methysergide, commonly used previously to treat migraine headache), beta-blockers, methyldopa and hydralazine.

RPF most commonly occurs in middle-aged men. It typically presents with the insidious onset of flank/abdominal pain. The appearance of bilateral proximal hydroureter and medial deviation of the ureters on ultrasound, CT or MRI is very characteristic of the disease, but further investigations may be needed to exclude other causes of urinary tract obstruction (e.g. malignancy). Treatment includes corticosteroids (to reduce the swelling) and, if necessary, surgical management (either stenting of the ureters, or surgically freeing them from the surrounding fibrotic tissue [ureterolysis]). The prognosis is generally good.

Options A, B and C are all unlikely given ultrasound findings that are highly suggestive of postrenal disease. Renal calculi may cause bilaterally obstructed ureters, but more often are found unilaterally. Furthermore, they most often present with acute, severe pain rather than with such an insidious onset. It would also be very unusual for there not to be dipstick haematuria if renal calculi were present.

Vaglio A, Salvarani C, Buzio C. Retroperitoneal fibrosis. Lancet 2006; 367(9506):241–251.

30. A IgA nephropathy

IgA nephropathy (also known as Berger's syndrome) is the most common primary glomerulonephritis in adults. It usually presents up to 3 days post-upper respiratory tract infection with recurrent episodes of haematuria. A similar pattern is seen in Henoch–Schönlein purpura, and is caused by IgA deposition within the glomerulus. Acute treatment is a 6-week course of oral corticosteroids, and long-term treatment Schistosoma the optimisation of blood pressure. Of those who receive a diagnosis, approximately 25% progress to end stage renal failure.

The time scale of the onset of symptoms differentiates this from post-streptococcal glomerulonephritis. The latter presents at least 1–2 weeks after an upper respiratory tract infection with a nephrogenic strain of *Streptococcus*, usually of Group A. Patients present with haematuria and oedema. Hypertension is present in 60–80%. Diuretics are used to treat any significant hypertension and oedema. Corticosteroids are not generally indicated. Specific therapy for streptococcal infection should be initiated.

Minimal change disease nearly always presents with a nephrotic picture and is most common in children. Membranous nephropathy can present in a variety of ways and has two peaks of incidence (patients in their 20s and 60s), it may be idiopathic, or secondary to other diseases (including malignancy, connective tissue diseases, hepatitis B or C), or drugs such as non-steroidal anti-inflammatories and gold.

Donadio JV, Grande JP. IgA nephropathy. N Eng J Med 2002; 347(10):738–748.

Chapter 12

Respiratory medicine

1. A 73-year-old man, a retired accountant, presented with a 3-month history of a dry, non-productive cough and back pain, which was worse on movement. He had a past history of ischaemic heart disease and atrial fibrillation. A plain chest X-ray revealed bilateral basal interstitial shadowing.

    What is the most likely diagnosis?

    A   Amiodarone toxicity
    B   Ankylosing spondylitis
    C   Sarcoidosis
    D   Silicosis
    E   Tuberculosis

2. A 58-year-old man, a farmer, presented to his general practitioner with fever, headaches and shortness of breath worsening over a 12-hour period. He was diagnosed with farmer's lung.

    What is the most likely causative agent for farmer's lung?

    A   *Aspergillus clavatus*
    B   Avian proteins
    C   *Micropolyspora faeni*
    D   *Penicillium frequentans*
    E   *Thermoactinomyces sacchari*

3. A 28-year-old homeless man presented with a 1-week history of progressively worsening neck stiffness and headache. He also described a dry cough for the past 1 month. He was apyrexial on admission, haemodynamically stable and had no rash. The rest of the examination was unremarkable. A CT head performed in the acute medical admissions unit showed no abnormality. A lumbar puncture was subsequently performed, with the following results:

    Investigations:

opening pressure	18 cm H_2O (5–18)
appearance	cloudy
protein	1.5 g/L (0.15–0.45)
glucose	2.0 mmol/L (3.3–4.4)
white cells	500 cells/mm³ (lymphocytes) (<5)
serum glucose	4.5 mmol/L (4.1–6.6)

Which of the following is the most in keeping with the results?

A   Bacterial meningitis
B   Cryptococcal meningitis
C   Normal cerebrospinal fluid
D   Tuberculous meningitis
E   Viral meningitis

4.   Which one of the following is the most likely cause of an increased transfer co-efficient (KCO)?

A   Arteriovenous malformation
B   Interstitial lung disease
C   Primary pulmonary hypertension
D   Pulmonary haemorrhage
E   Pulmonary oedema

5.   A 65-year-old woman presented with a 2-week history of pleuritic chest pain and shortness of breath on exertion. Six months ago, she was diagnosed with colon cancer, underwent surgical resection and had adjuvant chemotherapy. She was apyrexial and haemodynamically stable. A plain chest radiograph showed no abnormality but a CT pulmonary angiogram confirmed pulmonary embolism (PE).

What is the most appropriate anticoagulation regimen for this patient?

A   LMWH (low molecular weight heparin) for at least 3 months
B   LMWH for at least 6 months
C   Warfarin for at least 3 months
D   Warfarin for at least 6 months
E   Warfarin for at least 6 weeks

6.   A 46-year-old man with a history of sarcoidosis was seen in chest clinic. He was not taking any medications. A plain chest X-ray showed bilateral hilar lymphadenopathy with reticunodular infiltrates.

What stage of sarcoidosis does this correlate with?

A   Stage 0
B   Stage 1
C   Stage 2
D   Stage 3
E   Stage 4

7.   A 64-year-old man, a smoker, had a 2-month history of a dry cough but recently had started to bring up approximately a teaspoon of bright red blood every day. He had lost about 3 kg of weight over this period. He had also noted a dry mouth and increasing weakness in his legs and difficulty in getting up from a chair. However, this weakness improved with walking.

What is the most likely diagnosis?

A   Adenocarcinoma of the lung

    B Alveolar cell carcinoma of the lung
    C Large cell carcinoma of the lung
    D Small cell carcinoma of the lung
    E Squamous cell carcinoma of the lung

8. A 31-year-old man presented to the medical assessment unit with a non-productive cough lasting for 1 week. The previous week he had experienced headache, joint aches and generalised lethargy. There had been no foreign travel. He worked in an office. On admission, the patient had a temperature of 38.3°C and respiratory rate of 24 breaths per minute. He had bilateral lung crackles. There was an itchy, maculopapular rash with target lesions present on all his limbs. Plain chest X-ray showed bilateral patchy consolidation.

    What is the most likely causative organism?

    A *Chlamydia* spp.
    B *Klebsiella* spp.
    C *Legionella* spp.
    D *Mycoplasma* spp.
    E *Pneumococcal* spp.

9. Which one of the following is least likely to be associated with bronchiectasis?

    A Allergic bronchopulmonary aspergillosis (ABPA)
    B Human immunodeficiency virus (HIV)
    C Hypergammaglobulinaemia
    D Rheumatoid arthritis
    E Ulcerative colitis

10. Which one of the following therapies is not used in the management of obstructive sleep apnoea?

    A Acupuncture
    B Avoidance of alcohol and tobacco
    C CPAP (continuous positive airways pressure)
    D Imipramine
    E Tonsillectomy

11. A 26-year-old woman with a recent diagnosis of asthma had been taking increasing doses of her salbutamol inhaler. She was a non-smoker. Last month, her general practitioner started her on beclomethasone (400 μg), followed by salmeterol. Although her symptoms were improving after starting salmeterol, she still complained of wheezing and shortness of breath when exercising.

    What is the next most appropriate step in the management of her asthma?

    A Continue salmeterol and increase dose of beclomethasone to 800 μg
    B Continue salmeterol and start a trial of leukotriene receptor antagonist
    C Stop salmeterol and increase dose of beclomethasone to 600 μg
    D Stop salmeterol and increase dose of beclomethasone to 800 μg
    E Stop salmeterol and start trial of leukotriene antagonist

12. A 50-year-old woman visited her general practitioner with a 3-day productive cough. The general practitioner suspected a chest infection and started her on clarithromycin. Her past medical history included epilepsy, hypertension, gastro-oesophageal disease and a metallic mitral valve replacement. She normally took amlodipine, omeprazole, indomethacin, carbamazepine, warfarin and furosemide. At her next anticoagulation clinic appointment, she was found to have an international normalised ratio of 8 and the doctor noticed a large right knee haemarthrosis.

Which drug or combination of drugs is most likely to contribute to the increased risk of bleeding?

A   Clarithromycin only
B   Clarithromycin and omeprazole
C   Clarithromycin, omeprazole and carbamazepine
D   Clarithromycin, omeprazole and indomethacin
E   Clarithromycin, omeprazole, carbamazepine and indomethacin

13. A 23-year-old man, a Bangladeshi student, was admitted under the chest team with a 3-month history of cough, night sweats and weight loss. He had an old Bacillus Calmette–Guérin (BCG) scar on the right arm. A plain chest X-ray was unremarkable. CT chest, abdomen and pelvis and colonoscopy showed no abnormality. A Mantoux test was inconclusive. Tuberculosis (TB) was still suspected so a quantiferon test was requested.

Which one of the following best describes a quantiferon test?

A   Based on the enzyme-linked immunospot (ELISPOT) assay
B   Contraindicated in patients with previous BCG vaccines
C   Differentiates between latent and active TB
D   Quantifies interferon gamma from sensitised lymphocytes
E   Performed by intradermal injection of purified protein derivative (PPD)

14. A 23-year-old woman was admitted to the emergency department with an acute exacerbation of asthma. She was started on medical treatment but as she seemed to deteriorate, the intensive treatment unit team were asked to review the patient.

Which one of the following is the most likely characteristic feature of life-threatening asthma?

A $PaCO_2$ 4.0 kPa
B PaO_2 8.9 kPa
C   Peak expiratory flow rate (PEFR) 31% best or predicted value
D   Oxygen saturation 93%
E   Respiratory rate of 20 breaths per minute

15. A 28-year-old woman with a background of severe asthma and depression, presented with haemoptysis, worsening shortness of breath and wheeze. Blood tests performed in the outpatient clinic last month showed eosinophilia and positive perinuclear anti-neutrophil cytoplasmic antibodies (pANCA).

Which one of the following drugs is most closely associated with the diagnosis of her current condition?

A   Citalopram
B   Fluoxetine
C   Monteleukast
D   Prednisolone
E   Theophylline

16. A 23-year-old man with cystic fibrosis presented to the respiratory clinic with a 2-week history of coughing up bright red blood. He also described increased shortness of breath and reduced exercise tolerance. Six weeks ago, he had been admitted to hospital with an infective exacerbation of his chronic chest condition. Total IgE (1638) was elevated from his previous admission. Specific IgE to *Aspergillus fumigatus*-remained the same.

What is the most appropriate management plan?

A   Intravenous antibiotics only
B   Intravenous antibiotics and intravenous antifungals
C   Intravenous antibiotics, intravenous antifungal and short course of oral steroid
D   Intravenous antibiotics followed by long-term oral steroid
E   Intravenous antibiotics, intravenous antifungal, long-term steroids and long-term antifungal

17. A 63-year-old non-smoking woman presented to hospital with an infective exacerbation of bronchiectasis. She has had two similar episodes in the past year. On examination, her temperature was 38.1°C, pulse 100 beats per minute, blood pressure 112/72 mmHg, and respiratory rate 32 breaths per minute. There was widespread wheeze and crepitations on auscultation.

Which one of the following organisms is most closely associated with this syndrome?

A   *Haemophilus influenzae*
B   *Klebsiella*
C   *Mycoplasma avium* complex
D   *Pseudomonas aeruginosa*
E   *Staphylococcus aureus*

18. A 75-year-old woman presented with shortness of breath to the emergency department. A plain chest X-ray showed a left sided pleural effusion.

Which one of the following is not a cause of a transudate pleural effusion?

A   Acute glomerulonephritis
B   Cirrhosis
C   Myxoedema
D   Rheumatoid arthritis
E   Sarcoidosis

19. A 58-year-old non-smoking woman was referred to the outpatient clinic because plain X-ray and CT thorax showed a mass in the right upper zone suggestive of an aspergilloma. She was asymptomatic and otherwise well.

What is the most appropriate next step in management?

A   Aspergillus precipitins serology
B   Bronchoscopy and broncho-alveolar lavage
C   Observe and repeat plain chest radiograph in 3 months
D   Treat with antifungals for 3 months
E   Treat with a reducing dose of steroids for 3 months

20. Which one of the following best describes pulmonary surfactant?

A   Main component is DPCC (diphosphatidylcholine)
B   Only has hydrophilic molecules
C   Only has hydrophobic molecules
D   Phosphatidylglycerol forms more than 50% of the lipid in surfactant
E   Produced by type I respiratory alveolar cells

21. Which one of the following best describes alpha-1 antitrypsin enzyme?

A   A protein consisting of 284 amino acids
B   Located on chromosome 16
C   Only produced in the lungs
D   PIZZ is the normal genotype
E   Serum trypsin inhibitor

22. A 32-year-old man presented with a recent onset of cough and wheeze after starting a new job as a painter and decorator. His symptoms resolved during the weekends and when he travelled abroad for 1 week.

Which one of the following agents is most likely to be responsible for this condition?

A   Flout
B   Isocyanates
C   Latex
D   Organophosphates
E   Persulphates

23. A 72-year-old woman, a smoker with a background of chronic obstructive pulmonary disease (COPD), was being considered for lung volume reduction surgery (LVRS).

Which one of the following is a contraindication for this procedure?

A   Age of 73 years
B   Lung function FEV1 29% of predicted value
C   Predominantly upper lobe disease
D   Pulmonary hypertension (pulmonary arterial pressure [PAP] mean > 35 mmg)
E   Stopped smoking 5 months ago

24. A 62-year-old smoker with a 25-pack year history presented to clinic with suspected chronic obstructive pulmonary disease (COPD).

Which one of the following criteria is diagnostic of COPD?

A   FEV1 < 70% of predicted value and FEV1/FVC ratio < 80%
B   FEV1 < 70% of predicted value and FEV1/FVC ratio < 60%
C   FEV1 < 70% of predicted value and presence of respiratory symptoms
D   FEV1 > 80% of predicted value and presence of respiratory symptoms
E   FEV1 < 80% of predicted value and FEV1/FVC ratio < 70%

25. Which one of the following is least likely to be associated with pulmonary eosinophilia and pulmonary infiltrates?

A   Allergic bronchopulmonary aspergillosis (ABPA)
B   Churg–Strauss syndrome
C   Fibrosing alveolitis
D   Löffler's syndrome
E   Sulphasalazine

26. Which one of the following statements relating to cystic fibrosis (CF) is correct?

A   Autosomal dominant inheritance
B   The most common mutation is delta F506 of the cystic fibrosis transmembrane conductance regulator (CTFR) gene
C   The Liverpool Epidemic Strain (LES) is an aggressive strain of *Burkholderia cepacia* pathogen.
D   Pancreatic insufficiency occurs in all patients with CF
E   Sweat test chloride of greater than 60 mmol/L is considered a positive result in adults

27. A 32-year-old non-smoking female, had been recently diagnosed with pharyngitis. Following this she developed a 10-day history of flu like symptoms, increasing shortness of breath and a non-productive cough. Chest examination was normal, but she had maculopapular lesions on the trunk.

Chest X-ray: bilateral infiltrates.

What is the most useful diagnostic test?

A   Blood culture
B   Mycoplasma serology
C   Serum urea and electrolytes
D   Sputum culture
E   Urinary antigen for *Legionella*

28. A 21-year-old man with no past medical history was admitted to the emergency department with a left sided pneumothorax measuring 4 cm on a plain chest radiograph. The patient was haemodynamically stable with no shortness of breath.

What is the most appropriate management step?

A   Admit for observation for 24 hours
B   Aspiration of pneumothorax
C   Chest drain insertion after period of observation
D   Discharge home with a follow-up plain chest radiograph in 1–2 weeks
E   Immediate chest drain insertion

29. A 20-year-old woman attended to the emergency deparment with a 3-day history of worsening shortness of breath and wheeze. She had a background of asthma, with a best peak expiratory flow rate (PEFR) of 420 L/min. She was treated initially with oxygen via face mask, an ipratropium nebuliser, and continuous salbutamol nebulisers. Oral prednisolone was administered. On reassessment, examination revealed a respiratory rate of 36 breaths per minute and widespread expiratory polyphonic wheeze. PEFR was 180 L/min.

What is the most appropriate therapeutic next step in management?

A   Inhaled budesonide-formoterol
B   Intravenous hydrocortisone
C   Intravenous magnesium sulphate
D   Nebulised albuterol
E   Oral montelukast

30. A 42-year-old man with diagnosis of Kartagener's syndrome, presented to the outpatient respiratory clinic with worsening shortness of breath. He also complained of hearing loss. He had received four courses of oral antibiotics by his general practitioner over the past 2 months, but his symptoms still persisted.

Which one of the following is most closely associated with this condition?

A   Cardiomegaly
B   Glioblastoma multiforme
C   Otitis media
D   Recurrent pneumothoraces
E   Recurrent pulmonary emboli

Answers

1. A Amiodarone

The past history of atrial fibrillation and radiographic changes on a plain X-ray suggests that the correct answer is amiodarone. Although he has been complaining of back pain, the presentation of this is not consistent with ankylosing spondylitis, as changes would be expected in the upper zones. The following mnemonics may be used to differentiate between upper zone and lower zone lung changes.

Upper lobe fibrosis – *SACHETS-R*

Sarcoidosis
Ankylosing spondylitis
Coal workers pneumoconiosis
Histocytosis
Extrinsic allergic alveolitis
Tuberculosis
Silicosis
Radiation

Lower zone fibrosis – *ACID-L*

Asbestosis
Connective tissue disorders – systemic lupus erythematosus, rheumatoid arthritis,
Idiopathic pulmonary fibrosis
Drugs – amiodarone, bleomycin, sulphasalazine, nitrofurantoin
Lymphangitis carcinomatosis

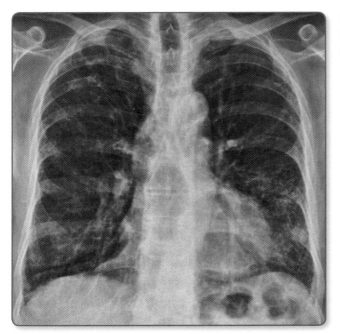

Figure 12.1 Chest X-ray demonstrating bibasal shadowing.

2. C *Micropolyspora faeni*

Extrinsic allergic alveolitis (EAA) is a process where inhalation of allergens results in a hypersensitivity reaction. **Table 12.1** shows the different types of EAA and causative agents.

Disease	Antigen	Exposure
Farmer's lung	*Micropolyspora faeni* *Thermoactinomyces vulgaris*	Handling mouldy hay
Bird fancier's lung	Avian protein	Handling birds, their feathers and excretions
Malt worker's lung	*Aspergillus clavatus*	Handling mouldy barley
Mushroom worker's lung	Thermophilic actinomycetes	Mould from mushrooms
Vaginosis	Thermophilic sacchari	Sugar cane (processors)
Suberosis	*Penicillium frequentans*	Handling mouldy cork dust

Table 12.1 Different types of extrinsic allergic alveolitis and their causative agents.

3. D Tuberculous meningitis

In view of the patient's background, the clinical suspicion of tuberculosis is high. **Table 12.2** differentiates the criteria for the various aetiologies of an abnormal cerebrospinal fluid. It will be important to investigate this patient further for tuberculosis affecting other organs, with a plain chest X-ray mandatory with this presentation. Further tests would include the Mantoux test and consideration of quantiferon or T spot testing.

CSF	Bacterial	Viral	Tuberculosis
Appearance	Cloudy	Clear	Cloudy/clear/fibrin web
Predominant cells	Polymorphs	Lymphocytes	Lymphocytes
Cell count/mm^3	90–1000	50–1000	10–1000
Protein (g/L)	>1.5	<1	1–5
Glucose mmol/L	< 50% of serum levels	> 50% serum levels	< 50% serum levels

Table 12.2 Features of cerebrospinal fluid (CSF) in different infective conditions.

4. D Pulmonary haemorrhage

The causes of **reduced** transfer co-efficient include:

- Arteriovenous malformation
- Interstitial lung disease
- Lymphangitis carcinomatosa
- Multiple pulmonary emboli
- Primary pulmonary hypertension
- Pulmonary oedema

The causes of **increased** transfer co-efficient include:

- Left to right shunts
- Polycythaemia
- Pulmonary haemorrhage
- Thoracic cage abnormalities

Hughes JM, Pride NB. In defence of the carbon monoxide transfer coefficient Kco (TL/VA). Eur Respir J 2001; 17(2):168–174.

5. A LMWH (low molecular weight heparin) for at least 3 months

The British Committee for Standards in Haematology has recently revised guidelines for venous thromboembolism (VTE) management. The recommendation is that as patients with cancer related VTE are at high risk of recurrence and LMWH has been shown to be more effective than warfarin in the first 6 months.

In non-cancer related VTE, patients with a proximal deep venous thromboembolism (DVT) or PE should be treated for at least 3 months with oral anticoagulants, aiming for an international normalised ratio 2.0–3.0. In distal or isolated DVT, treatment should be for at least 6 weeks with oral anticoagulation with a target range of 2.0–3.0.

Keeling D, et al. Guidelines on oral anticoagulation with warfarin, 4th edition. Br J Haematol 2011; 154 (3): 311–24.
Noble SI, et al. Management of venous thromboembolism in patients with advanced cancer: a systematic review and meta-analysis. Lancet Oncol 2008; 9(6):577.

6. C Stage 2

In sarcoidosis, chest X-ray changes correlate with four different stages:

Stage 1: Bilateral hilar lymphadenopathy
Stage 2: Bilateral hilar lymphadenopathy with reticunodular infiltrates
Stage 3: Bilateral pulmonary infiltrates
Stage 4: Diffuse reticunodualar changes consistent with fibrosis.

Stages on a plain chest X-ray can offer prognosis of the disease. Treatment for patients with known sarcoidosis will be determined by the clinical condition and radiographic changes. **Figure 12.2** is demonstrates bilateral hilar lymphadenopathy.

Patients with radiographic changes may not need to start treatment if they remain asymptomatic. Indications for treatment with prednisolone include onset of symptoms, hypercalcaemia or cardiac/neurological involvement.

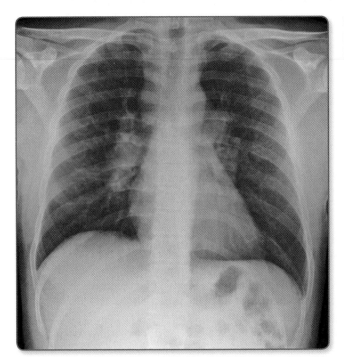

Figure 12.2
Bilateral hilar lymphadenopathy.

7. D Small cell carcinoma of the lung

This patient has the features and associations of Lambert–Eaton syndrome, which typically presents in small cell lung cancer. The description of weakness that improves with exercise is characteristic of Lambert–Eaton syndrome and unlike myasthenia gravis, there is increased strength post exercise. Other features of Lambert–Eaton syndrome include gait difficulty before eye symptoms, autonomic features and hyporeflexia on examination. Diagnosis is clinical, electromyography (EMG) and antibodies against voltage-gated calcium channels and along with investigation of the underlying lung cancer.

Successful treatment of the underlying malignancy usually leads to resolution of symptoms. However two means of treatment are also available. This is by improving the neuromuscular conduction (3,4-diaminopyridine and pyridostigmine) and immune suppression (prednisolone, intravenous immunoglobulin, steroid sparing agents), with 3,4-diaminopyridine and intravenous immunoglobulin being the most effective combination. Plasmapheresis may be an option, particularly in acute onset of symptoms.

Keogh M, Sedehizadeh S, Maddison P. Treatment for Lambert–Eaton myasthenic syndrome. Cochrane Database Syst Rev 2011; (2) CD003279.

8. D *Mycoplasma* species

This patient presents with a history suggestive of *Mycoplasma pneumoniae* infection, demonstrated by the dry cough and 'flu-like' symptoms and radiological changes. The organism tends to affect young adults and usually occurs in epidemics every 3–4 years. It would be important to analyse blood tests carefully to rule out haemolytic anaemia (as a result of cold agglutinins) and to check mycoplasma serology. Chest X-ray typically shows bilateral patchy consolidation (**Figure 12.3**).

A useful mnemonic, **MAGPIES**, may be used for the complications of mycoplasma pneumonia:

Meningoencephalitis
Autoimmune haemolytic anaemia
Guillain–Barré syndrome
Peri/Myocarditis, **p**eripheral neuropathies, (low) **p**latelets
Intravascular (disseminated intravascular coagulation)
Erythema multiforme, erythema nodosum
Stevens–Johnson syndrome

Treatment is usually with clarithromycin, erythromycin or a tetracycline.

Waites KB, Talkington DF. Mycoplasma pneumonia and its role as a human pathogen. Cl Clin Microbiol Rev 2004; 17(4):697–728.

9. C Hypergammaglobulinaemia

Bronchiectasis is the permanent dilatation of bronchi and bronchioles. Hypogammaglobulinaemia is a cause of bronchiectasis, not hypergammaglobulinaemia.

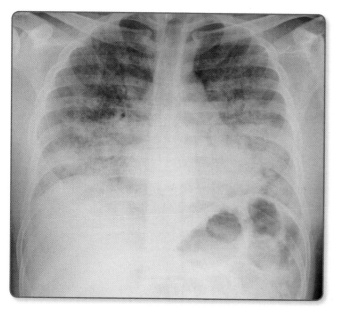

Figure 12.3 Chest X-ray showing bilateral patchy consolidation.

The causes of bronchiectasis may be divided into congenital and acquired,

*Congenital (mnemonic – **PICKY**)*

PrImary ciliary dyskinesia
Cystic fibrosis
Kartagener's syndrome
Young's syndrome

*Acquired (mnemonic – **ATROPHIC**)*

Allergic bronchopulmonary aspergillosis (ABPA)
Tuberculosis (post TB)
Rheumatoid arthritis, ulcerative colitis
Obstruction (distal to obstructed bronchus)
Post infective: pneumonia, measles, mumps, pertussis
Hypogammaglobulinaemia, **H**IV
Idiopathic
Chemical pneumonitis (inhalation of caustic chemicals)

Young's syndrome is rare condition comprising of bronchiectasis, reduced fertility and sinusitis.

10. D Imipramine

The main management goals after diagnosis of obstructive sleep apnoea (OSA) are:

- Weight reduction – over 80% of men diagnosed with OSA are obese
- Treatment of underlying medical conditions such as hypothyroidism and acromegaly
- Nocturnal continuous positive airways pressure (CPAP) via a nasal cannula
- Anterior mandible positioning devices – these have shown limited benefits
- Surgical procedures to relieve pharyngeal obstruction, e.g. tonsillectomy or in rare cases, tracheostomy.

Imipramine is a tricyclic antidepressant, which has been previously used for treatment of depression and cataplexy. Cataplexy is the sudden loss on muscle tone leading to collapse. Cataplexy is associated and a feature of narcolepsy. Imipramine is not first line treatment for cataplexy (or depression) due to its side effect profile, and has been replaced by venlafaxine, a selective serotonin reuptake inhibitor (SSRI).

Recent research has shown that acupuncture may play a role in the management of obstructive sleep apnoea. It has been demonstrated that a single session of manual acupuncture or electroacupuncture may have an immediate effect on reducing the number of nocturnal events in OSA.

Freire A, et al. Immediate effects of acupuncture on the sleep patterns of patients with obstructive sleep apnoea. Acupunc Med 2010; 28:115–119.

11. A Continue salmeterol and increase dose of beclomethasone to 800 µg

The British Thoracic Society (BTS) provide step-wise guidance to the management of asthma. This patient appears to still have symptoms of asthma, despite treatment with inhalers. The aim of asthma management is complete control of the disease. It is important that when using this guidelines to start at the step most appropriate to the severity of the patient's asthma. If it is thought that there is a lack of response to the treatment, compliance to medication should be assessed and alternative diagnoses should be considered.

Step 1: Intermittent mild asthma

- Use short-acting inhaled β_2-agonists, on an as required basis.

Step 2: Regular preventer therapy

- Add inhaled steroid 200–800 µg/day. It is suggested that 400 µg is a suitable initial dose for many patients
- Initiate at the dose of inhaled steroid, which is suitable for the severity of asthma

Step 3: Initial add-on therapy

- Add long-acting inhaled β_2-agonists (LABA)
- Evaluate the control of asthma:
  - if good response to LABA continue
  - if benefit from LABA but control still insufficient remain with LABA and raise the dose of inhaled steroid to 800 µg/day
  - if no response to LABA stop LABA and aim to increase the dose of inhaled steroid to 800 µg/day. If control at this stage remains insufficient, then consider trial of other therapies such as theophylline (slow release) or leukotriene receptor antagonists

Step 4: Persistent poor control

- Considering trial of increasing the dose of inhaled steroid up to 2000 µg/day
- Consider trial of initiation of a fourth drug, e.g. theophylline, leukotriene receptor antagonist (slow release) or β_2-agonists tablet

Step 5: Continuous or frequent use of oral steroids

- Start daily steroid tablet in the lowest possible dose to achieve adequate control
- Continue high dose of inhaled steroid at 2000 µg/day
- Evaluate other treatments to minimise use of steroid tablets and refer to a specialist

British Thoracic Society/Scottish Intercollegiate Guidelines Network (SIGN). British Guideline on the Management of Asthma. Edinburgh: SIGN, 2011.

12. D Clarithromycin, omeprazole and indomethacin

The cytochrome P450 group of enzymes are involved in drug metabolism and bioactivation. Clarithromycin and omeprazole are both cytochrome P450 inhibitors, thus they decrease the clearance of warfarin. This will cause a high international normalised ratio (INR) and increase the risk of bleeding. Carbamazepine, being a cytochrome P450 CYP3A4 enzyme inducer, increases the clearance of warfarin and so reduces the risk of bleeding. Indomethacin increases bleeding by inhibiting platelet function but has no effect on INR. Amlodipine and furosemide have no effect on INR levels.

Mnemonic for cytochrome P450 inducers: **PCBRASS**

- Phenytoin
- Carbamazepine
- Barbiturates
- Rifampicin
- Alcohol (chronic)
- Sulphonylureas
- Smoking

Mnemonic for cytochrome P450 inhibitors: **VIDEOCASE**

- Valproate
- Isoniazid
- Disulphiram
- Erythromycin (clarithromycin)
- Omeprazole
- Cimetidine
- Allopurinol
- Sulphonamides
- Ethanol (acute)

13. D Quantifies interferon gamma from sensitised lymphocytes

The diagnosis of tuberculosis may remain difficult to prove definitively, even when the clinical suspicion remains high. In many cases empirical treatment may be started. However, it is necessary to try to obtain a diagnosis.

Tuberculin skin testing (TST), or Mantoux test, has been traditionally used by assessing the reaction to an intradermal infection of purified protein derivative (PPD). However, there may be a high rate of false positive, including previous Bacillus Calmette–Guérin (BCG) vaccination, inability to detect recent tuberculosis, incorrect placement of PPD and incorrect readings of the reaction.

Quantiferon testing is one of the interferon gamma releasing assay (IGRA) blood tests. Quantiferon testing helps diagnosis in those clinically suspected with TB, where the Mantoux test fails to provide a reliable answer. The Quantiferon test can be used to diagnose both active and latent TB, but cannot differentiate between the two. It is based on the quantification of interferon gamma from sensitised lymphocytes from *Mycobacterium tuberculosis*. Interferon gamma is present in tuberculosis and is secreted in measurable amounts. The test involves a blood test followed by incubation of the blood with control and *Mycobacterium tuberculosis* antigens. This is then followed by detection of interferon gamma by ELISA.

The advantages of Quantiferon are that it can be performed by a single blood test, with results back within 24 hours. Also, it has a lower false positive rate than thiosulphate sulphurtransferase (TST) and is not subject to incorrect readings in TST. It can also be used in those patients previously vaccinated with BCG.

Option A describes T-SPOT. T SPOT is another interferon gamma releasing assay (IGRA) blood test, which detects interferon gamma produced by T cells in response to antigens specific to *Mycobacterium tuberculosis*, but uses a different overnight assay (ELISPOT vs ELISA).

Sester M, Sotgiu G, Lange C. Inteferon gamma release assays for the diagnosis of active tuberculosis: a systematic review and meta-analysis. Eur Respir J 2011; 37(1):100–111.

14. C Peak expiratory flow rate (PEFR) 31% best or predicted value

---

Moderate exacerbation of asthma
PEFR >50–75% predicted or best
Increasing symptoms
(no features of acute or life-threatening asthma)

↓

Acute severe exacerbation of asthma
PEFR 33–50% predicted or best
Heart rate >110 beats per minute
Respiratory rate > 24 breaths per minute
Inability to complete sentences in one breath

↓

Life-threatening asthma
PEFR < 33% predicted or best
$PaO_2 < 8$ kPa
$SpO_2 < 92\%$
Normal $PaCO_2$ (4.3–6.0 kPa)
Cyanosis
Silent chest
Poor respiratory effort
Exhaustion, reduced consciousness levels
Arrhythmia

↓

Near fatal
Increased $PaCO_2$ and requiring mechanical ventilation

British Thoracic Society/Scottish Intercollegiate Guidelines Network. British Guideline on the Management of Asthma. SIGN; 2011.

15. C Monteleukast

This patient has Churg–Strauss syndrome, which has been shown to be associated with leukotriene antagonists such as monteleukast. Monteleukast does not directly cause Churg–Strauss syndrome. Instead, it appears to be involved in the unmasking of the existing vasculitis.

Churg–Strauss typically features (late onset) asthma, eosinophilia and vasculitis. It can affect many organs, but commonly affecting lung, skin and peripheral nerves. An important blood test is for perinuclear anti-neutrophil cytoplasmic antibodies (pANCA), which is positive in the majority of cases, the condition responds to steroids, but other immunosuppressants such as azathioprine and cyclophosphamide may be required.

Wechsler ME, et al. Churg-Strauss Syndrome in patients receiving monteleukast as treatment for asthma. Chest 2000; 117(3):708–713.

16. E Intravenous antibiotics, intravenous antifungal, long-term steroids and long-term antifungal

This patient with cystic fibrosis most likely has had an episode of allergic bronchopulmonary aspergillosis (ABPA). It is often difficult to distinguish between an infective pulmonary exacerbation and ABPA, but in this case the symptoms of haemoptysis with raised total IgE immunoglobulins and a raised specific IgE to aspergillus fumigatus, are all highly suggestive of ABPA.

The management of these patients would be to cover for bacterial infection with intravenous antibiotics, but to also start intravenous antifungals and steroids. In the initial acute phase, intravenous steroids and intravanous antifungals would be used, along with tranexamic acid for the haemoptysis. However, once the acute episode has settled, it would be necessary to continue with a prolonged course of oral steroids and oral antifungals.

It is of course essential to also test sputum for microbiology and mycology and treat accordingly.

Aggarwal R. Allergic Bronchopulmonary Aspergillosis. Chest 2009; 135(3):805–826.

17. C Mycoplasma avium complex

The most common organism to be isolated from adults with bronchiectasis is *Haemophilus influenzae*. Other associated organisms include:

- *Pseudomonas aeruginosa*
- *Klebsiella*
- *Staphylococcus aureus*
- *Streptococcus pneumoniae*
- *Moraxella catarrhalis*
- *Aspergillus* species

Antibiotics, bronchodilators and chest physiotherapy remain the mainstay of treatment.

A sputum culture should be taken and empirical antibiotics started if no previous culture results are available. However, it is important in patients with bronchiectasis who have had multiple exacerbations (therefore use of antibiotics), that treatment is guided by sputum culture results. Antibiotic sensitivity (and resistance) varies between different pathogens and will therefore affect the response to treatment.

Duration of treatment is recommended as up to 14 days of oral antibiotics Intravenous antibiotics should be reserved for those who are unwell or who have failed to respond to oral treatment.

In addition, a significant number of patients may have chronic colonisation of *Staphylococcus aureus*. Persistent isolation of this pathogen (and/or *Pseudomonas aeruginosa*) should lead to the consideration of allergic bronchopulmonary aspergillosis (ABPA) or cystic fibrosis (in younger patients).

Pasteur MC, Bilton D, Hill AT. British Thoracic Society guideline for non-CF bronchiectasis. Thorax 2010; 65:i1–i58.

18. D Rheumatoid arthritis

This patient presents with a unilateral pleural effusion. **Figure 12.4** is a chest X-ray of a left-sided pleural effusion.

It is useful to determine whether this effusion is a transudate or exudate, which can be evaluated using Light's criteria. **Table 12.3** details the causes of each.

19. A Aspergillus precipitins serology

It is clearly not appropriate to observe and monitor this patient without further investigation into the cause of the abnormal radiological findings. Even if the images

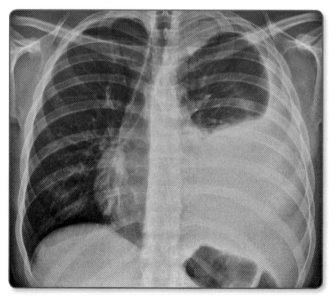

Figure 12.4 Chest X-ray of a left-sided pleural effusion.

Table 12.3

Transudate	Exudate
Common – 'CLAN'	*Common – 'PICC'*
Cirrhosis of liver	Pancreatitis
Left ventricular failure	Infection (bacterial, TB)
Acute glomerulonephritis	Cancer (primary or metastatic)
Nephrotic syndrome (other causes of hypoproteinaemia)	Connective tissue disorders (RA/SLE)
Uncommon – 'MEDS'	*Uncommon*
Myxoedema	Infection (fungal, viral)
Emboli (pulmonary)	Malignancy (haematological)
Dialysis	
Sarcoidosis	
RA, rheumatoid arthritis; SLE, systemic lupus erythematosus; TB, tuberculosis.	

Table 12.3 Causes of transudative and exudative pleural effusions.

are radiologically suggestive of an aspergilloma, it is important that malignancy and tuberculosis are excluded. A simple test would be to test serology for aspergillus precipitins along with sputum mycology and microscopy, cultures and sensitivities.

An aspergilloma is a clump of fungus, with *Aspergillus fumigatus* the most common species responsible. Aspergillus fungal spores are inhaled and thrive in the lung due to the moist environment. Aspergillomas may remain asymptomatic, but may lead to shortness of breath and haemoptyisis is people with underlying lung disease or additional co-morbidities.

Most cases of aspergillomas do not require treatment, but if significant haemoptysis occurs, then surgical resection or embolisation may be considered. Antifungals are ineffective.

Kousha M, Tadi R, Soubani AO. Pulmonary Aspergillosis: a clinical review. Eur Respir Rev 2011; 20(121):156–174.

20. A Main component is DPCC (diphosphatidylcholine)

Pulmonary surfactant is part of the innate immune host defence system. It is a lipoprotein that is produced and secreted by type II alveolar cells in the respiratory tract. It has two predominant roles. The first is to reduce the surface tension in the lung and also to act as a role in the defence against infection and inflammation by its ability to opsonise pathogens such as bacteria and viruses.

Pulmonary surfactant is composed of both hydrophilic and hydrophobic molecules. DPCC is a phospholipid and is a key molecule in pulmonary surfactant. Phosphatidylglycerol molecules form about 10% of the lipids in surfactant.

Wright JR. Pulmonary surfactant: first line of lung host defense. J Clin Invest 2003; 111(10):1453–1455.

21. E Serum trypsin inhibitor

Alpha 1 antitrypsin is a serum trypsin, or protease, inhibitor enzyme. The gene is located on chromosome 14. It protects tissues from neutrophil elastase. It is a single channel glycoprotein consisting of 394 amino acids and primarily produced in the liver.

Alpha 1 antitrypsin deficiency is characterised by early onset liver disease and lung disease. The most common abnormality is due to mutation of the SERPINA1 gene, giving rise to the Z allele, leading to a reduction in the serum levels of alpha one antitrypsin.

It is inherited in an autosomal recessive/co-dominant manner. Alleles are according to electrophoretic mobility as medium (M), slow (S) and very slow (Z) and Z types are due to single amino acid substitutions. The pathogenesis in emphysema is of increased cell turnover as a result of reduced pulmonary protection against protease breakdown.

The normal genotype is PiMM. Levels of alpha 1 antitrypsin are reduced by up to 60% in the PiSS, PiMZ and PiSZ. It is PiZZ where levels are less than 15 %, leading to early onset emphysema and liver cirrhosis.

Stoller JK, Aboussouan LS. Alpha1-antitrypsin deficiency. Lancet 2005; 365(9478):2225–2236.

22. B Isocyanates

This patient is most likely to have occupational asthma, as demonstrated by new onset symptoms at the start of a new job and resolution of these once away from work. Occupational asthma results in airway inflammation and bronchoconstriction secondary to hyper-responsiveness from a variety of allergens. Agents that are known to cause occupational asthma can be divided into high molecular weight (HMW) proteins that originate from vegetable and animal origins and low molecular weight (LMW) proteins.

Isocyanates are the most common causes of occupational asthma. They must be handled with caution. All work places and employers must adhere to the guidelines set out. It is important to demonstrate by peak flow measurements, changes at work and away from work. The diagnosis of occupational asthma is not only made on this basis, but in combination with other factors.

The alternative options may be responsible for occupational asthma, but occur less frequently. Flour can lead to occupational asthma in Baker's asthma. Additional investigations when suspicious of occupational asthma include formal pulmonary function tests, skin prick tests to common allergens, non-specific bronchial provocation tests and serum specific IgE levels.

Beach J, et al. A systematic review of the diagnosis of Occupational Asthma. Chest 2007; 131(2):569–578.

23. D Pulmonary hypertension (pulmonary arterial pressure [PAP] mean >35 mmg)

In patients who have had optimal medical treatment for chronic obstructive pulmonary disease, lung volume reduction surgery (LVRS) and lung transplantation, may be options for symptomatic relief. The aim of LVRS is to remove the least functional part of the lung, to improve airflow and gas exchange.

The National Emphysema Treatment Trial (NETT), a prospective, controlled multicentre study, randomised 1218 patients to either medical management or bilateral LRVS. The results confirmed that those selected for surgery, and in particular those with predominantly upper lobe disease, had a better outcome in terms of improved quality of life and functional status.

However, patients must be properly selected, due to the high-risk of morbidity and mortality with the procedure. Contraindications to the surgery are as follows:

- Lung function FEV1 < 20%
- DLCO (diffusion capacity of the lung for carbon monoxide) < 20%
- Smoker, or stopped smoking less than 4 months ago
- Angina, myocardial infarction within the last 6 months
- Pulmonary hypertension (PAP mean >35 mmg)

National Emphysema Treatment Trial Research Group. Patients at high risk of death after lung-volume-reduction surgery. N Engl J Med 2001; 345:1075–1083.

24. D FEV1 > 80% of predicted value and symptoms suggestive of chronic obstructive pulmonary disease (COPD)

All new patients suspected of COPD should undergo lung function testing with post bronchodilator spirometry to demonstrate obstructive airways disease. In addition, recommendations for baseline investigations include a plain chest radiograph, full blood count, and body mass index (BMI) calculation. Alternative diagnoses must be considered in those older patients where the FEV < 0.7, but with no symptoms suggestive of COPD and younger patients with COPD and with a FEV1 > 0.7. **Table 12.4** summarises three international guidelines on COPD, which all emphasise the importance of FEV1 percentages and post bronchodilator values, in the classification of COPD, rather than a single FEV1 measurement.

'Pack years' is a method of measuring how much an individual has smoked over a prolonged period of time. One pack year is the equivalent of smoking 20 cigarettes a day for one year. A way of calculating this is as follows:

$$\frac{\text{Number of cigarettes smoked per day} \times \text{number of years smoked}}{20}$$

American Thoracic Society/European Respiratory Society Task Force. Standards for the Diagnosis and Management of Patients with COPD [Internet]. Version 1.2. American Thoracic Society; 2004
NICE Guidelines. Chronic obstructive pulmonary disease: management of chronic obstructive pulmonary disease in adults in primary and secondary care. London: NICE; 2010

25. C Fibrosing alveolitis

Pulmonary eosinophilia details a group of conditions characterised by raised serum eosinophil levels and pulmonary infiltrates. **Figure 12.5** shows a typical chest X-ray of allergic bronchopulmonary aspergillosis (ABPA).

The following mnemonic categorises the different causes of pulmonary eosinophilia.

Table 12.4

FEV1 % predicted	Post broncho-dilator FEV1/FVC ratio	Severity		
		ATS/ERS (2004)	GOLD (2008)	NICE (2010)
		Post bronchodilator	Post bronchodilator	Post bronchodilator
>80%	>0.7	At risk*		
>80%	<0.7	Mild	Stage 1: Mild	Stage 1: Mild**
50–79%	<0.7	Moderate	Stage 2: Moderate	Stage 2: Moderate
30–49%	<0.7	Severe	Stage 3: Severe	Stage 3: Severe
<30%	<0.7	Very severe	Stage 4: Very severe***	Stage 4: Very severe***

*The 'at risk' group is described as patients (i) who smoke and have an exposure to pollutants, (ii) who have shortness of breath, cough or sputum production and (iii) family history of respiratory disease.
** Presence of symptoms is necessary for the diagnosis of mild COPD.
*** This classification may also be used for those patients who have a FEV1 < 50% with respiratory failure.

Table 12.4 Comparison of classification systems for chronic obstructive pulmonary disease (COPD).

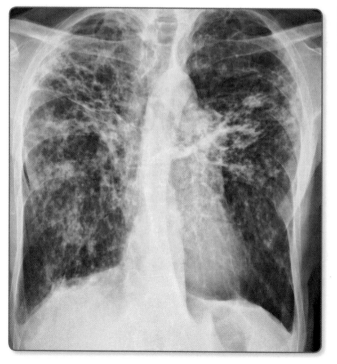

Figure 12.5 Allergic bronchopulmonary aspergillosis (ABPA).

Causes of pulmonary eosinophilia 'CHALETS'

Churg–Strauss syndrome
Hypereosinophilic syndrome
Allergic bronchopulmonary aspergillosis (ABPA)
Löffler's syndrome
Eosinophilic pneumonia (acute and chronic)
Tropical pulmonary eosinophilia
Sulphasalazine and other drugs (e.g. nitrofurantoin, phenytoin)

Hypereosinophilic syndrome is a persistent elevation of eosinophil for greater than 6 months (not explained by any other cause). Features include systemic symptoms such as fever, weight loss, in addition to lymphadenopathy and hepatomegaly. In approximately two-thirds of patients, there is also cardiac involvement as well as an increased risk of thromboembolism. Steroids are the mainstay of treatment.

Klion A. Hypereosinophilic syndrome: current approach to diagnosis and treatment. Ann Rev Med 2009; 60:293–306.

26. E Sweat test chloride of greater than 40 years is considered a positive result in adults

Cystic fibrosis (CF) follows an autosomal recessive pattern of inheritance. It affects males and females equally. In Caucasians, it affects approximately 1 in 2500 live births. The most common mutation is delta F508 gene of the CFTR (cystic fibrosis transmembrane conductor regulator) gene, but over 500 mutations have been identified. Diagnosis is made by detection of an abnormally high level of sweat chloride (>60 mmol/L) and also by genetic analysis.

The Liverpool epidemic strain (LES) is an aggressive form of *Pseudomonas aeruginosa*, which was discovered after recognising a drug resistant strain of *Pseudomonas aeruginosa* among cystic fibrosis patients. The LES strain is able to replace previous strain of *Pseudomonas* (superinfection) and can cause significant morbidity by affecting non-CF parents of CF patients.

Cystic fibrosis affects numerous systems and organs. It leads to pancreatic insufficiency in about 90% of patients resulting in the use of insulin. Distal intestinal obstruction syndrome (DIOS) is a common complication.

Cystic fibrosis related liver disease is now a recognised clinical problem and is a result of localised damage to intrahepatic bile ducts leading to portal tract fibrosis. The subtle early changes make the condition difficult to diagnosis until portal hypertension is well-established. Ursodeoxycholic acid is given to prevent the progression to significant cirrhosis. In those with portal hypertension, regular endoscopies are carried out to monitor oesophageal varices. Other complications of CF include arthritis, male infertility and vasculitis.

Rowland M, Charles GG, Ó'Laoide R. Outcome in cystic fibrosis liver disease. Am J Gastroenterol 2011; 106:104–109.

27. B Mycoplasma serology

The history of dry cough, pulmonary infiltrates and erythema multiforme is highly suggestive of *Mycoplasma pneumonia*. Mycoplasma serology is the diagnostic investigation of choice.

Complications of *Mycoplasma pneumonia* include haemolytic anaemia as a result of cold agglutinins. The following describes additional complications.

A useful mnemonic, **MAGPIES**, may be used for the complications of *Mycoplasma pneumonia*:

Meningoencephalitis
Autoimmune haemolytic anaemia
Guillain–Barré syndrome
Peri/Myocarditis, **p**eripheral neuropathies, (low) **p**latelets
Intravascular (disseminated intravascular coagulation),
Erythema multiforme, erythema nodosum
Stevens–Johnson syndrome

Waites KB, Talkington DF. *Mycoplasma pneumoniae* and its role as a human pathogen. J Clin Microbiol Rev 2004; 17(4):697–728.

28. B Aspiration of pneumothorax

This describes a primary presentation of pneumothorax, in an otherwise fit and well young patient. The current British Thoracic Society guidelines, published in 2010 recommend that patients with a pneumothorax measuring greater than 2 cm, with or without shortness of breath, should undergo aspiration using a 16–18 gauge cannula. If this results in the pneumothorax reducing to a size less than 2 cm and/or symptoms improve, then the patient can be discharged after observation for 2–4 hours. If the patient has an underlying lung condition, then this would warrant an insertion of a chest drain (secondary pneumothorax).

Figure 12.6 shows a left-sided pneumothorax measuring more than 4 cm and showing possibly early signs of tension. Tension pneumothoraces should be managed prior to a chest X-ray being performed, but this may not always occur clinically.

Macduff A, et al. Management of spontaneous pneumothorax. British Thoracic Society pleural disease guideline 2010. Thorax 2010; 65; ii18–ii31.

29. C Intravenous magnesium sulphate

There is a growing evidence base for the benefit of using intravenous magnesium sulphate as a bronchodilator in patients with severe acute asthma exacerbations that are slow to respond to conventional first-line therapies. Its mechanism of action remains poorly defined, but is thought to involve inhibition of calcium influx into airway smooth muscle cells. It has an excellent safety profile, but is contraindicated in renal failure. Hypermagnesemia is associated with muscle weakness and hypertension.

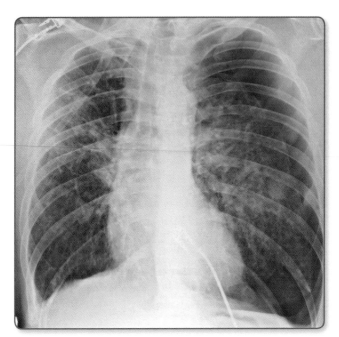

Figure 12.6 Left-sided pneumothorax.

Randomised controlled trials and meta-analyses have found conflicting evidence regarding the efficacy of inhaled corticosteroids in asthma exacerbations and most practitioners would not currently recommend their use, making option A incorrect. Pharmacokinetic research has demonstrated that oral prednisolone is rapidly absorbed (with peak plasma levels occurring approximately 1 hour after administration) and has almost complete bioavailability; trial data has confirmed that oral and intravenous corticosteroids are of similar efficacy in acute asthma (assuming that the patient is not vomiting), making option B incorrect. There is no strong evidence that any one nebulised short-acting β_2-agonist has better bronchodilator properties than any other, making option D incorrect. Montelukast (and other leukotriene receptor antagonists) are now well-established in the management of chronic asthma, but are not currently routinely used in the treatment of acute asthma, hence option E is incorrect.

Guidelines for the initial assessment and treatment and for ongoing management of those with acute asthma exacerbations have been published by professional bodies in the UK (British Thoracic Society/Scottish Intercollegiate Guidelines Network).

British Thoracic Society/SIGN Guidelines. British Guideline on the Management of Asthma. Scottish Intercollegiate Guidelines Network; 2011.

30. C Otitis media

Kartagener's syndrome, or primary ciliary dyskinesia, is an autosomal recessive disorder, characterised by the triad of bronchiectasis, situs inversus and chronic sinusitis. It is a rare condition, which is caused by a defect in cilia function resulting in impaired mucociliary clearance in the sinonasal and pulmonary passages, leading to the triad of features. Ciliary dysfunction also results in immotile sperm and otitis media.

Situs inversus is often diagnosed radiologically (see **Figure 12.7**) and the two features simplest to recognise on a chest X-ray is a right-sided cardiac apex and right-sided gastric air bubble. In addition, an ECG in such patients will be abnormal, revealing right axis deviation with negative P waves in leads I and aVL. There is usually no R wave progression in the chest leads and a dominant R wave in aVR.

Bronchiectasis is managed with physiotherapy, antibiotics (including pseudomonal coverage) and bronchodilators, along with supportive therapy. It is important to ensure that vaccinations are up to date.

Diagnosis of Kartagener's syndrome can be made through the assessment of cilia immotility, by evaluating cilia function, performing genetic studies or taking biopsies. A reduced nasal nitric oxide level is suggestive of this condition. In addition, bronchial or nasal (brush) biopsies are taken to calculate ciliary beat frequency as a screening tool and if this is reduced, then proceed to electron microscopy for diagnosis. Genetic testing for DNAI1 and DNAH5 can be carried out in specialist centres. If there is discrepancy in diagnosis in males, assessment of sperm motility is an option.

Pneumothoraces and pulmonary emboli may occur in these patients, but are not typical features of the condition.

Skeik N, Jabr FI. Kartagener syndrome. Int J Gen Med 2011; 4:41–43.
Al-Khadra AS. Mirror-Image Dextrocardia With Situs Inversus. Circulation 1995; 91:1602–1603.
Stannard WA, Chilvers MA, Rutman AR. Diagnostic testing of patients suspected of primary ciliary dyskinesia. Am J Respir Crit Care Med 2010; 181(4):307–314.

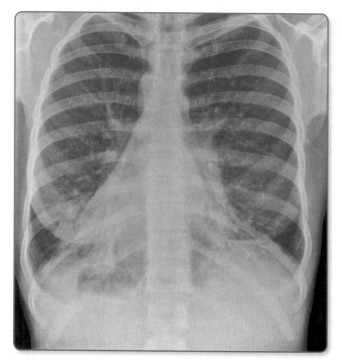

Figure 12.7 Chest X-ray showing situs inversus.

Chapter 13

Rheumatology

1. A 48-year-old woman presented with a 2-month history of lethargy, fatigue and pain affecting her knees, wrists and hands. She complained of early morning stiffness lasting for 2 hours. On examination, she had a temperature of 37.9°C. There was swelling of her right knee. On both hands there was swelling of her 2nd, 3rd and 4th metacarpophalangeal joints and a subcutaneous nodule on the extensor surface of the right elbow.

   Investigations:

haemoglobin	100 g/L (115–165)
mean cell volume	88.5 fL (80–96)
erythrocyte sedimentation rate	60 mm/1st hour (<20)
serum C-reactive protein	33 mg/L (<10)
serum creatine kinase	100 U/L (24–170)
rheumatoid factor	negative

   Which factor is most closely associated with a better prognosis?

   A Elevated C-reactive protein (CRP)
   B Elevated erythrocyte sedimentation rate (ESR)
   C Female sex
   D Negative rheumatoid factor
   E Presence of subcutaneous nodules

2. A 25-year-old woman with rheumatoid arthritis was planning to start a family with her husband.

   Which disease modifying anti-rheumatoid drug (DMARD) is contraindicated in pregnancy?

   A Azathioprine
   B Cyclophosphamide
   C Methotrexate
   D Prednisolone
   E Sulphasalazine

3. A 38-year-old woman was seen in the rheumatology clinic with pain in the small joints of both hands.

   Which blood test has the highest specificity as a marker for the diagnosis of rheumatoid arthritis?

   A Anti-cyclic citrullinated peptide (CCP) antibody
   B Anti-nuclear antibody (ANA)

C   Complement levels
D   C-reactive protein (CRP) and erythrocyte sedimentation rate (ESR)
E   Rheumatoid factor

4. A 70-year-old woman presented with a 3-month history of bilateral neck and
    shoulder pain. She described 2 kg weight loss over this time, early morning
    stiffness and increased lethargy. On examination, she had a temperature of 37.5°C.
    There was no wasting of her neck or shoulder muscles, but she had pain around
    the neck and shoulders on palpation, which was worse on shoulder abduction. She
    had a limited range of movement in her shoulders but no paresthesiae.

    Investigations:

haemoglobin	102 g/L (115–165)
mean cell volume	90.4 fL (80–96)
erythrocyte sedimentation rate	87 mm/1st hour (<20)
serum C-reactive protein	34 mg/L (<10)
rheumatoid factor	negative
anti-nuclear antibodies	negative

    What is the most likely diagnosis?

    A   Fibromyalgia
    B   Frozen shoulder
    C   Polymyalgia rheumatica
    D   Polymyositis
    E   Rheumatoid arthritis

5. A 40-year-old woman was referred to the rheumatology clinic with arthralgia and
    malaise. She also complained of dry mouth and gritty eyes.

    What is the most useful diagnostic investigation?

    A   Anti-double stranded DNA (dsDNA)
    B   Anti-nuclear antibody (ANA)
    C   Anti-Ro and anti-La
    D   Anti-topoisomerase I
    E   Rheumatoid factor

6. Which disease is not associated with rheumatoid factor?

    A   Hepatitis B
    B   Hepatitis C
    C   Sjögren's syndrome
    D   Systemic lupus erythematosus
    E   Systemic sclerosis

7. A 50-year-old woman was seen in the clinic with multiple episodes of bilateral
    ear pain and swelling over the last 2 years. She also described periodic episodes
    of joint pains mostly affecting her wrists and ankles. She was also being seen
    in ophthalmology clinic for recurrent episcleritis and scleritis. She only took

simple analgesia. On examination, she had bilateral auricular oedema and erythema but sparing the lobules and normal tympanic membranes. Weber's and Rinne's tests were normal. She had a saddle nose deformity and the bridge of her nose was tender to palpation. Examination of her joints revealed an asymmetric non-deforming arthropathy of her left elbow, left wrist and right ankle. Her chest was clear and heart sounds were normal with no added sounds.

Investigations:

haemoglobin	108 g/L (115–165)
mean cell volume	90 fL (80–96)
white cell count	6.5×10^9/L (4.0–11.0)
neutrophil count	3.3×10^9/L (2.5–7.0)
platelet count	250×10^9/L (150–400)
erythrocyte sedimentation rate	35 mm/1st hour (<20)
serum C-reactive protein	40 mg/L (<10)
anti-nuclear antibodies	positive
rheumatoid factor	negative

What is the most likely diagnosis?

A   Behçet's disease
B   Granulomatosis with polyangiitis (Wegener's)
C   Relapsing polychondritis
D   Rheumatoid arthritis
E   Systemic lupus erythematosus (SLE)

8. Which disease is least likely to be associated with human leucocyte antigen-B27 (HLA-B27)

A   Acute anterior uveitis
B   Ankylosing spondylitis
C   Enteropathic arthritis
D   Psoriasis
E   Reiter's syndrome

9. Which gene is most closely associated with Ehlers–Danlos syndrome?

A   ATP-binding cassette sub-family C member 6 (*ABCC6*)
B   Cartilage associated protein (*CRTAP*)
C   Collagen alpha-1 (V) chain (*COL5A1/COL5A2*)
D   Fibrillin-1 (*FBN1*)
E   Fibroblast growth factor receptor-3 (*FGFR3*)

10. Which drug is not a recognised cause of drug-induced lupus erythematosus?

A   Captopril
B   Hydralazine
C   Isoniazid
D   Simvastatin
E   Tacrolimus

11. Which feature is least likely to be associated with systemic lupus erythematosus (SLE)?

    A   Episcleritis
    B   Oral ulcers
    C   Pericarditis
    D   Seizures
    E   Thrombocytopenia

12. A 38-year-old woman presented to the clinic with painful discolouration of her fingers for the past 2 years. They changed colour from white to blue if she put her hands into cold water. She experienced dysphagia for solids and liquids for the past 6 months but had no associated weight loss. On examination, she had tight skin especially over her nose and fingers. There was also telangiectasia over her face.

What is the most appropriate next step in management?

    A   Atenolol
    B   Lisinopril
    C   Methotrexate
    D   Nifedipine
    E   Steroids

13. A 29-year-old-woman gave birth to her first child. She had a background of systemic lupus erythematosus (SLE). On examination by a paediatrician, the neonate was found to be bradycardic. Further investigations confirmed the diagnosis of neonatal congenital heart block.

Which autoantibodies are most likely to be detectable in this woman's serum?

    A   Anti-Jo-1 antibodies
    B   Anti-neutrophil cytoplasmic antibodies
    C   Anti-Ro (SSA) antibodies
    D   Anti-Sm antibodies
    E   Anti-U1 ribonucleoprotein (RNP) antibodies

14. A 71-year-old man presented with a 1-week history of worsening right sided headache and lethargy. He also noted pain on chewing and on combing his hair over the affected side. Over the past 24 hours, he had developed blurring of vision in his right eye. He had no other past medical history. On examination, it was difficult to palpate the right-sided temporal pulse.

Investigations:

    erythrocyte sedimentation rate   104 mm/1st hour (<20)

What is the most appropriate next step in management?

    A   Arrange for an urgent CT of the head
    B   Commence amitriptyline immediately

C Commence ibuprofen pending temporal artery biopsy
D Commence prednisolone immediately
E Review by an ophthalmologist

15. A 72-year-old woman presented with 6 months of progressive lethargy and generalised pain. She described the pain as an ache affecting all the muscles of her body. Her family described her mobility as worsening over this period, and said that she had become increasingly dependent on them for activities of daily living. She had no past medical history and took no regular medications. Examination revealed kyphosis and difficulty in standing up from sitting. Neurological examination was normal.

Investigations:

serum corrected calcium	2.1 mmol/L (2.2–2.6)
serum phosphate	0.6 mmol/L (0.8–1.4)
serum alkaline phosphatase	202 U/L (45–105)
serum gamma glutamyl transferase	42 U/L (4–35)
serum creatine kinase	140 U/L (24–170)
erythrocyte sedimentation rate	8 mm/1st hour (<30)

What is the most likely diagnosis?

A Fibromyalgia
B Osteomalacia
C Osteoporosis
D Paget's disease
E Polymyalgia rheumatica

16. A 42-year-old woman was referred to the rheumatology clinic because of a 1-year history of generalised muscle ache, paraesthesia in her hands and feet, and severe fatigue. Examination revealed tenderness on palpation over the occipital region, supraclavicular areas, and lower para-lumbar regions bilaterally. There was no evidence of rash, synovitis or deforming arthropathy, and neurological and gait examination were normal.

Investigations:

erythrocyte sedimentation rate	7 mm/1st hr (<20)
serum C-reactive protein	3 mg/L (<10)
serum creatine kinase	160 U/L (24–170)
plasma thyroid-stimulating hormone	1.0 mU/L (0.4–5.0)
plasma free T4	20 pmol/L (10–22)
serum 1,25-$(OH)_2$-cholecalciferol	50 pmol/L (43–149)
serum complement C3	72 mg/dL (65–190)
serum complement C4	22 mg/dL (15–50)
anti-nuclear antibodies	weakly positive (at 1:80 dilution)

What is the most likely diagnosis?

A   Ankylosing spondylitis
B   Fibromyalgia
C   Polymyositis
D   Sjögren's syndrome
E   Systemic lupus erythematosus

17. A 19-year-old man presented with recurrent arthralgia in the small joints of his hands. Examination of the hands revealed bilateral arachnodactyly and joint hyperextensibility. His arm span exceeded his height.

Which examination finding would suggest this man had homocystinuria rather than Marfan's syndrome?

A   Crowded teeth and high-arched palate
B   Downwards dislocation of the lens
C   Heterochromia of the irides
D   Pectus excavatum
E   Pes planus

18. A 25-year-old woman presented with a 4-week history of painful mouth ulcers. This was the third time this year that she had had this problem. On direct questioning, she also said that she had had similar ulcers on her vagina and these had resolved spontaneously. She had a previous medical history of recurrent anterior uveitis. She was originally from Lebanon but had recently settled in the UK. She was not on any medication and did not smoke or drink. On examination, she had aphthous ulcers on her buccal mucosa but nowhere else. Eye examination was normal.

What is the most likely diagnosis?

A   Behçet's disease
B   Crohn's disease
C   Familial mediterranean fever
D   Psoriatic arthropathy
E   Sarcoidosis

19. A 59-year-old woman presented with a 3-month history of weakness in her hips and a worsening rash. She had a background of non-small cell lung cancer, currently being treated with radiotherapy. She took no regular medications. Examination revealed proximal muscle weakness and tenderness, but no evidence of joint synovitis or deformity. There was no evidence of fatigability or other neurological deficit. Dermatological examination demonstrated a purple-coloured rash around the eyes, scaly plaques over the knuckles and elbows, and erythema over the upper chest.

Investigations:

serum creatine kinase   19,874U/L (24–170)

What is the most likely diagnosis?

A   Dermatomyositis
B   Inclusion body myositis
C   Lambert–Eaton syndrome
D   Psoriatic spondyloarthropathy
E   Systemic lupus erythematosus (SLE)

20. A 46-year-old woman presented with a three month history of generalised arthralgia, fatigue and rash. The woman had no past medical history and took no regular medications. She did not smoke or drink alcohol, but admitted to being a former intravenous drug user. She had palpable purpura on both legs, with examination of the hands demonstrating Raynaud's phenomenon but no evidence of joint synovitis or deforming arthropathy.

Investigations:

serum creatinine	220 mmol/L (140 mmol/L six months earlier) (60–110)
serum complement C3	96 mg/dL (65–190)
serum complement C4	3 mg/dL (15–50)
serum immunoglobulin G	9.6 g/L (6–13)
serum immunoglobulin A	2.4 g/L (0.8–3.0)
serum immunoglobulin M	6.3 g/L (0.4–2.5)
serum immunoglobulin E	40 kU/L (<120)
antineutrophil cytoplasmic antibodies	not detected
anti-nuclear antibodies	not detected
rheumatoid factor	724 kIU/L (<30)
hepatitis B surface antigen	negative
hepatitis B DNA	not detected
hepatitis C IgG	detected
HIV serology	negative
urine analysis	blood +2, protein +2

What is the most likely diagnosis?

A   Churg–Strauss syndrome
B   Cryoglobulinaemic vasculitis
C   Granulomatosis with polyangiitis (Wegener's)
D   Rheumatoid arthritis-associated vasculitis
E   Systemic lupus erythematosus (SLE)

21. A 55-year-old man underwent blood tests as a routine part of assessment for medical insurance. He felt well apart from some occasional lower back pain. His only past medical history of note was of gallstones. Examination was normal.

Investigations:

serum corrected calcium	2.4 mmol/L (2.2–2.6)
serum phosphate	1.2 mmol/L (0.8–1.4)

serum alkaline phosphatase	724 U/L (45–105)
serum gamma glutamyl transferase	49 U/L (4–35)
serum 1,25-$(OH)_2$-cholecalciferol	50 pmol/L (43–149)

What is the most appropriate next investigation?

A   Biliary tract ultrasound
B   Bone biopsy
C   Endoscopic retrograde cholangiopancreatography (ERCP)
D   Magnetic resonance imaging of the long bones
E   Pelvis X-ray

22. A 60-year-old man presented with a red, hot, swollen right knee which had prevented him from walking for the last 3 days.

Investigations:

| microscopy of joint aspiration | rhomboid-shaped crystals with positive birefringence under polarised light, no organisms seen on gram-staining |

Which underlying diagnosis is most strongly associated with this condition?

A   Chemotherapy
B   Chronic kidney disease
C   Haemochromatosis
D   Myeloproliferative disease
E   Thiazide diuretics

23. A 29-year-old man recently underwent investigation in the rheumatology clinic for recurrent lower back and heel pain. He was diagnosed with ankylosing spondylitis.

Which condition is this patient most at risk of developing?

A   Aortic stenosis
B   Basal pulmonary fibrosis
C   Blepharitis
D   Heart block
E   Minimal change nephropathy

24. A 62-year-old man attended the emergency department because of acute pain and weakness in his right heel. His only past medical history was a recent diagnosis of prostatitis, for which he had been taking a course of antibiotics for the past 10 days. There was no past history of musculoskeletal disease. Examination revealed swelling over the right heel and difficulty in plantar flexion at the ankle, consistent with Achilles tendon rupture.

Which antibiotic is this patient most likely to have been prescribed?

A   Amoxicillin
B   Cephalexin

    C   Ciprofloxacin
    D   Nitrofurantoin
    E   Trimethoprim

25. A 64-year-old woman sustained a Colles' fracture of the wrist. She had no past medical history and took no regular medications. After recovering, she underwent emission X-ray absorptiometry (DEXA):

Investigations:

	Lumbosacral spine	Hip
T-score	-1.2	-1.7
Z-score	-0.8	-1.4

What is the most likely diagnosis?

    A   Normal bone mineral density
    B   Osteoarthritis
    C   Osteopenia
    D   Osteopetrosis
    E   Osteoporosis

26. A 42-year-old man presented with 2 weeks of abdominal pain that occurred after meals. He also described a 2-month history of generalised myalgia, weight loss and rash, and had also recently noticed increased difficulty in walking. He was known to have chronic hepatitis B. Examination revealed generalised abdominal tenderness but no peritonism. There was a purpuric rash on the torso and limbs, and livedo reticularis was present on the shins. Neurological assessment demonstrated a peripheral neuropathy.

Investigations:

erythrocyte sedimentation rate	104 mm/1st hour (<15)
serum sodium	136 mmol/L (137–144)
serum potassium	4.8 mmol/L (3.5–4.9)
serum urea	9.2 mmol/L (2.5–7.0)
serum creatinine	184 mmol/L (96 mmol/L six months earlier) (60–110)
serum complement C3	68 mg/dL (65–190)
serum complement C4	22 mg/dL (15–50)
serum C-reactive protein	92 mg/L (<10)
antiglomerular basement membrane antibodies	negative
anti-neutrophil cytoplasmic antibodies	negative
anti-nuclear antibodies	negative
CT mesenteric angiogram	multiple microaneurysms within mesenteric arteries

What is the most likely diagnosis?

    A   Goodpasture's syndrome

B   Granulomatosis with polyangiitis (Wegener's)
C   Microscopic polyangiitis
D   Polyarteritis nodosa
E   Systemic lupus erythematosus (SLE)

27. A 38-year-old woman presented with a 5-day history of severe right-sided groin pain. The pain was present even at rest, but exacerbated by walking. She denied any trauma. She had a history of systemic lupus erythematosus (SLE), for which she had been taking prednisolone and hydroxychloroquine for 6 months. Examination of the hip revealed pain with movement in all directions, but no evidence of deformity. Both lower limbs were neurovascularly intact.

Investigations:

serum complement C3	84 mg/dL (65–190)
serum complement C4	24 mg/dL (15–50)
anti-double stranded DNA antibodies	52 U/mL (<73)
right hip X-ray	areas of bone lucency with surrounding sclerosis

What is the most likely diagnosis?

A   Arthritis secondary to lupus flare
B   Avascular necrosis of the hip
C   Meralgia paraesthetica
D   Osteoarthritis of the hip
E   Trochanteric bursitis

28. A 22-year-old man attended the genitourinary medicine clinic with 1 week of dysuria. He also described recent sore eyes and pain in both legs. His only past history was an episode of presumed gastroenteritis whilst abroad in Asia 3 weeks earlier, which had now resolved. He had not been sexually active for 4 months. On examination, there was balanitis and clear urethral discharge, but no evidence otherwise of skin or mucous membrane disease. Further examination confirmed bilateral knee arthritis and Achilles tendinitis, whilst ophthalmic assessment demonstrated bilateral conjunctival injection.

Investigations:

urethral swab	36 polymorphs/high power field, no organisms on microscopy, culture or polymerase chain reaction
urine analysis	no organisms detected on microscopy and culture
knee aspirate	inflammatory appearance to aspirate, but no evidence of crystals, and no organisms detected on microscopy and culture

What is the most likely diagnosis?

A   Ankylosing spondylitis
B   Behçet's disease
C   Coeliac disease
D   Disseminated gonococcal infection
E   Reactive arthritis

29. Which one of the following is the most consistently abnormal laboratory finding in adult onset Still's disease?

A   Eosinophilia
B   Hyperferritinaemia
C   Positive anti-nuclear antibodies
D   Positive rheumatoid factor
E   Raised alkaline phosphatase

30. A 68-year-old man presented with several months of worsening leg swelling. He had suffered from rheumatoid arthritis for the past 20 years, which had been difficult to control despite trying a number of disease-modifying and biologic agents. Examination revealed macroglossia, hepatomegaly and bilateral pitting leg oedema.

Investigations:

serum sodium	136 mmol/L (137–144)
serum potassium	4.8 mmol/L (3.5–4.9)
serum urea	7.4 mmol/L (2.5–7.0)
serum creatinine	168 mmol/L (60–110)
serum albumin	19 g/L (37–49)
urine dipstick	protein +3
abdominal ultrasound	smooth hepatomegaly with no focal lesions; unobstructed urinary tract; large, echogenic kidneys

What is the most appropriate next investigation?

A   Captopril renogram
B   CT kidney, ureter and bladder
C   Fat pad biopsy
D   Plasma alpha-fetoprotein
E   Plasma anti-cyclic citrullinated peptide

Answers

1. D Negative rheumatoid factor

The factors that predict poor prognosis in rheumatoid arthritis are summarised in **Figure 13.1**.

Bukhari M, et al. The performance of anti-cyclic citrullinated peptide antibodies in predicting the severity of radiologic damage in inflammatory polyarthritis: results from the Norfolk Arthritis Register. Arthritis Rheum 2007; 56(9):2929–2935.

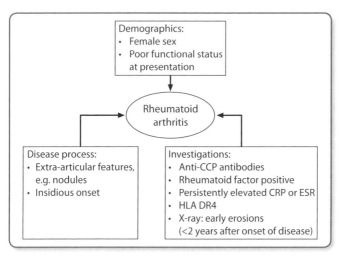

Figure 13.1 Factors that predict poor prognosis in rheumatoid arthritis. Anti-CCP, anti-cyclic citrullinated protein; CRP, C-reactive protein; ESR, erythrocyte sedimentation rate; HLA, human leucocyte antigen.

2. C Methotrexate

Prednisolone, despite having unwanted side effects like osteoporosis, diabetes mellitus and skin thinning, is the only drug not contraindicated in the control of rheumatoid arthritis compared to the other drugs. Azathioprine, cyclophosphamide and sulphasalazine are all relatively contraindicated and methotrexate is absolutely contraindicated. **Table 13.1** shows the side effects of the various disease modifying anti-rheumatoid drugs (DMARDs).

Chambers CD, et al. Human pregnancy safety for agents used to treat rheumatoid arthritis: adequacy of available information and strategies for developing post-marketing data. Arthritis Res Ther 2006; 8(4):215.

3. A Anti-cyclic citrullinated peptide (CCP) antibody

Both anti-CCP antibody and rheumatoid factor have been shown to be useful markers in the diagnosis of rheumatoid arthritis. Anti-CCP antibody has a sensitivity similar to rheumatoid factor (70–80%) with a much higher specificity of 90–95%. A meta-analysis of the diagnostic accuracy of anti-CCP antibody and

Table 13.1

Drug	Side effect
Azathioprine	May irreversibly affect male fertility by lowering sperm count
Cyclophosphamide	May irreversibly affect male fertility by lowering sperm count
Leflunomide	Contraindicated in pregnancy and whilst attempting conception because of risk of birth defects
Methotrexate	Contraindicated in pregnancy and whilst attempting conception because of risk of birth defects
Sulphasalazine	Transient aspermia

Table 13.1 Side effects of disease modifying anti-rheumatoid drugs.

rheumatoid factor for rheumatoid arthritis concluded that the former is more specific for the disease and may better predict erosive disease. It is especially useful in making a diagnosis of rheumatoid arthritis in rheumatoid factor negative patients.

Bas S, et al. Anti-cyclic citrullinated peptide antibodies, IgM and IgA rheumatoid factors in the diagnosis and prognosis of rheumatoid arthritis. Rheumatology 2003; 42(5):677.
Nishimura K, et al. Meta-analysis: diagnostic accuracy of anti-cyclic citrullinated peptide antibody and rheumatoid factor for rheumatoid arthritis. Ann Intern Med 2007; 146(11):797.

4. C Polymyalgia rheumatica

This patient has proximal muscle stiffness and tenderness so options C and D are the most likely. Fibromyalgia presents with a more widespread picture of muscular pain. **Table 13.2** shows the differences between polymyositis and polymyalgia rheumatica (PMR).

Miller M. Clinical manifestations and diagnosis of adult dermatomyositis and polymyositis. In: Basow DS (ed), UpToDate. Waltham, MA: UpToDate, 2010. http://www.uptodate.com (Last accessed 1 May 2012).

5. C Anti-Ro and anti-La

This patient's combination of xerostomia and xerophthalmia suggests Sjögren's syndrome, which is characterised by lymphocytic infiltration of the lacrimal and salivary glands causing reduced secretions. Anti-Ro and anti-La are present in primary Sjögren's syndrome; also rheumatoid factor and anti-nuclear antibodies are frequently present. Treatment involves the use of artificial tears to prevent corneal ulceration, artificial saliva and non-steroidal anti-inflammatory drugs (NSAIDs) for arthritis.

Kassan SS, Moutsopoulos HM. Clinical manifestations and early diagnosis of Sjögren syndrome. Arch Intern Med 2004; 164(12):1275.

Table 13.2

	Polymyositis	PMR
Muscle tender	Common	Common
Muscle wasting	Common	May occur
Proximal muscle weakness	Present	Absent
Headaches	Absent	May occur
Skin involvement	Present (30%)	Absent
Raised creatine kinase	Present	Absent
Anti-nuclear antibodies	Present (30%)	Absent
Rheumatoid factor	Present	Absent
Anti-Jo1 antibody	Present (20%)	Absent

Table 13.2 Differences between polymyositis and polymyalgia rheumatica (PMR).

6. A Hepatitis B

Rheumatoid factor is an IgM antibody that recognises the Fc portion of the IgG molecule to form complexes that contribute to the disease process in rheumatoid arthritis. 70% of people with rheumatoid arthritis are positive at disease onset. It is associated with more severe disease, e.g. joint destruction but, interestingly, does not correlate with disease activity. However, rheumatoid factor may be useful in patients on infliximab and etanercept because levels are reduced by these agents, thus reflecting reduced clinical disease activity. There are a number of diseases associated with positive rheumatoid factor:

- Sjögren's syndrome   70%
- Hepatitis C   40%
- Systemic sclerosis   30%
- Systemic lupus   20%
  erythematosus

Figure 13.2 illustrates how rheumatoid factor recognises the Fc portion of the IgG molecule.

Chen HA, et al. The effect of etanercept on anti-cyclic citrullinated peptide antibodies and rheumatoid factor in patients with rheumatoid arthritis. Ann Rheum Dis 2006; 65(1):35–39.

7. C Relapsing polychondritis

Relapsing polychrondritis (RP) is the only option that encompasses the combination of auricular chondritis, ocular inflammation, polyarthritis and nasal chondritis. Relapsing polychondritis is an episodic and progressive inflammatory condition involving cartilaginous structures, especially of the ears, nose and

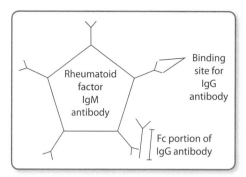

Figure 13.2 Rheumatoid factor binding to Fc portion of IgG antibody.

laryngotracheobronchial tree. Patients can present with a vast array of symptoms and see lots of different doctors in various clinics, and the episodic nature means that there is often a delay in diagnosis. The diagnostic criteria for RP include having three of the six listed clinical features:

- Bilateral auricular chondritis
- Non-erosive seronegative inflammatory polyarthritis
- Nasal chondritis
- Ocular inflammation
- Respiratory tract chondritis
- Audiovestibular damage

McAdam LP, et al. Relapsing polychondritis: prospective study of 23 patients and a review of the literature. Medicine 1976; 55:193.

Michet C. Diagnostic evaluation of relapsing polychondritis. In: Basow DS (ed), UpToDate. Waltham, MA: UpToDate. 2011. http://www.uptodate.com (Last accessed 1 May 2012).

8. D Psoriasis

Table 13.3 summarises the diseases associated with the various human leucocyte antigen (HLA) complexes.

Schur P, Thomson W. Human leukocyte antigens (HLA): a roadmap. In: Basow DS (ed), UpToDate. Waltham, MA: UpToDate, 2011. http://www.uptodate.com (Last accessed 1 May 2012).

9. C Collagen alpha-1 (V) chain (COL5A1 / COL5A2)

Ehlers–Danlos syndrome is a group of inherited connective tissue disorders caused by defects in collagen that share the common features of easy bruising, joint hypermobility and skin hyperelasticity/laxity. Treatment is supportive through physiotherapy, occupational therapy and monitoring of the cardiovascular system (to look for valvular heart disease, especially mitral valve prolapse).

Table 13.4 shows the disease associations of the genes.

Wenstrup RJ, et al. COL5A1 haploinsufficiency is a common molecular mechanism underlying the classical form of EDS. Am J Hum Genet 2000; 66(6):1766–1776.

Table 13.3

HLA	Disease associations
A3	Haemochromatosis
B5	Behçet's disease
B8	• Coeliac disease • SLE
B12	Behçet's disease with recurrent oral ulcers
B27	• Acute anterior uveitis • Seronegative spondyloarthropathies (can be remembered by the mnemonic **PEAR**): – **P**soriatic arthritis – **E**nteropathic arthritis – **A**nkylosing spondylitis – **R**eactive arthritis • Whipple's disease
Cw6	Psoriasis
DR2	• Goodpasture's disease • MS • Narcolepsy • SLE
DR3	• Coeliac disease • Dermatitis herpetiformis • PBC • Sjögren's syndrome • SLE
DR4	• Rheumatoid arthritis • Type I DM

DM, diabetes mellitus; MS, multiple sclerosis; PBC, primary biliary cirrhosis; SLE, systemic lupus erythematosus.

Table 13.3 Human leucocyte antigen (HLA) types and their disease associations.

Table 13.4

Gene	Disease association
ABCC6	Pseudoxanthoma elasticum
CRTAP	Osteogenesis imperfecta
COL5A1/COL5A2	Ehlers–Danlos syndrome (classical type)
FBN1	Marfan's syndrome
FGFR3	Achondroplasia

Table 13.4 Disease associations of various genes.

10. E Tacrolimus

A useful mnemonic to remember the causes of drug-induced lupus is **SCAMPIS**:

- **S**ulphasalazine
- **C**aptopril/**C**hlorpromazine
- **A**ntiepileptic – phenytoin
- **M**inocycline
- **P**rocainamide
- **I**soniazid
- **S**tatins

Schur P, Burton R. Drug-induced lupus. In: Basow DS (ed), UpToDate. Waltham, MA: UpToDate, 2011. http://www.uptodate.com (Last accessed 1 May 2012).

11. A Episcleritis

The American College of Rheumatology established 11 criteria for systemic lupus erythematosus (SLE) in 1982, which were revised in 1997 as a classificatory tool to standardise the definition of SLE in clinical trials. For the purpose of trials, a person has SLE if he/she has at least 4 out of 11 criteria. These features can be remembered by the mnemonic **DOPAMIN RASH**:

Discoid rash
Oral ulcers
Photosensitivity
Arthritis
Malar rash

Immunological disorder – anti-ds (double-stranded) DNA antibodies, anti-smith antibodies

Neurological disease – seizures or psychosis

Renal disease

ANA positive

Serositis – pleuritis, pericarditis

Haematological abnormalities – anaemia, thrombocytopenia

SLE patients can get keratoconjunctivitis but rarely episcleritis, which is more common in rheumatoid arthritis .

Hochberg MC. Updating the American College of Rheumatology revised criteria for the classification of systemic lupus erythematosus. Arthritis Rheum 1997; 40(9):1725.

12. D Nifedipine

This lady most likely has limited cutaneous systemic sclerosis (formerly known as CREST syndrome), which is characterised by:

- **C**alcinosis
- **R**aynaud's phenomenon
- o**E**sophageal disorders

- Sclerodactyly
- Telangiectasia

This patient's main problem is Raynaud's phenomenon due to vasospasm. The initial treatment would be to keep warm and wear gloves. Drug treatment would be calcium channel blockers such as nifedipine or diltiazem. If these drugs are not tolerated then angiotensin II receptor blockers such as losartan or angiotensin-converting enzyme (ACE) inhibitors could be used. Failing that, intravenous vasodilators like prostacyclin analogues, e.g. iloprost, can be tried. In severe cases, sympathectomy can be an option. Beta-blockers should be avoided as they can make the symptoms worse. Incidentally, calcium channel blockers could help with dysmotility syndrome which might be the cause of her dysphagia.

Thompson AE, et al. Calcium-channel blockers for Raynaud's phenomenon in systemic sclerosis. Arthritis Rheum 2001; 44(8):1841.

13. C Anti-Ro (SSA) antibodies

Anti-Ro (SSA) antibodies are detectable in the serum of up to 60% of patients with systemic lupus erythematosus (SLE) and up to 90% of those with Sjögren's syndrome. In pregnant women with SLE who have detectable anti-Ro antibodies, up to 25% of neonates will have transient cutaneous lupus, and approximately 2% will have congenital heart block. The presumed mechanism is that the anti-Ro antibody crosses the placenta and binds to the atrioventricular (AV) node, generating an immune response and localised injury as it does so. There is also evidence for an association between anti-La (SSB) antibodies and neonatal heart block, but it remains unclear as to whether this is related to the fact that anti-La is found only very rarely without anti-Ro also being present, or via a direct mechanism.

Anti-nuclear cytoplasmic antibody (ANCA), anti-Sm antibody and anti-U1 ribonucleoprotein (RNP) are detectable in the serum of less than 40% of patients with SLE, with none of them having any relationship to neonatal congenital heart block. Anti-U1 RNP is of more use in helping to diagnose mixed connective tissue diseases. Anti-Jo-1 is not present in the serum in patients with SLE, but is useful in diagnosing polymyositis and dermatomyositis.

Brucato A, et al. Pregnancy outcomes in patients with autoimmune diseases and anti-Ro/SSA antibodies. Clin Rev Allergy 2011; 40(1):27–41.

14. D Commence prednisolone immediately

The scenario is highly suggestive of temporal arteritis/giant cell arteritis (GCA). The 'gold standard' for making the diagnosis of GCA is through temporal artery biopsy; however, obtaining a biopsy should not delay treatment, and international guidelines advise clinicians with a strong suspicion of the diagnosis to commence corticosteroid treatment immediately (see references). There are a number of justifications for this:

- Temporal artery biopsy is not a test with a very high sensitivity. A number of explanations are given for this, not least the fact that GCA manifests as 'skip lesions' (i.e. affects 'patchy' areas of the artery). It is estimated that up to 9% of temporal artery biopsies give 'false negative' results.

- Visual loss in one eye is found in up to 20% of patients with GCA at the time of diagnosis, with anterior ischaemic optic neuropathy being the most common reason. Such visual loss is usually minimally reversible, but rapid treatment with high-dose glucocorticoid therapy may help to induce remission of the vasculitis, and therefore prevent further loss of acuity or extension of the vasculitis into the other eye.

Given that a temporal artery biopsy may take some time to arrange, it seems prudent to commence corticosteroids immediately in a scenario such as this.

Ezeonyeji AN, Borg FA, Dasgupta B. Delays in recognition and management in giant cell arteritis: results from a retrospective audit. Clin Rheumatol 2011; 30(2):259–262.
Mukhtyar C, et al for the European Vasculitis Study Group. EULAR recommendations for the management of large vessel vasculitis. Ann Rheum Dis 2009; 68:318–323.

15. B Osteomalacia

Osteomalacia arises through the defective mineralisation of bone with calcium and phosphate. Any condition causing either a deficiency in calcium and phosphate intake/metabolism or excessive loss may cause osteomalacia, but the majority of cases relate to defective vitamin D metabolism (**Figure 13.3**), including:

- Reduced vitamin D production, e.g. through inadequate sunlight exposure, poor diet, or malabsorptive disease.
- Failure of metabolism of vitamin D from inactive to active forms, i.e. lack of 1-α-hydroxylase activity in chronic kidney disease.

Immigrants to Western countries from from sunnier climates (such as Africa and Asia) are particularly at risk of osteomalacia for several reasons, including impaired vitamin D production (secondary to a lack of sunlight exposure), and through the dietary consumption of phytates (which impair calcium absorption).

The clinical presentation is typically of vague generalised pain. Examination may reveal kyphosis. This patient's difficult in standing up from sitting down is suggestive of proximal myopathy, another characteristic clinical finding. Patients may also first present with fractures.

Although bone biopsy is the diagnostic gold standard, osteomalacia is usually diagnosed from characteristic radiological and biochemical features:

- Radiologically – the characteristic radiological findings are called Looser's zones (also known as 'pseudofractures'). These are narrow radiolucent lines with sclerotic borders, most characteristically found in the neck of femur and pelvis. They represent previous stress fractures which have been repaired with poorly-mineralised osteoid.
- Biochemically – serum calcium and phosphate are low or low-normal, whilst alkaline phosphatase (ALP) tends to be raised, reflecting the secondary hyperparathyroidism that occurs in response to calcium deficiency. Serum vitamin D concentration may also be measured.

Treatment is of the underlying cause (e.g. vitamin D supplementation), and with supplementation of calcium and phosphate.

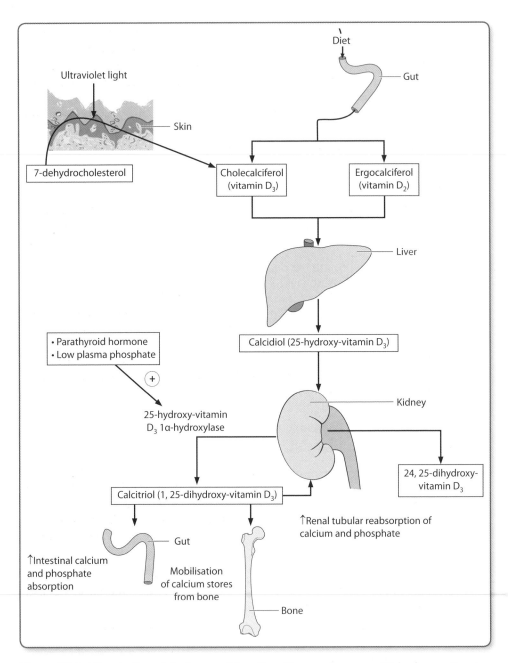

Figure 13.3 Vitamin D metabolism and function. The renal enzyme 25-hydroxy-vitamin D31α-hydroxylase converts calcidiol into calcitriol, the activated form of vitamin D3; in its absence, calcidiol is metabolised to the relatively inactive 24, 25-dihydroxyvitamin D3. 1α-hydroxylase activity is reduced in chronic kidney disease and when phosphate levels are high, but is increased by parathyroid hormone.

Fibromyalgia and osteoarthritis are both possible with this history, but neither is associated with proximal myopathy or changes in bone biochemistry. Polymyalgia rheumatica may present with proximal myopathy and raised ALP, but the normal erythrocyte sedimentation rate makes this unlikely. Paget's disease is also associated with a raised ALP, but this is normally much higher than the level here (usually several times greater than the upper limit of normal), and is not typically associated with reduced serum calcium or phosphate.

Gifre L, et al. Osteomalacia revisted. Clin Rheumatol 2011; 30(5):639–645.

16. B Fibromyalgia

Fibromyalgia should be considered early in the differential diagnosis of any patient with chronic widespread muscular pain and fatigue without another obvious explanation, but should only be made as a 'diagnosis of exclusion' because of a wide range of mimics for these symptoms.

Fibromyalgia can resemble rheumatological disorders, and the weakly positive anti-nuclear antibody (ANA) may initially make the candidate think of option D or E; however, up to 5% of the healthy population may have ANA detectable at these weak titres. Similarly, normal inflammatory markers and the absence of features of sacroiliitis, peripheral arthritis or enthesitis make ankylosing spondylitis unlikely. The normal creatine kinase excludes myositis, whilst the normal vitamin D level and thyroid function tests help to exclude metabolic conditions that can present with similar symptoms (i.e. osteomalacia, hypothyroidism).

Goldenberg DL. Diagnosis and differential diagnosis of fibromyalgia. Am J Med 2009; 122 (12):S14–S21.

17. B Downwards dislocation of the lens

There are a wide variety of clinical features that may be found in a patient with Marfan syndrome. Homocystinuria is one of the key differential diagnoses for Marfan syndrome because of their overlapping clinical features. **Table 13.5** illustrates the major features of the two diseases. The different pattern of lens dislocation in Marfan syndrome and homocystinuria is one of the key means by which the two diseases may be differentiated.

The most widely used diagnostic criteria for Marfan syndrome are the Ghent criteria. These use a combination of clinical and genetic factors to assess the likelihood of the patient having Marfan syndrome.

Loeys BL, et al. The revised Ghent nosology for the Marfan syndrome. J Med Genet 2010; 47:476–485.

18. A Behçet's disease

Behçet's disease is a vasculitis of uncertain aetiology. It is most commonly found in those from the 'sillk route', i.e. a region starting at countries in the Eastern Mediterranean, passing through Turkey, and extending as far east as Japan. There is a wide variety of associated clinical findings, but the most common clinical feature is recurrent painful oral ulceration. An added difficulty in making the diagnosis is the

Table 13.5

		Marfan's syndrome	Homocystinuria
Pathogenesis/diagnosis		• Usually autosomal dominant, with mutations principally in the fibrillin-1 gene. ~25% of mutations are de novo • Diagnosis made by genetic analysis in affected families, otherwise via diagnostic criteria	• Autosomal recessive disease caused through deficiency of cystathionine β-synthase • Usually diagnosed through blood/urine assays in neonatal screening
Organs affected	Cardiac	• Dilatation of the ascending aorta, with risk of aortic regurgitation or aortic dissection • Mitral valve prolapse or regurgitation	No structural involvement of heart itself, but association with: • Recurrent thrombosis • Accelerated atherosclerosis
	Ocular	• Ectopia lentis – usually *upwards* and *outwards* lens dislocation • Heterochromia of the irides and blue sclera • Retinal detachment	• Ectopia lentis – usually *downwards* dislocation of the lens
	Skeletal	• Crowded teeth and high-arched palate • Arm span exceeding height • Arachnodactyly of digits/hyperextensibility of joints • Pectus excavatum or carinatum • Pes planus	• Similar skeletal features to Marfan's syndrome • Propensity to generalised osteoporosis
	Other	• Dural ectasia (i.e. enlargement of the neural canal) • Normal intellect	• Intellectual disability • Skin changes, e.g. livedo reticularis
Treatment		No specific treatment; focus on management of individual organ disease, i.e. • Regular echocardiograms for monitoring of aortic valve disease, with aortic root/valve replacement if progressive disease • Regular ophthalmological follow-up	No specific treatment, but up to 50% show an improvement of symptoms with pyridoxine supplementation

Table 13.5 Similarities and differences between Marfan's syndrome and homocystinuria.

lack of a specific diagnostic test – elevated inflammatory markers are normally the only supportive laboratory finding. A number of different diagnostic criteria have been suggested, with the most commonly used one being from the International Study Group for Behçet's disease:

- **Must have** recurrent oral ulceration at least three times within the past 12 months without any other explanation.
- **Plus at least two of the following:**
  - Recurrent genital ulceration.
  - Eye lesions, e.g. anterior or posterior uveitis, retinal vasculitis.
  - Skin lesions, e.g. erythema nodosum, papulopustular lesions, acneiform nodules.
  - Positive pathergy test, i.e. hyper-reactivity and sterile pustule formation at the site of minor trauma.

Other possible clinical features may be neurological (e.g. sterile meningo-encephalitis, brain stem syndromes), gastrointestinal (e.g. colonic ulceration) or vascular (e.g. migratory thrombophlebitis).

Crohn's disease may be associated with recurrent mouth ulceration indistinguishable from Behçet's and eye disease, but the lack of gastrointestinal features in this patient makes this diagnosis unlikely. Sarcoidosis and psoriatic arthropathy can both present as multi-systemic disorders, but neither have any strong association with either mouth ulcers or pathergy. This patient has the right demographic details for familial Mediterranean fever but none of the characteristic clinical findings, such as acute abdominal pain, fever, arthralgia or serositis.

International Study Group for Behçet's disease. Criteria for diagnosis of Behçet's disease. Lancet 1990; 335 (8697):1078–1080.

19. A Dermatomyositis

Inclusion body myositis affects distal rather than proximal muscles. Lambert–Eaton syndrome is an autoimmune condition associated with lung cancer that is characterised by fatigability; however, the condition is primarily a disease of nerve rather than muscle, and cannot explain the presence of myositis (as implied by the elevated creatine kinase [CK] level). Both psoriasis and systemic lupus erythematosus (SLE) may cause both skin and musculoskeletal disease, but neither could account for the periorbital rash or degree of proximal myositis found here.

The description given is characteristic of dermatomyositis. This is a rare autoimmune condition with a strong association with a number of malignancies as well as certain medications (e.g. penicillamine). As well as proximal myopathy, patients may display a wide range of skin features, including:

- Heliotrope rash – a purple-coloured rash found in both periorbital regions, often accompanied by periorbital oedema
- Gottron's papules – these are scaly plaques found over the extensor surfaces, especially the metacarpophalangeal joints and elbows
- Shawl sign – the presence of erythema in a photosensitive, V-shaped distribution over the anterior neck and upper torso

- Nail changes – in particular, periungual telangiectasia (i.e. dilated nail-fold capillaries)

Certain patients develop pulmonary involvement, caused through intercostal/diaphragmatic muscle weakness and/or an autoimmune interstitial lung disease.

Anti-synthetase antibody (anti-Jo-1) may be detected in those who develop interstitial lung disease but not in other affected patients. A number of different antibodies to extractable nuclear antigens may also be detected in certain patients, including anti-U1 ribonucleoprotein and anti-PM-Scl. CK may be measured serially during treatment, with reducing levels indicative of the success of therapy. However, the key investigation for confirming the diagnosis is muscle biopsy. Electromyography and skin biopsy may also be useful.

The mainstay of treatment is corticosteroid therapy, which normally induces a swift remission. Other immunomodulatory agents – including methotrexate, azathioprine and ciclosporin – may be required as additional therapies.

Note that polymyositis is the same as dermatomyositis aside from the skin manifestations.

Dalakas MC, Hohlfeld R. Polymyostitis and dermatomyositis. Lancet 2003; 362 (9388):971–982.

20. B Cryoglobulinaemic vasculitis

The clinical findings and abnormal blood tests suggest a multi-system disease with an autoimmune basis, such as a primary rheumatological disease or a systemic vasculitis. The strongly positive rheumatoid factor may initially suggest option D; however, rheumatoid vasculitis almost always occurs in the context of long-standing, severe rheumatoid arthritis, which is not the case here. Serum anti-nuclear antibody (ANA) is detected in the vast majority of patients with systemic lupus erythematosus (SLE), and is absent here, excluding option E. Options A and C may both present with an acute vasculitic illness; however, no description is given of the other features often associated with these diseases, e.g. asthmatic symptoms in Churg–Strauss disease, or upper airway disease in granulomatosis with polyangiitis (Wegener's). In addition, the reduced complement levels and absence of detectable anti-neutrophil cytoplasmic antibodies (ANCA) are also inconsistent with these diagnoses.

The correct answer is B. Cryoglobulins are immunoglobulins present within the circulation that precipitate in the cold and can produce vasculitis. There is a very strong association between cryoglobulinaemic vasculitis and hepatitis C; this patient's serology confirms that she is infected with hepatitis C, which she may have contracted through her former intravenous drug use. Other associated disorders include rheumatological diseases (e.g. Sjögren's syndrome, rheumatoid arthritis) and certain malignant haematological conditions (including lymphoproliferative disorders and paraproteinaemias).

Cryoglobulinaemic vasculitis presents classically with a triad of arthralgia, cutaneous vasculitis and glomerulonephritis. There may be any of a number of additional features which reflect associated microvascular disease (e.g. Raynaud's phenomenon, mononeuritis multiplex). The disease is immunologically complex, with the form occurring secondary to hepatitis C associated with the production of a monoclonal IgM rheumatoid factor and consumption of the C4 complement component. The key diagnostic test is detection of serum cryoglobulins – this is a technically difficult laboratory assay, as it relies on a blood sample being transferred immediately from the patient to the laboratory whilst being kept at body temperature throughout to prevent premature immunoglobulin precipitation. Treatment depends upon the underlying aetiology, but includes the use of interferon-alpha and immunosuppressive therapies (e.g. cyclophosphamide).

Ferri C, Mascia MT. Cryoglobulinaemic vasculitis. Curr Opin Rheumatol 2006; 18(1):54–63.

21. E Pelvis X-ray

This man most likely has Paget's disease. This is a disorder characterised by focal excessive bone remodelling, resulting in deformed bones with a high propensity to fracture. Although patients tend to first present with symptoms resulting from bone disease, many patients with the condition are in fact asymptomatic, and diagnosed incidentally via abnormal blood tests or radiographs performed for other reasons. Characteristic clinical features include:

- Bone disease – includes bone pain, deformity (e.g. tibial bowing), or with pathological fractures. Paget's most often affects the axial skeleton, with the pelvis, long bones, lumbar spine and skull being the sites usually affected.
- Neurological disease – this may reflect either bony compression of cranial nerves (e.g. deafness through vestibular nerve involvement) or the spinal cord (e.g. paraparesis resulting from vertebral disease).
- Cardiac failure – high output cardiac failure may development secondary to the increased cardiac output required to support deformed, thickened bones.
- Osteosarcoma – this occurs in rare cases.

This man has the typical biochemistry of Paget's disease, i.e. normal serum calcium and phosphate levels, accompanied by a very elevated alkaline phosphatase (ALP) level, reflecting excessive osteoblastic activity. Although osteomalacia is also a cause of a raised ALP, it is usually not elevated to the extent seen here, and also tends to be associated with reduced plasma calcium and phosphate levels. In addition, the normal vitamin D level also makes osteomalacia unlikely. The presence of a normal gamma-glutamyl transpeptidase (GGT) makes it unlikely that the elevated ALP reflects hepatic cholestasis, meaning that there is no indication for biliary ultrasound or endoscopic retrograde cholangiopancreatography (ERCP).

Paget's disease may be first suggested through characteristic changes on plain radiograph, namely bone expansion with alternating areas of osteosclerosis and bone thinning. MRI of bone is not helpful in making the diagnosis, and bone biopsy is an invasive test that is usually only indicated if there is diagnostic uncertainty. This man's lower back pain may suggest pagetic involvement of the lower vertebrae or pelvis, and a simple radiograph of the pelvis would be the most appropriate next investigation here. If Paget's disease was suspected from the radiograph but confirmation was needed, the appropriate next test would be a radionuclide bone scan. Bone scans are very sensitive for pagetic lesions, showing these areas as 'hot spots'. Such scans are also useful for differentiating pagetic lesions from those of metastatic malignant disease.

Whyte MP. Paget's disease of bone. N Eng J Med 2006; 355:593–600.

22. C Haemochromatosis

Acute gout and pseudogout have different risk factors, reflecting their different aetiologies. These are summarised – along with other distinguishing features in **Table 13.6**.

This patient's presentation and joint aspiration results confirm that he has pseudogout. Haemochromatosis has a well-described association with pseudogout but – in contrast to the other options given – is not a risk factor for gout.

Lillicrap M. Crystal arthritis: contemporary approaches to diseases of antiquity. Clin Med 2007; 7(1):60–64.

23. D Heart block

Ankylosing spondylitis (AS) is a seronegative disease that classically first presents in individuals less than 30 years of age as inflammatory back pain for at least three months focused on the sacroiliac region. It is one of the group of seronegative spondyloarthropathies, other causes of which are psoriatic arthropathy, reactive arthritis and enteropathic arthritis. There is no single investigation which confirms the presence of AS, although magnetic resonance imaging is particularly useful for helping to detect sacroiliitis.

Symptomatic sacroiliitis is the most common clinical manifestation of AS, although there are also a wide variety of extra-articular manifestations that may be found. These may be remembered as the **nine A s**, i.e.:

- **A**rthritis – peripheral arthritis affects approximately 15% of patients
- **A**ortic regurgitation
- **A**trio-ventricular conduction defects – often high level heart block
- **A**pical pulmonary fibrosis – reflecting costovertebral rigidity
- **A**nterior uveitis – affecting up to 40% of patients
- **A**chilles tendonitis – plus other forms of enthesitis, such as plantar fasciitis
- **A**tlanto-axial subluxation
- Ig**A** nephropathy
- **A**myloidosis – as a consequence of chronic inflammatory disease

Option D is the only one that has a strong association with AS, making this the correct answer.

Dougados M, Baeten D. Spondyloarthritis. Lancet 2011; 377(9783):2127–2137.

24. C Ciprofloxacin

Case-control studies have demonstrated that patients treated with fluoroquinolones have a small but significant increased risk of tendinopathy or tendon rupture.

Table 13.6		
	Gout	**Pseudogout**
Risk factors	May be idiopathic, but any factor that increases urate stone formation, i.e. Increased production of uric acid: • Myeloproliferative/ lymphoproliferative disorders • Chemotherapy Decreased excretion of uric acid: • Lack of activity of xanthine oxidase – either primary deficiency, or drug-related (e.g. allopurinol) • Chronic renal failure • Increased production of organic acids, i.e. starvation or dehydration, exercise, any other acute physiological stress • Drugs (remember as **'PACED'** – pyrazinamide, aspirin [or allopurinol], ciclosporin, enalapril [plus other ACE inhibitors], diuretics [especially thiazides])	• Idiopathic • Familial • Prior joint trauma • Haemochromatosis • Hyperparathyroidism • Hypomagnesaemia • Hypophosphatasia • Hypothyroidism
Distribution	• Acutely, typically presents as monoarthritis of the first metatarsophalangeal joint	• Acutely, typically presents as mono- or oligoarthritis. Most often knee or wrist, but may also occur in shoulder or elbow
Microscopy	• Monosodium urate crystals • Needle-shaped • Negative birefringence under polarised light	• Calcium pyrophosphate crystals. • Rhomboid-shaped • Positive birefringence under polarised light

ACE, angiotensin-converting enzyme.

Table 13.6 Similarities and differences between gout and pseudogout.

The population at greatest risk are those above 60 years of age, those also taking corticosteroid therapy, and patients who have been taking fluoroquinolones for a median of eight days prior to the onset of tendon damage. None of the other antibiotics listed have any significant association with tendon disease.

Khaliq Y, Zhanel GG. Fluoroquinolone-associated tendinopathy: a critical review of the literature. Clin Infect Dis 2003; 36 (11):1404–1410.

25. C Osteopenia

The World Health Organisation (WHO) provides definitions for the diagnosis of osteoporosis. These are based upon bone mineral density (BMD) results, established from dual-energy X-ray absorptiometry (DEXA) scans:

- T-score:
  - This is the difference (expressed as number of standard deviations) between the patient's BMD, and that of a young adult female reference population. The value of this score helps define whether a patient has osteoporosis or not.
  - T-score greater than 1: normal
  - T-score between 1 and -2.5: osteopenia
  - T-score less than 2.5: osteoporosis
  - T-score less than 2.5 and at least one fragility fracture: severe osteoporosis

- Z-score:
  - This is the difference (expressed as number of standard deviations) between the patient's BMD, and that of an age-matched population.
  - Z-scores cannot be used for making the diagnosis of osteoporosis, but indicate whether the bone mineral density is appropriate for the patient's age.
  - Specifically, Z-scores less than 2 are below the expected level for age, and should prompt investigation as to metabolic causes of bone disease.

This woman has T-scores all between 1 and 2.5, meaning that she has generalised osteopenia.

Note that DEXA cannot be used to diagnose osteoarthritis, making option B incorrect.

World Health Organisation. Assessment of fracture risk and its application to screening for postmenopausal osteoporosis. Report of a WHO Study Group. World Health Organization technical report series 1994; 843:1–129.

26. D Polyarteritis nodosa

A disease that affects multiple organ systems associated with a raised erythrocyte sedimentation rate is suggestive of an underlying vasculitis. Goodpasture's syndrome is associated with pulmonary haemorrhage and positive anti-glomerular basement membrane antibody – neither is present here. Similarly, the majority of cases of granulomatosis with polyangiitis (Wegener's) and microscopic polyangiitis are associated with respiratory disease and positive anti-nutrophil cytoplasmic antibodies (ANCA-typically cANCA and pANCA respectively), making both unlikely. The negative anti-nuclear antibody (ANA) and normal complement levels are inconsistent with systemic lupus erythematosus.

This patient has polyarteritis nodosa (PAN). This is a systemic vasculitis that particularly affects medium-sized muscular arteries, although may affect small vessels too. The aetiology is unclear, but there is a recognised strong association between PAN and hepatitis B infection. Vasculitic lesions are triggered by the deposition of immune complexes within the arterial endothelium, which is accompanied by neutrophilic infiltration into the arterial tunica media. This process over time results in aneurysmal dilatation of affected arteries, necrotising inflammation and eventual vessel occlusion.

A wide variety of different organ systems may be affected by the disease, as described in **Table 13.7.**

The American College of Rheumatology has established diagnostic criteria for PAN, which has clinical, radiological and histological components. The radiological criterion is the detection of microaneurysms on angiography, whilst the histological factor is the presence of polymorphonuclear cells in medium-sized arteries on biopsy of a relevant site. Typical sites for biopsy include the sural nerve, kidney, muscle, or puerperal lesions. Treatment is with immunosuppressive therapy, including corticosteroids and cyclophosphamide.

Lightfoot RW. The American College of Rheumatology 1990 criteria for the classification of polyarteritis nodosa. Arthritis Rheum 1990; 33 (8):1088–1093.

27. B Avascular necrosis of the hip

Meralgia paraesthetica and trochanteric bursitis are two common causes of acute hip pain in adults; however, neither can account for the radiological abnormalities found

Table 13.7	
Organ system	**Specific features**
Rheumatological	Arthralgia and myalgia
Neurological	Various forms of neuropathy
Dermatological	Puerperal or urticarial rashes
	Livedo reticularis
Gastrointestinal	Gastrointestinal pain/bleeding may result from microaneurysm rupture
Genitourinary	Renal arterial involvement may give renal infarcts and glomerulonephritis
	Orchitis may also occur
Cardiovascular	Cardiac disease, including congestive cardiac failure
	Accelerated peripheral vascular disease
General features	Include fever and weight loss

Table 13.7 Features of polyarteritis nodosa.

in this patient. Subchondral sclerosis is one of the characteristic radiological findings of osteoarthritis, but none of the other associated radiological features are described. The young age of the patient also makes osteoarthritis unlikely. Hip arthritis would be an unusual manifestation of active lupus but has been described; however, the normal complement and anti-dsDNA titres suggest that this patient's lupus is well-controlled, making option A unlikely. In addition, the history is atypical for a lupus flare, with arthritis in lupus tending to be symmetrical, polyarticular and transient.

The correct answer is therefore B. Avascular necrosis (also known as osteonecrosis or osteonecrosis dissecans) is a disease characterised by disruption to the bone vasculature, with eventual complete mechanical failure of bone and joint destruction. The pathogenesis is unclear, but there are a large number of aetiological factors, often divided up into traumatic and atraumatic causes. The atraumatic causes may be remembered as **PICKLES**:

- **P**regnancy, **p**rocoagulant disorders, **p**ancreatitis
- **I**diopathic
- **C**orticosteroid use – the single strongest risk factor, particularly long courses at high dose; also **C**aisson's disease ('the bends')
- **K**idney – chronic kidney disease itself, along with kidney (and other solid organ) transplantation
- **L**upus – plus antiphospholipid syndrome
- **E**thanol, i.e. alcohol excess
- **S**ickle cell disease – especially HbSS disease

This woman's systemic lupus erythematosus and prolonged corticosteroid use clearly make her at particularly high-risk of the disease.

The most common presentation of avascular necrosis of the hip is with groin pain exacerbated by movement and weight bearing. The initial investigation is usually a hip X-ray – this may be normal in the earliest stages, but may show a combination of radiolucency and sclerosis as the disease progresses. Patients normally progress from plain radiograph to MRI of the hip, as this is the most sensitive imaging modality for making the diagnosis. Treatment varies according to the extent of damage at the time of diagnosis; in the worst cases, patients will need to be immediately considered for joint replacement.

Malizos KN, et al. Osteonecrosis of the femoral head: etiology, imaging and treatment. Eur J Radiol 2007; 63(1):16–28.

28. E Reactive arthritis

Reactive arthritis is defined as the development of inflammatory arthritis from days to weeks after an infection elsewhere in the body. It was previously called Reiter's syndrome. The pattern of the arthritis is variable, although tends to be a monoarthritis or asymmetrical oligoarthritis focused on the lower limbs. There may also be evidence of enthesitis, such as Achilles tendinitis. Although a 'classic triad' is often described of urethritis, conjunctivitis and arthritis, many patients present with only one or two of these features. Other extra-articular features include circinate balanitis, keratoderma blenorrhagica (waxy, yellow-brown plaques found on the soles of the feet), dystrophic nails or mouth ulcers.

It seems likely that recent gastroenteritis has precipitated his illness. A number of different organisms have been linked with reactive arthritis, those with the strongest association being:

- *Campylobacter jejuni*
- *Salmonella* spp.
- *Shigella* spp.
- *Yersinia* spp.
- *Chlamydia trachomatis*

In many cases of reactive arthritis, the triggering organism is not directly detectable (e.g. by stool culture or urethral swab) at the time of presentation. In such situations, serological tests may be employed (e.g. anti-*Campylobacter* antibodies) to help confirm the precipitating infection. Joint aspiration may also be appropriate to help exclude septic arthritis or crystal arthropathy. X-rays may be useful in recurrent disease, but contribute little in the acute setting. Other non-specific findings include raised plasma inflammatory markers. As with other seronegative spondyloarthropathies, human leucocyte antigen (HLA)-B27 is present in up to half of patients with the disease, but this is not a useful test in isolation in helping to make the diagnosis.

There are no fixed specific diagnostic criteria for reactive arthritis, and it is important to exclude disease mimics. Ankylosing spondylitis is also characterised by eye disease and inflammatory arthritis, but tends to first present with several months of sacroiliitis rather than acute peripheral oligoarthritis. The lack of oral ulceration makes Behçet's disease unlikely. Crohn's disease and ulcerative colitis can cause a form of seronegative spondyloarthropathy, but non-inflammatory bowel diseases (such as coeliac disease) do not have this association. Disseminated gonococcal disease may present with arthritis and tenosynovitis, but also tends to cause pustular skin lesions; furthermore, if this was the diagnosis here, the gonococcal organism would likely have been detected by the microbiological investigations.

Treatment of reactive arthritis is with rest, non-steroidal anti-inflammatory drugs (NSAIDs), intra-articular corticosteroids and – in particularly severe cases – disease-modifying anti-rheumatic agent (DMARD) therapy. There is ongoing debate about whether antibiotics to treat the precipitating infection are of any benefit; current evidence suggests that they may shorten the course of disease only where *Chlamydia trachomatis* has been the trigger.

Rihl M, et al. Infection and musculoskeletal conditions: reactive arthritis. Best Practice & Research. Clin Rheumatol 2006; 20(6):1119–1137.

29. B Hyperferritinaemia

Adult-onset Still's disease (AOSD) is a rare systemic inflammatory disorder of unclear aetiology. The most typical presentation is with recurrent spikes of fever, arthritis, and a transient maculopapular rash, although this is highly variable between patients. Other possible features include recurrent pharyngitis, lymphadenopathy, hepatosplenomegaly, and pleural and pericardial effusions.

Table 13.8

Laboratory	Test	Details
Haematology	Leucocyte count	Usually $> 10 \times 10^9$/L, with $\geq 80\%$ neutrophils
	Platelet count	Elevated
	Haemoglobin	Hb < 10 g/dL in over 60% of patients
	ESR	Significantly raised
Biochemistry	Ferritin	Often hugely raised (may be in the order of several thousands), reflecting ferritin's role as a marker of the acute-phase response*
	Liver function tests	Elevated transaminases found in a large proportion of patients, but no consistent finding of changes in ALP
	C-reactive protein	Significantly raised
Immunology	ANA	Typically negative, although weakly detect-able in $\leq 10\%$ of patients
	Rheumatoid factor	

*The percentage of ferritin that is glycosylated has been shown to be lower in AOSD than other rheumatological diseases, which may aid in making the diagnosis.

ALP, alkaline phosphatase; ANA, anti-nuclear antibodies; ESR, erythrocyte sedimentation rate.

Table 13.8 Laboratory findings in adult-onset Still's disease.

One difficulty in diagnosing AOSD is the large number of disease mimics, and extensive investigation is first required to exclude other causes. Another complexity is the lack of highly specific clinical or laboratory features. However, certain abnormal laboratory findings are found consistently, which may be helpful in making the diagnosis when found in combination, and are summarised in **Table 13.8.**

Neutrophilia may be found in AOSD but not eosinophilia. Autoantibodies are typically negative in the condition. AOSD is characterised by elevation of transaminases rather than alkaline phosphatase. Hyperferritinaemia is by far the most consistent laboratory abnormality in AOSD.

Efthimiou P, et al. Diagnosis and management of adult onset Still's disease. Ann Rheum Dis 2006; 65(5):564–572.

30.　C Fat pad biopsy

Patients with chronic inflammatory disease risk developing secondary (AA) amyloidosis. This is since ongoing inflammation is associated with prolonged production of serum amyloid A (AA) protein (an acute phase reactant), fibrils of which become progressively deposited in a range of extracellular tissues over time. Many inflammatory conditions have been associated with secondary amyloidosis – both rheumatological (e.g. seronegative diseases) and otherwise (e.g. bronchiectasis, Crohn's disease, etc.) – but rheumatoid arthritis is the condition with the strongest association. In contrast, systemic/primary (AL) amyloidosis is a plasma cell dyscrasia associated with overproduction of monoclonal immunoglobulin light chains. Several different forms of hereditary amyloidosis also exist.

AA amyloidosis may affect a number of different organs and so present in a variety of different ways (**Figure 13.4**). This patient's nephrotic syndrome suggests that he has very marked renal amyloid deposition. The ultrasound findings of large, echogenic kidneys are also characteristic of renal amyloid. The presence of hepatomegaly in this setting implies that he has hepatic amyloidosis too.

The diagnosis of AA amyloidosis is usually confirmed on biopsy. Although this patient appears to have renal and hepatic amyloid, the risk of significant bleeding post-renal/liver biopsy is much higher in patients with amyloid, hence these may not be the most appropriate biopsy sites. Subcutaneous fat pads and rectal tissue are most often biopsied, since the site is easily accessible (both for tissue sampling and control of post-procedure bleeding), and also since these tissues tend to have a high amyloid load. Characteristic biopsy findings are red-green birefringence when stained with Congo red and viewed under cross-polarised light.

Biopsy is also key to diagnosing other forms of amyloidosis. In addition, protein electrophoresis and/or bone marrow examination is helpful in diagnosing AL amyloidosis, whilst hereditary forms of amyloid may be diagnosed through gene mutation analysis. One other useful test is serum amyloid P (SAP) scintigraphy,

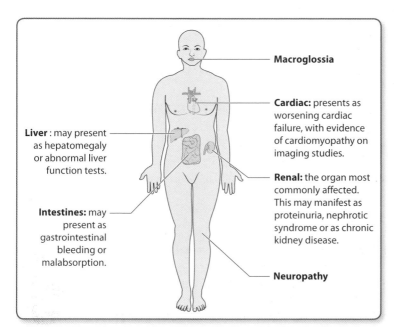

Figure 13.4 Organ systems affected by AA amyloidosis.

Macroglossia

Cardiac: presents as worsening cardiac failure, with evidence of cardiomyopathy on imaging studies.

Liver : may present as hepatomegaly or abnormal liver function tests.

Renal: the organ most commonly affected. This may manifest as proteinuria, nephrotic syndrome or as chronic kidney disease.

Intestines: may present as gastrointestinal bleeding or malabsorption.

Neuropathy

a nuclear medicine scan that can highlight organs where amyloid has been deposited.

AA amyloidosis is best treated by attempting to control the underlying inflammatory disease, whilst AL amyloidosis is usually treated with combination chemotherapy. Hereditary amyloidosis may require treatment with liver transplantation.

Obici L, et al. Susceptibility to AA amyloidosis in rheumatic diseases: a critical overview. Arthritis Rheum 2009; 61 (10):1435–1440.

Chapter 14

Tropical, infectious and sexually transmitted diseases

1. A 42-year-old man with diabetes and end stage renal failure recently underwent a renal transplant. His inpatient bed was in close proximity to building works on another part of the hospital. Soon after returning to the ward, he had started to develop increasing shortness of breath, fever and some mild confusion. Infection was thought to be the most likely cause of his symptoms.

   What is the most likely causative organism?

   A *Aspergillus fumigatus*
   B *Blastomyces dermatitidis*
   C *Coccidioides immitis*
   D *Escherichia coli*
   E *Mycobacterium tuberculosis*

2. A 23-year-old Ghanaian woman presented to the outpatient clinic with patches of hypopigmentation on her abdomen. She had visited Ghana last year on a family holiday and had been otherwise well. Apart from the skin patches, which were approximately 1 cm in diameter, there were no other abnormal findings. She was started on a course of topical steroids, but in spite of this, the rash spread. Wood's lamp examination revealed a yellow fluorescence.

   What is the most likely causative organism?

   A *Candida albicans*
   B *Cryptococcus neoformans*
   C *Epidermophyton floccosum*
   D *Pityrosporum orbiculare (Malassezia)*
   E *Trichophytum rubrum*

3. A 27-year-old man, presented to his general practitioner with a 7 day history of fever, lethargy, and vomiting. He had also noticed his urine becoming darker in colour. He had returned to the UK 10 days ago from a canoeing vacation in the USA. On examination, there was no rash, but he was jaundiced and had suffused conjunctivae.

What is the most likely causative organism?

A   *Borrelia afzelii*
B   *Borrelia burgdorferi*
C   *Brucella melitensis*
D   *Leptospira interrogans*
E   *Rickettsia typhi*

4.   What is the most likely causative organism of erysipelas?

A   *Staphylococcus aureus*
B   *Staphylococcus epidermidis*
C   *Streptococcus pyogenes*
D   *Streptococcus sanguinis*
E   *Streptococcus viridans*

5.   Which one of the following is the most likely example of a live attenuated vaccine?

A   Diphtheria
B   Influenza
C   Rabies
D   Tetanus
E   Yellow fever

6.   What is the most likely mechanism of action of sulphonamides?

A   Block cell wall synthesis
B   Inhibit bacterial protein synthesis
C   Inhibit DNA synthesis
D   Inhibit enzymes converting para-aminobenzoic acid into folic acid
E   Interact with structure of cell wall

7.   A 21-year-old man attended the sexual health clinic with a history of dysuria associated with urethral discharge. He was confirmed to have *Chlamydia trachomatis.*

What is the most appropriate treatment?

A   Azithromycin
B   Cephalexin
C   Flucloxacillin
D   Metronidazole
E   Penicillin V

8.   A 34-year-old woman presented to the medical assessment unit with a 7-day history of shortness of breath, fever, myalgia and a non-productive cough. Two days ago, she arrived back from a holiday in Greece.

Investigations:

white cell count	15.3×10^9/L (4–11)
lymphocytes	0.9×10^9/L (1.5–4.0)

neutrophils	15.1×10^9/L (1.5–7.0)
platelets	265×10^9/L (150–400)
sodium	128 mmol/L (137–144)
potassium	4.7mmol/L (3.5–4.9)
urea	7.1mmol/L (2.5–7.0)
creatinine	92 μmol/L (60–110)
C-reactive protein	186 mg/L (<5)
chest X-ray	consolidation in the left lower lobe

What is the most useful diagnostic investigation?

A   Blood cultures
B   Cold agglutinin test
C   CT of the thorax
D   Sputum cultures
E   Urinary antigen test

9. A 26-year-old man, a security guard, presented to hospital following a dog bite on the right hand. He had no known allergies. He was afebrile and haemodynamically stable. Examination revealed four 1 cm wounds on the hypothenar aspect of the right hand.

What is the most appropriate treatment for this patient?

A   Augmentin
B   Ciprofloxacin
C   Doxycycline and metronidazole
D   Erythromycin
E   No antibiotics required

10. A 20-year-old male student had returned from a 2-month backpacking trip to Chile. He described a 1-week history of general malaise, lethargy and fever. On examination, he had bilateral swollen eyelids.

What is the most likely causative organism?

A   *Brugia malayi*
B   *Necator americanus*
C   *Trypanosoma brucei*
D   *Trypanosoma cruzi*
E   *Wuchereria bancrofti*

11. A 26-year-old woman presented to her general practitioner with an ulcer on the right arm. She had recently returned from a backpacking trip to southern India. She had no other symptoms and had no significant past medical history, nor any known drug allergies. On examination, the centre of the ulcer was necrotic and black. Wound culture revealed gram-positive rod-like bacilli.

What is the most appropriate initial treatment?

A   Amikacin
B   Clindamycin

    C   Gentamicin
    D   Metronidazole
    E   Penicillin

12. A 38-year-old man presented with a 4-week history of headache, fevers and general malaise. He had recently moved to the UK from Malta. He had no cough or other symptoms. On admission to the medical assessment unit, he was found to have a temperature of 38.3°C, pulse 120 beats per minute, blood pressure 109/61 mmHg and oxygen saturation of 97% on room air. Abdominal examination revealed mild hepatosplenomegaly.

Investigations:

chest X-ray	normal
blood culture	gram-negative coccobacilli in Castaneda's medium

What is the most likely causative organism?

    A   *Borrelia burgdorferi*
    B   *Bordetella pertussis*
    C   *Brucella melitensis*
    D   *Corynebacterium* species
    E   *Listeria* species

13. A 43-year-old woman with a history of sarcoidosis survived an out of hospital ventricular fibrillation cardiac arrest and had an implantable cardiac defibrillator (ICD) inserted. Two weeks later she presented with pyrexia, and was found to also have elevated inflammatory markers.

Investigations:

chest X-ray	normal
pulmonary function tests	normal
urine culture	normal
transthoracic echocardiogram	2 × 3 cm vegetation on the right ventricular ICD lead with preserved left ventricular function

What is the most appropriate next step in management?

    A   Extract ICD immediately
    B   High resolution CT chest
    C   Start intravenous antibiotics immediately
    D   Take multiple sets of blood cultures and extract ICD
    E   Take multiple sets of blood cultures and immediately start intravenous antibiotics

14. A 24-year-old woman presented with offensive smelling, vaginal discharge. The discharge was a grey fluid with no blood. She first noticed this about 4 weeks ago

but felt too embarrassed to seek medical advice until now. Her menstrual cycles were regular and currently she was not currently sexually active.

What is the most likely type of infection?

A   Bacterial vaginosis
B   *Candida*
C   Chlamydia
D   Gonorrhoea
E   *Trichomonas vaginalis*

15. A 18-year-old man was admitted to hospital with increasing drowsiness. He was known to have anaphylactic reaction to penicillin the in the past. Examination revealed a purpuric rash affecting both lower limbs.

Which one of the following is the most appropriate treatment for this patient?

A   Ceftriaxone
B   Chloramphenicol
C   Erythromycin
D   Gentamicin and metronidazole
E   Rifampicin

16. A 42-year-old woman presented to the medical admissions unit with fevers, vomiting and headache. She had recently returned from a 6-week trip to Sierra Leone and started to feel unwell during the last day of her trip. She was not taking malaria prophylaxis and had no known drug allergies. On examination, her temperature was 38.4°C, but she was haemodynamically stable.

Investigations:

white cell count	12.0×10^9/L (4–11)
neutrophils	10.1×10^9/L (1.5–7.0)
platelets	65×10^9/L (150–400)
C-reactive protein	34 mg/L (<5)
international normalised ratio	1.1 (<1.4)
random glucose	4.8 mmol/L (4.4–6.1)

normal renal function

blood film	6% parasitaemia with *Plasmodium falciparum*

What is the most appropriate initial treatment?

A   Intravenous artesunate
B   Intravenous quinine
C   Oral atovaquone
D   Oral chloroquine
E   Oral quinine

17. A 29-year-old woman presented with 10-day history of fevers, night sweats and general malaise. She had recently returned to the UK from the Congo. She was 5 months pregnant. Blood film: 1% parasitaemia with *Plasmodium falciparum*.

What is the most appropriate treatment?

A   Atovaquone plus proguanil
B   Doxycycline
C   Mefloquine
D   Primaquine
E   Quinine plus clindamycin

18. A 30-year-old sexually active homosexual man presented with a 2-week history of anal itching and discharge of pus. He had no drug allergies. Testing was positive for *Neisseria gonorrhoea*, and chlamydia was negative.

What is the most appropriate treatment?

A   Azithromycin and ceftriaxone
B   Benzylpenicillin
C   Cefixime and metronidazole
D   Ciprofloxacin and doxycycline
E   Doxycycline

19. A 63-year-old woman presented with a 3-day history of bloody diarrhoea with very loose stools, opening her bowels 7–8 times per day. She had just returned from a 10-day cruise on the Nile. On examination, she had a temperature of 38.5°C and a blood pressure of 87/43 mmHg. She was treated with intravenous fluids. Stool cultures were positive for gram-negative rod-like bacilli.

What is the most likely causative organism?

A   *Bacillus cereus*
B   *Campylobacter jejuni*
C   *Shigella* species
D   *Staphylococcus aureus*
E   *Yersinia enterocolitica*

20. A 23-year-old HIV positive Caucasian man, presented to the clinic with a skin rash affecting all his limbs for the past 2 weeks. On examination, he had purple plaques on the anterior aspect of his legs and arms but no other findings. The clinical suspicion was that this was Kaposi's sarcoma.

What is the most likely causative virus?

A   Cytomegalovirus-8
B   Human herpes virus (HHV)-3
C   HHV-5
D   HHV-8
E   Human T-lymphotropic virus (HTLV)-1

21. A 54-year-old man complained of a 2-week history of fevers, malaise and headaches. He was bitten by a rat whilst on holiday in China and had just returned to the UK. On examination, there was an indurated and ulcerated lesion at the site

of the bite on his right leg. In addition, there was a large maculopapular, violaceous rash on the trunk.

Which one of the following is the most likely cause?

A   *Bartonella clarridgeiae*
B   *Bartonella henselae*
C   Parapox virus
D   *Spirillum minor*
E   *Streptobacillus moniliformis*

22. A 45-year-old woman presented with gross haematuria. She had travelled to Malawi 3 months ago and had been well during her trip. She admitted to swimming in the lakes whilst there.

Investigations:

urine analysis	blood +++
malaria blood films	negative

What is the most likely diagnosis?

A   Amoebiasis
B   Dengue fever
C   Schistosomiasis
D   Typhoid
E   Yellow fever

23. A 35-year-old Bangladeshi man was diagnosed with pulmonary tuberculosis 4 weeks ago. He attended the respiratory clinic with worsening headaches. CT head scan showed no tuberculosis abscess or deposits, however lumbar puncture was suggestive of meningeal tuberculosis.

What is the most appropriate management plan?

A   Isoniazid, ethambutol, rifampicin and pyrazinamide for 8 months
B   Isoniazid, ethambutol, rifampicin for 6 months
C   Isoniazid, ethambutol, rifampicin, pyrazinamide and prednisolone for 12 months
D   Isoniazid, ethambutol, rifampicin, pyrazinamide and streptomycin for 8 months
E   Isoniazid, rifampicin and streptomycin for 8 months

24. Which one of the following is least likely to be associated with Lyme disease?

A   Bell's palsy
B   Cerebellar ataxia
C   Cranial nerve VII palsy
D   Erythema marginatum
E   Heart block

25. A 32-year-old HIV positive man presented with a 1-week history of worsening confusion and diplopia. He denied any headache. There was no history of trauma. Examination revealed no evidence of meningism but did suggest gait ataxia.

Investigations:

CD4 count	4×10^{6}/L (430–1690)
HIV-1 viral load	1.8×10^{6} viral copies/mL
MR brain	bilateral high intensity signals in the periventricular and subcortical
regions, consistent with demyelination.	No evidence of raised intracranial pressure or space-occupying lesion

What is the most likely diagnosis?

A   Cerebral toxoplasmosis
B   Cerebral tuberculoma
C   Multiple sclerosis
D   Progressive multifocal leucoencephalopathy
E   Subdural haematoma

26. Which one of the following bacteria is least likely to be associated with overwhelming post splenectomy infection?

A   *Haemophilus influenza*
B   *Mycobacterium tuberculosis*
C   *Neisseria meningitidis*
D   *Pseudomonas aeruginosa*
E   *Streptococcus pneumonia*

27. What is the most appropriate treatment for hydatid disease?

A   Albendazole
B   Amphotericin
C   Ciprofloxacin
D   Itraconazole
E   Metronidazole

28. A 21-year-old man complained of loose stools for the past 2 weeks. There was no blood but he was opening his bowels up to 6 times per day. He also had associated intermittent abdominal pain, nausea and 4 kg weight loss. He had just arrived back from a trip to Russia and presented to the emergency department due to ongoing symptoms.

What is the most appropriate initial treatment?

A   Albendazole
B   Ciprofloxacin
C   Mebendazole
D   Metronidazole
E   Paromomycin

29. A 19-year-old man attended the sexual health clinic. He had developed multiple warts on the shaft of his penis a couple of months ago and recently these had become itchy.

What is the most appropriate treatment?

A   Cauterisation
B   Cryotherapy
C   Topical acyclovir
D   Topical podophyllum
E   Topical salicylic acid

30. Which one of the following is a nucleoside analogue that inhibits reverse transcriptase?

A   Efavirenz
B   Indinavir
C   Nevirapine
D   Ritonavir
E   Zidovudine

Answers

1. A *Aspergillus fumigatus*

This patient has acquired the fungus *Aspergillus fumigatus*, which is usually found in decaying organic matter and soil. The fungus attacks immunocompromised individuals, leading to aspergillosis and is a well-recognised cause of post-transplant infection. Building works are a source of the aspergillus through the release of dust and spores. Once the diagnosis has been made, management includes reducing the dose of immunosuppression and the use of antifungals such as voriconazole.

Blastomyces dermatitidis leads to blastomycosis, found commonly in northern and midwest United States and Canada in various environments, but typically appears in rivers and lakes.

Coccidioides immitis is a fungus found in soil in southwest United States and Mexico, leading to coccidioidomycosis or 'valley fever'. It presents with a rash and generalised flu-like symptoms.

It is unlikely that *Mycobacterium tuberculosis* infection has developed over the short-time period. In addition, recipients would have been screened extensively for latent (and active tuberculosis) prior to the renal transplantation.

Pappas PG, et al. Invasive fungal infections among organ transplant recipients: results of the transplant-associated infection surveillance network (TRANSNET). Clin Infect Dis 2010; 50 (8):1101–1111.

2. D *Pityrosporum orbiculare (Malassezia)*

Pityrosporum orbiculare is a member of the genus of yeast termed *Malassezia*. It is more widespread in humans and typically affects the skin and is a common cause of seborrhoeic dermatitis. In opportunistic infections, the organism can lead to hypopigmentation (typically on the trunk) and therefore this patient should be investigated further for an immunocompromised state. The use of a topical steroid cream has exacerbated the rash, which is a feature of fungal infections.

Infection with *Candida albicans* is more frequent and typically does not cause hypopigmentation of the skin.

Epidermophyton floccosum is an anthropophilic dermatophyte, which can lead to tinea pedis, tinea corporis and onychomycosis. There is increased prevalence in hot and humid climates, with an incubation period of 5–10 days.

Trichophytum rubrum is the most common cause of tinea pedis (athlete's foot) and dermatophytosis (ringworm), thriving in moist areas where people walk barefoot. Treatment is initially with topical antifungal agents such as miconazole. Oral agents such as terbinafine, itraconazole and fluconazole may be used in resistant cases.

Gupta AK, et al. Skin diseases associated with *Malassezia* species. J Am Acad Dermatol 2004; 51(5):785–798.
Bell-Syer SE, Hart R, Crawford F. Oral treatments for fungal infections of the skin of the foot. Cochrane Database Syst Rev 2002; (2):CD003584.

3. D *Leptospira interrogans*

These are the classical features of leptospirosis. It is important to note that there is no rash, thereby eliminating a number of the other options.

Leptospira interrogans is one of the zoonotic spirochaete species responsible for leptospirosis. Spirochaetales are a family of organisms, which belong to the gram-negative family of bacteria.

There is usually a history of recreational (water sports) or occupational (sewage workers) exposure. Leptospirosis results from the transmission of *Leptospira interrogans* in contaminated water and presents with headaches, fever, myalgia and neck stiffness for approximately 4–7 days. This may then progress to vasculitis, meningitis (Canicola fever) and jaundice with renal impairment and proteinuria (Weil's disease). Other systemic manifestations include severe pulmonary haemorrhage syndrome, perimyocarditis, and rarely cardiac failure.

Diagnosis is made through blood cultures, urine cultures, serology and polymerase chain reaction testing.

Treatment is with penicillin, doxycycline and tertracycline along with supportive measures. In some regions, prophylactic doxycycline may be given to those participating in water sports/activities.

Borellia burgdorferi and *Borellia afzelii* are responsible for Lyme disease.

McBride AJ, et al. Leptospirosis. Curr Opin Infect Dis 2005; 18(5):376–386.

4. C *Streptococcus pyogenes*

Erysipelas is an acute bacterial skin infection due to *Streptococcus pyogenes* infection. Points of entry include trauma to the skin, or as a result from psoriasis, eczema or fungal infections of the skin. Treatment of choice is with penicillin.

Streptococci can be divided in α and β subtypes (**Figure 14.1**).

Bisno AL, Stevens DL. Streptococcal infections of skin and soft tissues. N Engl J Med 1996; 334: 240–246.

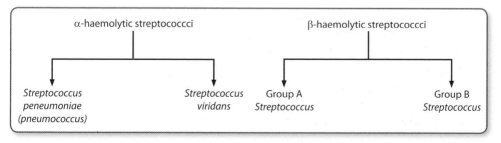

Figure 14.1 Classification of *Streptococcus* species.

5. E Yellow fever

The following categorise the different forms of vaccinations:

Live attenuated vaccines: **'BOOMY'**

Bacillus Calmette–Guérin (BCG)
Oral polio
Oral typhoid
Measles, mumps, rubella (MMR)
Yellow fever

Inactivated preparations:

Influenza
Rabies
Hepatitis A

Fragmented:

Hepatitis B
Pertussis
Diphtheria

Table 14.1

Antimicrobial classification	Example of antibiotics	Mechanism of action
Penicillin	Benzylpenicillin	Inhibit cell wall synthesis
Quinolones	Ciprofloxacin Levofloxacin Moxifloxacin	Inhibit bacterial DNA synthesis
Sulphonamides	Trimethoprim Sulphadiazine	Competitively inhibit enzymes converting para-aminobenzoic acid into folic acid
Tetracyclines	Tetracycline doxycycline Minocycline	Inhibit bacterial protein synthesis
Cephalosporin	Cephalexin (1st generation) Cefuroxime (2nd generation) Ceftazidime (3rd generation)	Inhibit cell wall synthesis
Macrolide	Clarithromycin Erythromycin Azithromycin	Inhibition of bacterial protein synthesis

Table 14.1 Mechanism of action of antibiotics.

6. D Inhibit enzymes converting para-aminobenzoic acid into folic acid

Table 14.1 Summarises the mechanism of action of each of the antimicrobial groups.

7. A Azithromycin

The treatment for chlamydia is either azithromycin 1 g in a single dose or doxycycline 100 mg twice daily for 7 days. Azithromycin may be the preferred agent if the patient has a history of poor compliance and unpredictable follow-up appointment attendance.

It has been shown that azithromycin and doxycycline are equally effective in treating chlamydia, with no difference in the outcomes.

Antibiotics are only part of the treatment. It is important to encourage patients to adhere to safe sexual practices and to take a detailed sexual history, screening and treating any partners who may be positive for chlamydia. It is essential that the treatment is prompt, as delays can lead to significant complications such as pelvic inflammatory disease and subfertility or infertility.

Lau CY, Qureshi AK. Azithromycin versus doxycycline for genital chlamydial infections: a meta-analysis of randomized clinical trials. Sex Transm Dis 2002; 29:497–495.

8. E Urinary antigen test

The recent return from abroad, along with features of pneumonia and hyponatraemia, are highly suggestive of Legionnaire's disease. The features of *Legionella pneumophila* are 'flu like' symptoms, non-productive cough, and shortness of breath. Hepatitis, renal failure, hyponatraemia and confusion are extra-pulmonary manifestations.

Diagnosis is by urinary or serological antigens. It is useful to check electrolytes and liver function. Treatment is with macrolides such as clarithromycin and/or fluoroquinolone if no treatment response. Treatment may be required for up to three weeks.

Ricketts K, Joseph CA, Yadav R. Travel-associated legionnaire's disease in Europe in 2008. Euro Surveill 2010; 15(21):19578.

9. A Augmentin

This patient has a significant injury from the dog bite and requires antibiotics. Although in 15–20% of patients infection occurs, it is important to give antibiotic prophylaxis. It is essential to make an initial assessment, to rule out any muscular or nerve injury, irrigate the wound and administer tetanus prophylaxis.

The following organisms are commonly found in dog bites.

Staphylococcus aureus
Pasteurella
Streptococcus species

Corynebacterium
Eikenella corrodens
Capnocytophaga canimorsus

The recommended management of an uncomplicated wound is treatment with 3–7 days of prophylactic antibiotics. In those with frank cellulitis or significant infection, a prolonged course is recommended lasting a minimum of 2 weeks.

Augmentin is the first line treatment in dog bites. If the patient is penicillin allergic, then doxycycline (+/– metronidazole) is used (except for pregnant patients and children). Other possible antimicrobials include erythromycin, clindamycin and intramuscular ceftriaxone (for those where compliance is an issue).

Presutti RJ. Bite wounds. Early treatment and prophylaxis against infectious complications. Postgrad Med 1997; 101:243–4,246–52,254.

10. D *Trypanosoma cruzi*

This patient demonstrates the features of acute Chagas' disease. The causative organism is *Trypanosoma cruzi* and is transmitted by triatomine insects. It is common in Central and South America. Other forms of transmission include consuming contaminated foods and blood transfusion. It is estimated that approximately 10 million people in South America are infected with the parasite.

The disease progression can be divided into acute and chronic phases.

The acute phase is characterised by infection lasting for 1–3 weeks and non-specific features, which may not be attributed specifically to Chagas' disease such as lethargy, general. One of the more recognisable features is swelling of the eyelids (Romana's sign). This is a result of the bite and subsequent itching and swelling.

The chronic phase of the infection may develop after a latent period of months or years. Significant complications include:

- Megacolon
- Megaoesophagus
- Cardiomyopathy
- Arrhythmias

Treatment is with antiparasitic agents such as benznidazole and nifurtimox. It has been shown that treatment leads to eradication of parasites in 60–85% of patients. In the chronic phase of the disease, symptomatic control is required, along with managing complications such as cardiomyopathy and heart failure.

Le Loup G, Pialoux G, Lescure FX. Update in treatment of Chagas disease. Curr Opin Infect Dis 2011; 24(5):428–434.

11. E Penicillin

This is a description of an eschar and along with the culture results, is in keeping with infection with *Bacillus anthracis*, or anthrax.

Anthrax predominantly affects three systems. The most common is the cutaneous form leading to a black necrotic ulcer, which occurs in 95% of cases and responds well to high doses of penicillin. Those infections that are resistant to penicillin can be treated with ciprofloxacin or doxycycline. If a case of bioterrorism attack is suspected, up to 60 days of antibiotics may be required, rather than 7–10 days if the condition is acquired naturally.

Bacillus anthracis affecting the pulmonary system is associated with high mortality rates and has been considered as a possible agent for bioterrorism. Presentation follows inhalation of anthrax spores resulting in pulmonary oedema, leading to cardiogenic shock. Incubation period is normally less than 1 week, but can be as much as up to 2 months. It usually presents with non-specific symptoms for 2–5 days, then an abrupt onset of respiratory distress and development of cardiogenic shock within 24–36 hours. Treatment for pulmonary anthrax should be commenced once there is a clinical suspicion and is usually with ciprofloxacin or doxycycline, and another two antimicrobial agents. Due to potential for rapid deterioration, management should be in an intensive care setting, with appropriate precautions for infection control.

Gastrointestinal anthrax, is the rarest form of the infection. Its features include nausea, vomiting and abdominal pain. Ascites can develop rapidly over a period of 24–72 hours, followed by shock. Management adheres to the same principles as pulmonary anthrax.

Swartz MN. Recognition and management of anthrax – an update. N Engl J Med 2001; 345: 1621–1626.

12. C *Brucella melitensis*

Brucellosis is a group of infections resulting from gram-negative coccobacilli, acquired when humans handle animal carcasses or ingest unpasteurised milk. The following are commonly found species:

Brucella abortus – from cattle
Brucella melitensis – from sheep and goat
Brucella suis – from pig

Brucella melitensis, also known as 'Malta fever', is primarily the result of ingesting unpasteurised milk (mainly from sheep) or in occupational exposure in those working with animals. It occurs more frequently in Mediterranean, Middle East and South American regions.

Symptoms may be present from days to months and include fever, malaise, weight loss. Lymphadenopathy and hepatosplenomegaly may be present. Less commonly, orchitis, meningoencephalitis, endocarditis and osteomyelitis may occur.

Treatment is with either oral doxycycline or rifampicin antibiotics. If resistant to this treatment or the patient is critically unwell, aminoglycosides should be used.

Corynebacterium and *Listera* are gram-positive organisms.

Pappas G, et al. Brucellosis. N Engl J Med 2005; 352:2325–2336.

13. D Take multiple sets of blood cultures and extract ICD

This patient most likely has a device related infection, following insertion of an implantable cardiac defibrillator (ICD). This is becoming more prevalent, as more pacemakers and defibrillators are inserted.

This patient has features of bacterial endocarditis, with a vegetation on the ICD lead. Therefore, the infection should be managed aggressively. It is important to take multiple sets of peripheral blood cultures (ideally six) and the device should subsequently be extracted. At the time of extraction, further cultures should be taken from the lead tip, to help isolate organisms responsible for the infection. Following this, management will differ according to individual circumstances; however, in most cases blood cultures should be confirmed prior to starting antibiotic treatment. Once a prolonged course (minimum 6 weeks) has been completed, re-insertion should be considered.

The common organisms responsible for cardiac device related infections can be remembered using the following mnemonic.

'PACKS'

Pseudomonas aeruginosa
Staphylococcus Aureus
Coagulase-negative staphylococci
Klebsiella pneumonia
Serratia marcescens

Sohail MR, et al. Management and outcome of permanent pacemaker and implantable cardioverter-defibrillator infections. J Am Coll Cardiol. 2007; 49:1851–1859.

14. A Bacterial vaginosis

The history and symptoms are suggestive of bacterial vaginosis. **Table 14.2** summarises the differences between various causes of vaginal discharge.

Table 14.2	
Condition	**Symptoms**
Bacterial vaginosis	Grey/white discharge with 'fishy' odour
Candida	Thick white discharge, with pruritus
Trichomonas vaginalis	Yellow/green offensive discharge 'Strawberry' cervix
Chlamydia	Can often be asymptomatic. Otherwise features include dysuria, dyspareunia and possibly clear discharge
Gonorrhoea	Can often be asymptomatic. Otherwise pruritus, thick yellow/green discharge, dysuria, abdominal pain, dyspareunia

Table 14.2 Different causes of vaginal discharge.

Bacterial vaginosis can be diagnosed using the Amsel criteria, and remembered by the mnemonic 'PACT':

- **p**H(vaginal) > 4.5
- **A**ddition of potassium chloride, offensive 'fishy' odour
- **C**lue cells on microscopy
- **T**hin grey/white discharge

Treatment is with oral or vaginal metronidazole and clindamycin.

Amsel R, et al. Nonspecific vaginitis. Diagnostic criteria and microbial and epidemiologic associations. Am J Med 1983; 74 (1):14–22.

15. B Chloramphenicol

In patients suspected of bacterial meningitis, it is important to administer antibiotics immediately and if the patient is deteriorating or unwell, this should be given prior to performing a lumbar puncture.

In non-penicillin allergic patients, intravenous or intramuscular benzylpenicillin should be administered.

Contacts of the patient should be given prophylactic antibiotics.

16. A Intravenous artesunate then oral therapy

Approximately 1500–2000 cases of malaria are diagnosed every year in the UK. Around 75% of cases are due to *Plasmodium falciparum* and can be associated with significant morbidity and mortality if not treated promptly.

Non-falciparum malaria is usually caused by *Plasmodium vivax*, although a small number are caused by *Plasmodium ovale* and *Plasmodium malaria*.

Diagnosis of malaria cannot be ruled out until three blood films are performed with thick and thin films. Newer rapid diagnostic tests can be used for *Plasmodium falciparum*, but are less reliable at diagnosing other species.

In those with no complications, *Plasmodium falciparum* can be treated with oral quinine, atovaquone plus proguanil or co-artemether. Quinine is highly effective, but poorly tolerated when given as a prolonged course, therefore it is always prescribed with another agent, usually doxycycline.

In those who are critically unwell or who have a high parasite count (greater than 2%), intravenous artesunate should be started until the patient has clinically improved and can tolerate oral preparations. The intravenous treatment should be for a minimum of 24 hours. The World Health Organisation (WHO) recommendations (2010) state that intravenous artesunate should be used in preference to quinine in those with severe malaria, due to the widespread presence of quinine resistance.

World Health Organization (WHO). Guidelines for the treatment of malaria, 2nd edition. Geneva: WHO, 2010.

17. E Quinine plus clindamycin

Plasmodium falciparum in pregnancy is associated with significant co-morbidities both for the mother and the fetus. The patient should be admitted to the high dependency or intensive care unit, depending on the clinical state. Diagnosis may be difficult, as parasites may be sparse in the peripheral blood, and can collect around the placenta.

First-line treatment is with quinine, and as doxycycline should not be used in pregnancy, this should be substituted with clindamycin. Primaquine is also contraindicated in pregnancy.

World Health Organization (WHO). Guidelines for the treatment of malaria, 2nd edition. Geneva: WHO, 2010.

18. A Azithromycin and ceftriaxone

Although this patient tested positive for *N. gonorrhoea*, it is not clear if co-infection with other conditions is present. Therefore, recommendations are to treat both for gonorrhoea and chlamydia in high-risk patients. It is likely in this case that compliance may be a problem: attempts should be made to minimise the length of treatment and to try and to a regimen where once only administration can be achieved: Therefore, intramuscular ceftriaxone as a single dose along with a one-off dose of azithromycin should be sufficient. The patient should be counselled to inform his sexual partner(s) and encouraged to attend a follow-up appointment, for the results of his other investigations.

Recommendations are:

> Ceftriaxone 250 mg intramuscular (IM) as a single dose
>
> or
>
> Cefixime 400 mg oral as a single dose
>
> or
>
> Spectinomycin 2 g IM as a single dose

AND

> Azithromycin 1 g orally as a single dose
>
> or
>
> Doxycycline 100 mg twice daily for 7 days
>
> In those allergic to penicillin:
>
> Spectinomycin 2 g IM as a single dose.

Quinolones such as ciprofloxacin cannot be recommended due to high levels of resistance worldwide.

Bignell C, Fitzgerald M. UK national guideline for the management of gonorrhoea in adults. Int J STD AIDS 2011; 22:541–547.

19. C *Shigella* species

This scenario describes a case of shigellosis or shigella dysentery. There are four species of *Shigella*:

- *Shigella sonnei*
- *Shigella dysenteriae*
- *Shigella boydii*
- *Shigella flexneri*

Shigella dysentery may present with abdominal cramps and nausea along with loose stools mixed with blood, pus and mucous. The condition develops over a period of 12 – 72 hours. It is commonly transmitted following consumption of contaminated salads and water.

Table 14.3 summarises different causes of traveller's diarrhoea.

Treatment includes supportive management with intravenous fluids and maintaining balanced electrolytes. Antibiotic treatment should be commenced with a positive culture result. Ciprofloxacin is the first line treatment, but increasing resistance to *Shigella dysenteriae* means that other quinolones, cephalosporins and azithromycin may be used as alternatives.

Niyogi SK. Shigellosis. J Microbiol 2005; 43(2):133–143.

Table 14.3		
Organism	**Incubation period**	**Clinical features**
Escherichia coli	12–72 hours	Commonest in travellers. Nausea and abdominal cramps. Loose, watery diarrhoea
Bacillus cereus	1–6 hours	Severe vomiting and diarrhoea. Toxin from rice and meat
Shigella	12–96 hours	Bloody diarrhoea. Results from faecal–oral transmission
Staphylococcus aureus	2–7 hours	Toxin from dairy or meat products. Severe vomiting. Short incubation period
Campylobacter jejuni	1–10 days	Preceded by flu-like symptoms, followed by abdominal cramps and bloody diarrhoea
Giardia	1–2 weeks	Prolonged, non-bloody diarrhoea
Vibrio cholera	1–5 days	Profuse, watery diarrhoea. Not common in travellers
Entamoeba histolytica	Days to months	Mild diarrhoea to dysentery with blood and mucus

Table 14.3 Causes of traveller's diarrhoea.

20. D HHV-8

Kaposi's sarcoma is the most common malignancy associated with HIV infection Kaposi's sarcoma is associated with the human herpes virus (HHV-8). It usually presents with purple plaques (can be pruritic) on skin and mucosa and may metastasise to lymph nodes.

Confirmation of diagnosis is by biopsy. Treatment can either be targeting locally or providing systemic agents. In addition, a significant proportion may respond to treatment of the underlying immunosuppression, with antiretroviral agents.

The lesion can be also be targeted with radiation therapy, intra-lesional chemotherapy, topical retinoids and cryotherapy. Systemic treatments include the use of interferon and systemic chemotherapy.

Mesri EA, Cesarman E, Boshoff C. Kaposi's sarcoma and its associated herpesvirus. Nat Rev Cancer 2010; 10(10):707–719.

21. D *Spirillum minor*

This patient has rat bite fever. The two bacteria which are responsible for this disease are *Spirillum minor* (spirillary fever known as 'Sodoku') and *Streptobacillus moniliformis* (Haverhill fever). The two conditions are relative uncommon, but *S. minor* occurs more commonly in Asia, whilst *S. moniliformis* occurs more commonly in the USA. The incubation period for spirillary fever is 1 day to 6 weeks, with most cases occurring at 14–18 days. It is characterised by a relapsing/remitting fever and an indurated and ulcerated lesion to the side of the bite. There are often violaceous and/or red macules on the skin.

Diagnosis is by identifying the organism from blood, lymph node aspirates, or from bite wounds. Using Giemsa silver (stain used in detection for malaria or other parasites) or Wright's stain (stain to help differentiate blood cell types).

Treatment is with penicillin, erythromycin or tetracyclines.

Streptobacillus moniliformis presents in a similar manner, but more typically presents with myalgia, joint pain, headaches, nausea and vomiting. There are maculopapular and petechial rashes, which occurs in the extremities, mainly the hands and the feet. Complications include septic arthritis, endocarditis, meningitis and hepatitis.

Bartonella clarridgeiae and *Bartonella henselae* are associated with cat-scratch disease. Orf is caused by the parapox virus and transmitted to humans by contact with infected sheep or goats.

Booth CM, Katz KC, Brunton J. Fever and a rat bite. Can J Infect Dis 2002; 13(4):269–272.

22. C Schistosomiasis

Travellers who go swimming in freshwater lakes, particularly in Africa, are at risk of developing schistosomiasis (bilharzia).

Schistosomiasis is a common parasitic infection, with the *S. haematobium* type prevalent in Africa, *S. mansoni* in South America and *S. japonicum* in the Far East. It develops following exposure to fresh water infested with larvae that penetrate the skin and travel towards the bladder, bowel and liver.

In the acute phase (within 24 hours of exposure), the patient develops cercarial dermatitis or 'swimmer's itch' as a result of acute penetration of the larvae. Katayama's fever is more serious and occurs around 4–8 weeks after initial infection and is characterised by an immune mediated complex reaction – dyspnoea, urticaria and cough.

In the chronic phase of the condition a number of organs are affected (**Table 14.4**).

Treatment is with praziquantel. Metrifonate has been shown also to be effective, but is not currently licensed for use.

Ross AG, Bartley PB, Sleigh AC. Schistosomiasis. N Engl J Med 2002; 346:1212–1220.
Danso-Appiah A et al. Drugs for treating urinary schistosomiasis. Cochrane Database Syst Rev 2008 (3): CD000053.

23. C Isoniazid, ethambutol, rifampicin, pyrazinamide and prednisolone for 12 months

In pulmonary tuberculosis, the treatment is with four agents for 6 months, then 2 agents for an additional 2 months. The mnemonic '**SPIRE TIR**' may be used:

'**SPIRE**'

SIX months
Pyrazinamide
Isoniazid
Rifampicin
Ethambutol

Then:

'**TIR**'

TWO months
Isoniazid
Rifampicin

In those with evidence of meningeal involvement, treatment should be for a total of 12 months and the addition of a glucocorticoid. If the treatment includes rifampicin,

Table 14.4	
Urinary tract	Large-volume haematuria as eggs pass through, leading to fibrosis and calcification of the bladder
Bowel and liver	Haemorrhagic polyps and colitis, hepatosplenomegaly
Cardiac	Pulmonary hypertension
Neurological	Paraparesis and convulsions

Table 14.4 Clinical manifestations of schistosomiasis.

the dose should be higher (due to up-regulation of CP450 enzyme), around 20–40 mg (regular dose is 10–20 mg). For this patient, CT head did not show evidence of tuberculous meningitis. Although imaging cannot rule this out, MR would have been the preferred imaging modality.

National Institute for Clinical Excellence (NICE). NICE Guidelines. Tuberculosis: clinical diagnosis and management of tuberculosis, and measures for its prevention and control. Clinical Guideline 117. London: NICE, 2011.

24. D Erythema marginatum

Lyme disease is caused by the spirochete *Borrelia burgdorferi*. It is acquired by a tick bite and presents with flu like symptoms and erythema migrans. Complications can be serious including cardiac (heart block) and neurological, that may develop over a period of weeks to months.

Neurological complications are as follows:

'EMMA BC'

Encephalitis
Meningitis
Mononeuritis multiplex
Ataxia (cerebellar)
Bell's palsy
Cranial nerve palsies

Management of uncomplicated Lyme disease is with oral doxycycline. If evidence of neurological/cardiac complications, then intravenous ceftriaxone may be used, along with supportive measures and correction of abnormalities (e.g. pacemaker for heart block).

25. D Progressive multifocal leucoencephalopathy

Progressive multifocal leucoencephalopathy (PMLE) is a rapidly progressive demyelinating disorder of the central nervous system caused by the reactivation of the human polyoma virus, JC virus. JC virus normally manifests as an asymptomatic infection in childhood that remains latent in lymphoid tissue thereafter; however, profound immunosuppression – such as that found in advanced HIV infection – allows the virus to reactivate and attack oligodendrocytes (the cells responsible for myelin synthesis within the central nervous system).

The MRI finding of periventricular and subcortical white matter lesions in the absence of raised intracranial pressure or space-occupying lesions is very typical of PMLE. Although multiple sclerosis can give similar neuroimaging findings, this seems less likely within the clinical context presented. Cerebral toxoplasmosis and tuberculoma are common disorders in those with poorly controlled HIV disease, but they would tend to be associated with space occupying lesions/mass effect.

Symptoms of PMLE reflect the underlying white matter disease, and include cognitive deficit, motor impairment (e.g. hemiparesis), ataxia, aphasia and visual symptoms such as hemianopia and diplopia. There is poor correlation between the severity of clinical disease and the burden of disease suggested by neuroimaging. Although the definitive means of diagnosis is brain biopsy, the increasing sophistication of imaging and significant morbidity associated with biopsying means that this is becoming less necessary. JC virus polymerase chain reaction testing on cerebrospinal fluid samples may be a helpful assay, but many immunocompromised patients without PMLE and some healthy individuals may have positive results, limiting its usefulness.

Without treatment, PMLE usually quickly progresses to dementia, coma and death. Although there is no specific treatment for JC virus, initiation or optimisation of antiretroviral therapy is associated with a significantly improved prognosis; nevertheless, prognosis even then remains at less than 2 years.

Tan CS, Koralnik IJ. Progressive multifocal leucoencephalopathy and other disorders caused by JC virus: clinical features and pathogenesis. Lancet Neurol 2010; 9(4):425–437.

26. B *Mycobacterium tuberculosis*

Overwhelming post splenectomy infection (OPSI) is a rare but fatal condition which occurs due to overwhelming sepsis following splenectomy. However, the encapsulated bacterium *Streptococcus pneumonia* is the most frequently associated organism and along with *Haemophilus influenza* and *Neisseria meningitidis*, account for the majority of infections.

The following mnemonic describes the different organisms for OPSI

'EGG PACE'

Encapsulated bacteria: *S. pneumonia, H. influenza, N. meningitidis*
Gram negative: *P. aeruginosa, Klebsiella sp., Salmonella sp.*
Group B streptococci

Plasmodium species
Aureus (Staphylococcus)
Capnocytophagia canimorsus
Enterococcus species

For a planned a splenectomy, the patient should be vaccinated at least 2 weeks before with the following vaccines:

- Pneumococcal
- Haemophilus influenza Type B
- Influenza
- Meningococcal serogroup C

Following emergency splenectomy, vaccinations should be administered at least 14 days after the procedure.

Antibiotic prophylaxis with penicillin V or erythromycin is recommended for a minimum of two years after a splenectomy or in children, until they reach the age of 16.

Davies JM, Barnes R, Milligan D. Update of guidelines for the prevention and treatment of infection in patients with an absent or dysfunctional spleen. Clin Med 2002; 2: 4403.

27. Albendazole

The life cycle of *Echinococcus granulosus* involves a definitive host (dogs) and intermediate hosts such as sheep, goats and pigs. Humans are incidental hosts as they play no role in the transmission cycle. The adult tapeworm inhabits the small intestine of the definitive host and lays its eggs. These eggs are then expelled in the faeces. From here, the eggs can be ingested by the intermediate or incidental host. Following ingestion, the eggs hatch and the parasite migrates through the intestinal mucosa to the liver and other viscera via the blood and lymphatics. Soon after this a fluid-filled cyst develops. Human to human transmission does not occur because two mammalian species are necessary for completion of the life cycle.

Hydatid disease is common in the Far East, Middle East and Africa, and often occurs in sheep farming regions. The majority of cysts remain asymptomatic, but may cause abdominal discomfort, fevers, hepatomegaly, jaundice, and cholangitis. The cysts can migrate to the lungs, causing dyspnoea, cough and haemoptysis.

Treatment of hydatid cysts is with either albendazole or mebendazole. Albendazole is much more effective in treating liver cysts and is usually given for 28 days.

28. Metronidazole

Giardiasis is caused by flagellate protozoa, which is spread via the faecal oral route. Giardiasis is associated with significant morbidity if the patient has underlying immunosuppression.

The patient may be asymptomatic. Other features are bloating, abdominal cramps, flatulence, abdominal pain and explosive diarrhoea.

Diagnosis is made by examining for cysts and trophozoites in stool samples. The most sensitive test is performing ELISA test.

First-line treatment is with oral metronidazole. Other agents such as tinidazole may be used. If a patient is pregnant, then paromomycin should be given.

29. Topical podophyllum

Condylomata acuminata or genital warts are caused by the human papilloma virus (usually serotypes 6 and 11).

Treatment of a solitary keratinised wart is with cryotherapy. If multiple non-keratinised warts are present, then the choice of treatment is topical podophyllum. For genital warts resistant to treatment, imiquimod can be used as a second line-treatment.

British Association of Sexual Health and HIV (BASHH). National guidelines for the management of genital herpes. London: BASHH, 2007.

30. Zidovudine

Zidovudine was the first antiretroviral drug and is a nucleoside analogue reverse transcriptase inhibitor (NRTI).

Nucleoside analogue reverse transcriptase inhibitors (NRTI) **'DELTAZ'**:

- **D**idanosine
- **E**mtricitabine
- **L**amivudine
- **T**enofovir
- **A**bacavir
- **Z**idovudine

Non-nucleoside reverse transcriptase inhibitors (NNRTI) **'ERNE'**:

- **E**favirenz
- **R**ilpivirine
- **N**evirapine
- **E**travirine

Protease inhibitors (PI) **'SAFARID'**:

- **S**aquinavir
- **A**mprenavir
- **F**osamprenavir
- **A**tazanavir
- **R**itonavir
- **I**ndinavir
- **D**arunavir

Highly active antiretroviral treatment (HAART) usually consists of two NRTIs and one protease inhibitor (PI) or non-neucleoside reverse transcriptase inhibitor (NNRTI).

Each medication is associated with a variety of side effects.

Hammer SM, et al. Antiretroviral treatment of adult HIV infection JAMA 2008; 300:555–570.

Index

Note: Page numbers in **bold** or *italic* refer to tables or figures respectively.

cuong.dang ∂ pat.uhsink